T0289620

Food Security and Nutrition

Food Security and Nutrition

Editor: Reagan Perry

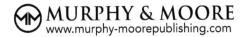
MURPHY & MOORE
www.murphy-moorepublishing.com

www.murphy-moorepublishing.com

ⓜ MURPHY & MOORE

Cataloging-in-Publication Data

Food security and nutrition / edited by Reagan Perry.
    p. cm.
Includes bibliographical references and index.
ISBN 978-1-63987-724-9
1. Food security. 2. Food supply. 3. Nutrition. 4. Diet. I. Perry, Reagan.
TX357 .F66 2023
641.3--dc23

Murphy & Moore Publishing
1 Rockefeller Plaza,
New York City,
NY 10020, USA

ISBN 978-1-63987-724-9

Contents

Preface

Food and nutrition security (FNS) is achieved when adequate food is available and is accessible to individuals in terms of quantity, quality, safety, and socio-cultural acceptability. At the same time, individuals should consume it to live a healthy and happy life. Food security is a broad concept that includes availability, accessibility, utilization and stability of food. The stability of these elements varies in their nature, causes and effects at the macro, meso and micro levels. FNS is associated with a number of overlapping concerns that hinder the development of individuals and societies. Prominent among these issues are gender, livelihoods and poverty, in addition to conflicts, crises and natural disasters. This book elucidates the concepts and innovative models with respect to food and nutrition security. Different approaches, evaluations, methodologies, and advanced studies on FNS have been included herein. The book is appropriate for students seeking detailed information in this area of study.

This book unites the global concepts and researches in an organized manner for a comprehensive understanding of the subject. It is a ripe text for all researchers, students, scientists or anyone else who is interested in acquiring a better knowledge of this dynamic field.

I extend my sincere thanks to the contributors for such eloquent research chapters. Finally, I thank my family for being a source of support and help.

Editor

Born to Eat Wild: An Integrated Conservation Approach to Secure Wild Food Plants for Food Security and Nutrition

Teresa Borelli [1,*], Danny Hunter [1], Bronwen Powell [2], Tiziana Ulian [3], Efisio Mattana [3], Céline Termote [1], Lukas Pawera [4,5], Daniela Beltrame [6], Daniela Penafiel [7,8], Ayfer Tan [9], Mary Taylor [10] and Johannes Engels [1]

1   Alliance of Bioversity International and CIAT, via dei Tre Denari 472/a, 00054 Rome, Italy;
     D.Hunter@cgiar.org (D.H.); C.Termote@cgiar.org (C.T.); j.engels@cgiar.org (J.E.)
2   Center for International Forestry Research, Penn State University, State College, PA 16802, USA;
     bxp15@psu.edu
3   Royal Botanic Gardens Kew, Wakehurst, Ardingly, West Sussex RH17 6TN, UK; t.ulian@kew.org (T.U.);
     E.Mattana@kew.org (E.M.)
4   Faculty of Tropical AgriSciences, Czech University of Life Sciences Prague, Kamýcká 129,
     16500 Praha-Suchdol, Czech Republic; paweralukas@gmail.com
5   The Indigenous Partnership for Agrobiodiversity and Food Sovereignty,
     c/o Alliance of Bioversity International and CIAT, Via dei Tre Denari 472/a, 00054 Rome, Italy
6   Biodiversity for Food and Nutrition Project, Ministry of the Environment, Brasília-DF 70068-900, Brazil;
     dani.moura.oliveira@gmail.com
7   Escuela Superior Politécnica del Litoral, Centro de Investigaciones Rurales–FCSH,
     Campus Gustavo Galindo-km. 30.5 vía Perimetral, Guayaquil 090112, Ecuador; ddpenafi@espol.edu.ec
8   Faculty of Medicine, Universidad de Especialidades Espíritu Santo, Samborondon 091650, Ecuador
9   Aegean Agricultural Research Institute, Menemen, Izmir P.O. Box 9 35661, Turkey; ayfer_tan@yahoo.com
10   Environmental Studies, University of the Sunshine Coast, Maroochydore, QLD 4556, Australia;
     maryt@oxalis.plus.com
*   Correspondence: t.borelli@cgiar.org

Abstract: Overlooked in national reports and in conservation programs, wild food plants (WFPs) have been a vital component of food and nutrition security for centuries. Recently, several countries have reported on the widespread and regular consumption of WFPs, particularly by rural and indigenous communities but also in urban contexts. They are reported as critical for livelihood resilience and for providing essential micronutrients to people enduring food shortages or other emergency situations. However, threats derived from changes in land use and climate, overexploitation and urbanization are reducing the availability of these biological resources in the wild and contributing to the loss of traditional knowledge associated with their use. Meanwhile, few policy measures are in place explicitly targeting their conservation and sustainable use. This can be partially attributed to a lack of scientific evidence and awareness among policymakers and relevant stakeholders of the untapped potential of WFPs, accompanied by market and non-market barriers limiting their use. This paper reviews recent efforts being undertaken in several countries to build evidence of the importance of WFPs, while providing examples of cross-sectoral cooperation and multi-stakeholder approaches that are contributing to advance their conservation and sustainable use. An integrated conservation approach is proposed contributing to secure their availability for future generations.

Keywords: wild food plants; food security; nutrition data; multi-sectoral collaboration; policy; conservation

1. Introduction

The practice of consuming wild food plants (WFPs) is as old as human prehistory. Early humans obtained their food by hunting, fishing and gathering these plants, or parts of plants (e.g., stems, roots, flowers, fruits, leaves, buds, and seeds), that were safe for human consumption. It was not until 10,000 years BC that people started settling into more permanent homesteads and domesticating plant species (mostly carbohydrate-rich staples) while maintaining some hunter-gatherer activities and collecting WFPs from the wild [1,2]. This still holds true for some traditional horticultural societies today (e.g., the Machiguenga in South America) [3]. All of the plants we now call domestic crops were once WFPs, altered by human manipulation to achieve domestication by selecting more favorable plant traits. With plant domestication and farming came also the development of weeds; that is, unwanted plant species in cultivated fields, and many of the WFPs consumed today include relatives of today's crops.

Today, the term "wild" is mostly taken to indicate species that grow spontaneously in self-sustaining populations outside cultivated areas, in field margins, forests, woodland, grassland, and wetlands (e.g., paddy fields), independently of human activity [4]. However, the distinction between "wild" and "cultivated" or "domesticated" is not so clear-cut and many WFPs fall somewhere in between these extremes depending on the degree of human intervention and management. For example, they can grow spontaneously in areas that are or have been themselves cultivated [4,5], or, as in the case of the "quelites" greens in Mesoamerica (e.g., the genus *Amaranthus*, *Chenopodium*, *Porophyllum*, *Portulaca*, *Crotalaria*, and *Anoda*), they have become the focus of systematic in situ management practices such as "selective harvesting" and "let standing", with important repercussions on plant communities [6]. Another known management practice is that of "encouraging growing" recorded by Cruz-Garcia [7] in the Peruvian Amazon along the deforestation border. Surveys revealed that, out of 30 wild food plant species identified, 20 are actively managed by local farmers and that most are transplanted from the forest to their agricultural fields for easy access. From these, 57% of the species are classified as weeds, yet are perceived by farmers to play a role in food security, particularly with increasing deforestation and reduced availability of food plants [7].

In this review paper, the term "wild food plants" is extended to all those food plants (herbs and spices included) that are also semi-domesticated, in addition to economically important non-timber forest food products, such as açaí berries and Brazil nuts [8]. As they are often wild relatives of domesticated species, WFPs have potential for domestication and can provide a pool of genetic resources for hybridization and selective breeding [9].

2. The Importance of Wild Food Plants Today

WFPs continue to play a vital role in the subsistence of many human populations particularly when the availability of food crops is scarce, when household budgets are insufficient to buy enough food or when access to markets is challenging [5,8,10–16]. Wild foods are also integral to traditional food systems and have nutritional and cultural value for many indigenous peoples [4,5,17,18]. Deeply connected to their land, indigenous peoples, who represent 5% of the global population [19], are often the sole custodians of rich and diverse knowledge relating to plant uses and traditional food systems and to local food biodiversity existing within the ecosystems they inhabit [18]. Traditional communities also have better ecological knowledge about local environments and their customary users, making monitoring and regulating of natural resources easier [20].

Although the caloric contribution of WFPs to people's diets is generally low compared to staple foods [21], these species contribute to diet diversification in many geographical settings where otherwise monotonous diets may prevail [22–26]. Wild foods (both plants and non) provided between 1% and 19% of the iron consumed, between 5% and 45% of the calcium and between 0% and 31% of the vitamin A equivalents (RAE) in the diets of women and children in studies from Benin, Tanzania, and the Philippines [21]. These neglected biological resources have, in fact, been shown to contain equally, if not higher amounts, of nutrients than more widely available commercial crops [5,27–29], and, if properly assessed and managed, could be introduced in national food and nutrition security and sovereignty strategies that focus on nutrient adequacy rather than quantity of staples, while being culturally acceptable.

WFPs could also be central to efforts directed at empowering local market actors as well as reducing the distance between consumers and producers and the overreliance on globalized value chains. Although, recent research by Kinnunen et al. [30] highlights the unfeasibility of localizing production for important global staples such as rice, maize and temperate cereals, there is increasing evidence that the local trade of minor crops, traditional varieties, and WFPs has potential to empower communities and increase livelihoods in rural areas, particularly of women and youth [31,32]. Meanwhile, the COVID-19 crisis has revealed the vulnerability of our global food systems to disease-related disruptions and shocks [33–35]. For example, the imposed travel restrictions on people and goods as a result of the lockdowns are causing logistical bottlenecks in food supply chains [36]. Given the national and international trade restrictions, long supply chains are struggling to cope with the rise in food demand for non-perishable food supplies [37], while short supply chains are suffering due to the closing of informal and local open-air markets [38], where the majority of the world's population still obtains fruits, horticultural, and other perishable products [37,39]. At the same time, the pandemic has opened up opportunities for a new food system paradigm that supports local self-sufficiency and domestic agricultural production and sees home and community gardens, traditional agroecosystems, and farmers' markets as essential services [38,40]. With food shortages affecting specialized, high value horticultural crops [41], people are turning to traditional vegetables and WFPs as a sustainable source of food, vitamins and nutrients [42], not to mention for herbal ingredients, traditional medicine formulations or new biopharmaceuticals [38,43,44].

This paper builds mainly on the authors' own efforts being undertaken in several countries to provide evidence of the role of WFPs in supporting nutrition and livelihood security. This paper also provides examples of cross-sectoral cooperation and multi-stakeholder approaches that are contributing to the better conservation and use of WFPs, including by fostering linkages between in and ex situ conservation. In the case of WFPs, "use" includes the various practices and activities involved in (i) domesticating wild species; (ii) the management of wild species and their habitats in and around production systems to promote the delivery of ecosystem services; and (iii) the introduction of wild species into production and consumption systems, for example by creating demand for the species, and regulating their harvesting in the wild. Lastly, details will be provided of a proposed integrated conservation approach that focuses on local interventions based on traditional food systems.

2.1. Diversity (Geographical Use) and Contribution to Diets

The use of WFPs in many countries is confirmed by national contributions to the recent "State of the World's Biodiversity for Food and Agriculture"—"SOWBFA"—of the Food and Agriculture Organization of the United Nations [45]. Of 91 countries reporting information for compiling the report, 69 nations reported a total of 1955 wild plant species that contribute to food security and nutrition in their respective countries, as well as making diets healthier and more diverse. However, as the examples provided by the authors and recently published papers [46] demonstrate, the number is probably much higher and these species remain largely unreported in national statistics, as does the actual contribution of these biological resources to national economies in many parts of the world [47]. Table S1 in the Supplementary materials lists the wide range of plant families that encompass the edible wild and semi-cultivated plant species researched by the authors and mentioned in the text as contributing to food and nutrition security. The list, as the review carried out by the authors, is by no means exhaustive and could undoubtedly include more.

2.1.1. Africa

As part of the MGU Useful Plants Project (UPP) managed by the Royal Botanic Gardens, Kew, UK, institutional partners working alongside local communities in Botswana, Kenya, Mali, South Africa, and Mexico identified 615 species used for food across the five countries [48]. Information on seed conservation, propagation and traditional uses has been published for 48 of them and is now available on the internet [49]. In Africa, the species included the baobab (*Adansonia digitata)*, the mongongo tree (*Schinziophyton rautanenii*), and the morama bean (*Tylosema esculentum)* [49]. Research undertaken by Bioversity International in the early 1990s has documented 210 African leafy vegetables in Kenya alone [50]. These are wild or semi-domesticated species that are grown mostly for household consumption or traded informally, but which have seen a revival particularly in urban and peri-urban areas [51]. In Western Kenya, between 23 and 42 African leafy vegetables continue to be consumed by local communities depending on the district. Eleven species, including amaranth (*Amaranthus* spp.), spider plant (*Cleome gynandra*), and African nightshades (*Solanum* spp.) were selected for further research as part of the African Leafy Vegetables program from 1996 to 2004 (Bioversity International and EIARD, 2013; Gotor and Irungu, 2010) [51,52] as well as for the Biodiversity for Food and Nutrition Project [28,53]. In addition to filling the nutrient gap, a cost of diet study carried out in Eastern Baringo, Kenya, has shown that wild plant species, especially vegetables, are able to significantly reduce (by 30–70%) the cost of a nutritious meal for women and children aged 6 to 23 months in hypothetically-modeled lowest cost nutritious diets [54].

2.1.2. South America

In Ecuador, one of the top seven mega diverse countries in the world, wild edible fruits and plants collected from a diverse range of habitats play a fundamental role in traditional diets, particularly for the indigenous communities living in forest areas. Studies in the country by Penafiel et al. [55,56], documenting local knowledge on the use of WFPs among the Andean indigenous communities of Guasaganda (Cotopaxi) and the Andean Kichwa mothers of Arosemena Tola (Napo), recorded the culinary use of 49 and 10 WPFs, respectively. Brazil also contains vast amounts of wild food plant diversity [57]. Some of this diversity is of national and regional relevance, e.g., Brazil nut (*Bertholletia excelsa*) and açaí (*Euterpe oleracea*), but most is of local value and its potential nutritional and economic value remains unexplored and unexploited [58]. The "Plants for the Future (PPF) Initiative", a prioritization exercise undertaken by the Ministry of the Environment that set out to explore the wealth of Brazil's plant biodiversity, has identified a considerable number of wild species of nutritional value and market potential. Across the country's five eco-regions, out of 78 native undervalued edible plant species, 49 are found exclusively in the wild (mostly fruits and nuts) [28]. Mostly found in forest areas, the species are managed by family farmers or harvested from the wild by local communities using traditional practices. The link between local communities and nature is such that the Brazilian ministries of Agriculture, Environment, and Social Development have coined the term "sociobiodiversity" to describe these traditionally managed biodiversity-derived goods that are sold in local markets, provide incomes and improve the livelihoods of traditional communities, while protecting biodiversity and the environment.

2.1.3. The Mediterranean

In the Mediterranean, WFPs are still common in traditional cuisine and are widely consumed locally [59,60]. In their compendium of gathered Mediterranean food plants, Rivera et al. [61] identified approximately 2300 different WFPs and fungi taxa in this region alone, of which 1000 are strictly used locally. As part of the Biodiversity for Food and Nutrition (BFN) project, Turkey prioritized 42 wild edible plants for further research [28] out of hundreds of known species [59,62,63], while across Morocco, Nassif and Tanji [64] compiled a list of 246 wild plant species used as food. While many WFPs are only used occasionally or in small regional areas, some are central to Moroccan diets and culinary traditions. Aromatic herbs such as thyme (*Thymus* spp.), mint (*Mentha* spp.), and sage (*Salvia* spp.) are the most widely consumed wild plants; however, they contribute little to the diet in terms of energy (kcal) and nutrients because they are used as condiments [65]. Wild leafy vegetables, on the other hand, are a seasonally important component of Moroccan diets, particularly in rural Morocco where 86% of households reported consuming wild leafy vegetables (WLVs) on a regular basis [66]. Some of the most commonly consumed WLVs (many of which are also consumed in Turkey and other Mediterranean countries) include mallow (*Malva* spp.), purslane (*Portulaca oleracea*), goosefoots (*Chenopodium* spp.), docks and sorrels (*Rumex* spp.), fennel (*Foeniculum* sp. cf *F. vulgare*), golden thistle (*Scolymus hispanicus*), and watercress (*Nasturtium officinale*). They are commonly served as a cooked salad or side dish, eaten in moderate portion sizes (approximately 50 g per meal). Argan oil (*Sideroxylon spinosum*), capers (*Capparis spinosa* and *C. decidua*), acorns (*Quercus* spp.), and the fruits of the strawberry tree (*Arbutus unedo*) as well as jujube (*Ziziphus jujube*), mulberry (*Morus* spp.), and blackberry (*Rubus* spp.) are other commonly consumed plant products in this region [64,65,67].

2.1.4. Asia Pacific

The consumption of WFPs and food trees makes a significant contribution to human health in the Pacific region [68]. In "Food Plants of Papua New Guinea, A Compendium" [69], Bruce French produces a list of food plants, many of which are sourced from the wild, including root crops and staples, legumes, green leafy and other vegetables, nuts, fruits and what are categorized as "minor foods and flavorings". For example, the kernel of wild *karuka* (*Pandanus brosimos*), endemic to Papua New Guinea (PNG), is eaten by about one-third of the rural population [70], particularly by communities living at high altitudes. When the fruit matures, villagers migrate to high altitudes to harvest the fruit and extract the nuts. Nuts have not been recorded in the main highland markets, but it is possible that they are sold in some high-altitude locations [71]. PNG and surrounding region are also one of the few places in the world where communities obtain the majority of their carbohydrate staple from a wild food plant: sago [72,73].

In Niue (Polynesia), the traditional processing of wild arrowroot (*Tacca* spp.) is still an ongoing practice. Starch processed from the root is a local delicacy used to make local puddings and breads [74]. Thaman [75] lists 60 WFPs used in Fiji, noting that these plants play an important role as emergency or famine foods when extreme climatic events disrupt cultivation. Among these are wild marine seaweeds such as sea grapes (*Caulerpa racemosa*), known as nama, and other edible seaweeds that are still widely consumed. "The Guide to the Common Edible and Medicinal Sea Plants of the Pacific Islands" provides an insight into marine WFPs and the benefits that can be gained from their use [76].

In the mosaic tropical landscape of West Sumatra, Indonesia, composed predominantly of rice fields, home gardens, cacao agroforestry, and forests, with the help of local communities, the Food, Agrobiodiversity and Diet (FAD) project has identified 85 WFPs [77]. In this region, WFPs are consumed less than in the past, and the FAD project aimed to raise knowledge and awareness of wild foods by organizing workshops, traditional food competitions, and sharing community materials such as illustrations, posters, and community guidebooks, on food plants for nutrition and health [78].

2.2. Income Generation

In many parts of the world, WFPs are not only harvested for subsistence [79–81]. Gathered in excess, they are sold in local markets to generate income, thereby contributing to the household economies of gatherers and collectors, usually women, or to bolster the incomes of migrants and unemployed moving from rural to urban areas [82]. For example, in the Chimanimani communities living in the Trans-Frontier Conservation Area in Mozambique, the fruits of *Uapaca kirkiana* and *Strychnos madagascariensis* are sold for a reasonable profit and represent an important source of income outside the maize harvest season (March to May) [83]. In their review paper, Hickey et al. [84] showed that 50% of almost 8000 households sampled in forested areas of 24 developing countries across Asia, Africa, and Latin America derived their income from wild food collection. The study also highlighted that the sale of plant foods contributed 2.3% to total household income across the study sites on three continents, the proportion increasing to 2.8% in Africa and Latin America, particularly in poorer households.

In parts of Turkey, where WFPs are central to traditional cooking, wild edibles are sold unprocessed in local markets and processed (e.g., pickled, canned, or frozen) in district markets or supermarkets via wholesalers and middlemen [85]. In 2012, in the Pacific Island States of Fiji, Samoa, and Tonga the yearly production and revenue from the harvesting and sales of the seaweed *Caulerpa racemosa* was valued at USD 266,492 [86]. However, the true extent of this revenue is not always available. For example, a recent European assessment established the value of collected non-wood forest products, mainly food plants, at € 19.5 billion with value per hectare rising to € 77.8, and ten times above the official European estimates [87]. Many markets for WFPs are informal, and market players may hold back information because of illicit harvesting in local conservation areas [82]. Data about geographic and temporal distribution, production cost, quantity harvested, and price is also often limited. Increased profits can often lead to overexploitation of WFPs and negative outcomes for the entire community [20]. To avert this possibility, participatory research is key to establish sustainable management guidelines and harvest rates, and to monitor the ecological impacts of increased use [83].

2.3. Threats to WFPs

Despite the realization of the potential use of WFPs in food security and poverty reduction strategies, the SOWBFA, along with other recent global reports [46], warn us that this precious diversity is fast disappearing, particularly in forest habitats [88,89]. Land use changes (e.g., conversion to agriculture, change in agricultural practices and infrastructure development), habitat destruction (resulting from timber harvesting, fuelwood collection, grazing, and forest fires) and overharvesting collectively account for 62% of the threats reported to WFPs in SOWBFA, which mostly grow beyond the limit of protected areas [45,90,91]. The SOWBFA used the Sampled Red List Index for Plants of the International Union for Conservation on Nature (IUCN) [92] to determine that, of a total 822 WFP species considered across 7 different classes, 73% are currently at low risk of extinction (Figure 1), with some classes highly threatened in the wild (e.g., WFPs that are derived from conifers and cycads). However, the IUCN Red List Index for Plants includes global conservation assessments for only one third (31%) of known WFPs. Local assessments for many WFPs that are currently excluded from the IUCN assessment paint a very different story indicating the need to consider community perceptions when ascribing risk class (Table 1). Furthermore, an assessment of the comprehensiveness of conservation of 1587 WFP taxa (including cereals, fruit, and nuts), carried out by the International Center for Tropical Agriculture (CIAT) as part of a larger study to identify conservation gaps for useful plants, shows that only 3.3% of WFPs are sufficiently conserved ex situ, i.e., in gene banks or in other living plant repositories, while 89.1% require urgent off-site conservation measures given the impending threats to their existence [93]. Their continued use in diets, when accompanied by careful sustainable management by the communities consuming them, and protection of WFP habitats, on the other hand, seems to have ensured their momentary conservation in situ, in the natural habitats in which they grow. Of the WFP taxa analyzed 42.1% are sufficiently conserved, 46.7% deserve medium priority and 11.1% require stepping up conservation measures [93]. Nonetheless, Khoury et al. [93] caution against the overreliance on protected areas for the long-term conservation of these species. Rapidly warming temperatures and habitat destruction can alter the species' geographic distribution, driving them across the artificially designated boundaries of many protected areas in pursuit of favourable growing conditions [94].

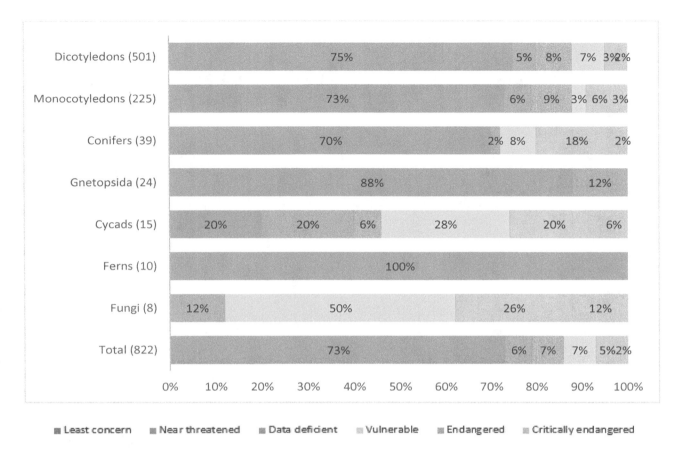

Figure 1. Number of WFPs and fungi on the IUCN Red List of Threatened Species classified by class and risk category Source: IUCN Red List 2017. Adapted from FAO [45].

Given that many WFPs grow in agricultural systems (as weeds, in hedge rows, as wild trees in agroforestry systems, and in small forest patches [5,21]), agricultural change, including intensification, more pesticide use and removal of trees can threaten the existence of these biological resources [12,14,95]. Food production systems that pollute the environment by using large quantities of fertilizers, pesticides, and herbicides, are also major causes of biodiversity loss [45,88,96]. Applying chemical herbicides in rice fields or agroforestry plots, for example, leads to the reduced availability of WFPs in West Sumatra, Indonesia [77]. WFPs that survive aerial spraying with herbicides are contaminated by these harmful substances, making them unfit for human consumption, while pesticides wipe out many of the pollinators needed for plant reproduction.

Overharvesting can also be an important pressure on non-timber forest products, including wild foods [97]. This is the case for Morocco and Turkey. Morocco is the twelfth global exporter of medicinal and aromatic plants, a trade that places extensive harvesting pressure on many of the species traditionally used as herbs [98]. A rapid vulnerability assessment carried out by Lamrani-Alaoui and Hassikou identified six species that grow across wide areas of Morocco's government owned forests (*Thymus satureioides, Lavandula dentata, Origanum compactum, Origanum elongatum, Salvia rosmarinus* and *Fraxinus dimorpha*) as needing urgent conservation, restoration, and sustainable management measures [98].

Table 1. Local threat assessments carried out in partnership with local communities have identified increasing dangers to the survival of nutritious and locally important WFPs. A selection from the authors' project sites is provided along with suggested measures for conservation and sustainable use.

Country	Species Name	Local Name	Edible Use	Main Nutritional Benefits	Habitat	Threat Status (IUCN, Community to Other)	Threats/Suggestion for Conservation	Photo
Brazil	*Astrocaryum aculeatum*	Tucumã	Fruit pulp	Rich in vitamin A as well as lauric, myristic and oleic acid [99]	Amazon rainforest	No IUCN assessment	Habitat loss—deforestation/ Preserve natural habitats	Credit: J. Camillo
	Euterpe edulis	Jussara	Fruit pulp consumed as puree, palm heart (discouraged)	The fruit is rich in antioxidants [99]	Dense shady forest (Atlantic forest)	No IUCN assessment, listed as Vulnerable in the Red Book of Brazilian Flora [100]	Habitat loss—deforestation, overharvesting of palm heart/ Preserve natural habitats	Credit: A. Popovkin
	Butia eriospatha	Butiá	Fruit pulp, seed	Good source of fiber, potassium, and vitamin C (equivalent to levels found in oranges) [99]	Highland mixed shady forests (Araucaria forest), around 800–900 m elevation	IUCN—Vulnerable	Habitat loss—deforestation/ Preserve natural habitats	Credit: G. Lopes
	Dipteryx alata	Baru nut	Fruit/Nut	High in fiber; the nut is high in quality protein [99]	Tropical savannah (Cerrado)	IUCN—Vulnerable	Habitat loss—deforestation/ Preserve natural habitats	Credit: J. Camillo
	Hancornia speciosa	Mangaba	Fruit	Excellent source of vitamin C, folates and a good source of carotenoids and vitamin E [99]	Scrublands (Caatinga) and barren lands in central Brazil	No IUCN assessment	Habitat loss—deforestation/ Preserve natural habitats	Credit: J. Camillo

Table 1. *Cont.*

Country	Species Name	Local Name	Edible Use	Main Nutritional Benefits	Habitat	Threat Status (IUCN, Community to Other)	Threats/Suggestion for Conservation	Photo
Ecuador	Vasconcellea microcarpa (Carica microcarpa)	Col de monte	Leaves	N/A	Forest	IUCN—Least concern	Deforestation/Nutrition education needed	Credit: X. Scheldeman
	Pouteria multiflora	Logma	Fruit	N/A	Forest	No IUCN assessment	Deforestation/Nutrition education needed	Credit: IKIAM
	Hypolepis hostilis	Garabato yuyo	Leafy green vegetable (fern)	N/A	Forest	No IUCN assessment	Loss of traditional food culture /Use as complementary food for infants	Credit: IKIAM
	Plukenetia volubilis	Sachainchi	Nut	Good source of lipids, proteins, and essential amino acids (e.g., cysteine, tyrosine, threonine, and tryptophan), vitamin E and polyphenols [101]	Home garden	No IUCN assessment	Loss of traditional food culture /Use as complementary food for infants	Credit: IKIAM
Fiji/ Samoa	Caulerpa racemosa	Nama, Limu	Sea vegetable	Contains proteins, fiber, minerals, vitamins, polyunsaturated fatty acids, and bioactive anti-oxidants [102]	Near reefs, in shallow waters	No IUCN assessment	Unsustainable harvesting, storm surges, cyclones	Credit: N.Hobgood

Table 1. *Cont.*

Country	Species Name	Local Name	Edible Use	Main Nutritional Benefits	Habitat	Threat Status (IUCN, Community to Other)	Threats/Suggestion for Conservation	Photo
Kenya	*Cleome gynandra*	Spider plant, Ofsaga, saga, liSaga, lisaka	Leaves used as vegetables [103]	High in β-carotene, folic acid, vitamin C, calcium and a good source of vitamin E, iron [104]	Roadsides, field margins, semi-domesticated	No IUCN assessment	No organized collecting missions	Credit: BFN Kenya
	Amaranthus tortuosus	Amaranth, Ekichabo, Dodo	Leaves used as vegetables and seed crushed for flour	Good source of proteins, fibers, calcium, iron, riboflavin, niacin and vitamin C and an excellent source of lysine [104]	Roadsides, field margins, semi-domesticated	No IUCN assessment	No organized collecting missions	Credit: BFN Kenya
	Chorchorus olitorius	Jute mallow, murere	Leaves used as vegetables	High levels of β-carotene, vitamin C, folic acid, calcium and iron [104]	Roadsides, field margins, semi-domesticated	No IUCN assessment	No organized collecting missions	Credit: C. Kerr
Morocco	*Nasturtium officinale*	Watercress, Gernouch	Leafy vegetable	Rich in vitamin K, vitamin A, vitamin C, vitamin B6, manganese, calcium, and folate [105]	Springs, river edges, irrigation canals	IUCN—Least Concern	Paving of irrigation canals may decrease community access, changing diet and preference and leading to decreased use	Credit: M. Lavin
	Malva sylvestris	Mallow, Tibi, Khobiza, Bakola houra	Leafy vegetable	Strong antioxidant properties, rich in phenols, flavonoids, carotenoids, and tocopherols, alpha-linolenic acid and minerals [106]	Fields, field margins, along irrigation canals and roads	IUCN—Least Concern	Changing diet and preferences may lead to decreased use	Credit: B. Powell

Table 1. *Cont.*

Country	Species Name	Local Name	Edible Use	Main Nutritional Benefits	Habitat	Threat Status (IUCN, Community to Other)	Threats/Suggestion for Conservation	Photo
	Sideroxylon spinosum	Argan	Edible oil	Good source of linoleic and oleic fatty acids. Rich source of tocopherol (vitamin E) [107]	Dry forests from the Atlantic coast to 800 m elevation	IUCN criteria at national level—Vulnerable [108]	Social-ecological systems change driven by commodification and globalization	Credit: B. Powell
Niue	*Tacca leontopetaloides*	Kai Niue	Root starch	Good source of carbohydrate, also contains vitamin C, fat, and protein [109]	Uncultivated land	IUCN Least Concern	General lack of information	Credit: B. Dupont
Papua New Guinea	*Pandanus brosimos*	Karuka	Fruit (boiled) & extracted nut	Good source of protein and oil especially for highland communities [71]	Forest, high altitudes	No IUCN assessment	No known threat, but general lack of information	Credit: Green Dean
	Scolymus hispanicus	Golden thistle, Şevketi bostan	Roots and young leaves	Rich in dietary fiber, magnesium and calcium [105,110]	Disturbed habitats and fallow fields	No IUCN assessment	Overharvesting/ domestication programs initiated	Credit: BFN Turkey
Turkey	*Eremurus spectabilis*	Foxtail lily, Çiriş otu	Shoots, buds and young leaves	Rich in antioxidants and minerals [111]. High in vitamin C [112]	Dry and stony grazed hillsides	No IUCN assessment	Overharvesting/ domestication programs initiated	Credit: K.D. Zinnert

Table 1. *Cont.*

Country	Species Name	Local Name	Edible Use	Main Nutritional Benefits	Habitat	Threat Status (IUCN, Community to Other)	Threats/Suggestion for Conservation	Photo
West Sumatra, Indonesia	*Elateriospermum tapos*	Tapuih	Seeds consumed raw or fermented	Rich in protein and unsaturated fatty acids [113]	Forest/agroforest	No IUCN assessment	Perceived as rare by local communities/Preserve forest and multi-strata agroforests	Credit: L. Pawera
	Mangifera foetida	Ambacam, Bacang	Fruits consumed raw or cooked	Rich in vitamins A and C [114]	Forest, agroforest, homegardens	IUCN -Least Concern	Perceived as rare by local communities/Preserve forests and multi-strata agroforests	Credit: L. Pawera
	Diplazium esculentum	Pakis, Pahu	Young shoots as a vegetable, cooked	Rich in vitamin B9 (folate) [114]	Forests, wetlands	IUCN—Least concern	Relatively common/Preserve forests and wetlands	Credit: L. Pawera
	Ipomoea aquatica	Kangkung air, Kangkuang liar	Leaves and stems as a vegetable, cooked	Rich in Iron and provitamin A [114]	Rivers, ponds, rice fields	No IUCN assessment	Threatened by overuse of herbicides/Reduce the use of herbicides and keep clean water bodies	Credit: L. Pawera

Exacerbating these problems in the different geographies are the uncertain effects of climate change, which in many countries is expected to lead to increased variability in seasonality, temperatures and precipitations and increased incidence of hurricanes and wildfires [89]. Climate change is also predicted to severely impact cultivated plants, affecting crop production in specific geographic locations [115], stripping nutrients from staple crops [46,116] and making WFPs all the more important for food and nutrition security. Although generally highly adaptable and often more drought tolerant than cultivated crops, WFPs, as many useful plants, are also not fully resistant to climate change [116]. In the past, many WFPs survived major climatic fluctuations, but thematic studies on the implications of future climate change suggest important impacts on the ability of wild species to survive. This includes WFPs, particularly in tropical regions where economies are already fragile and capacity may be inadequate to protect these species effectively [94,116]. One key impact that could threaten WFP use is the likely shifts in both WFP geographic ranges and phenological changes in ripening times. This could create mismatches with traditional knowledge and practices of the communities that traditionally harvest them [117].

At present, there are very few formal systematic efforts that support and regulate the conservation and sustainable use of WFPs [118]. A sample survey of some of the most recent National Biodiversity Strategies and Action Plans (NBSAPs) submitted to the CBD as part of the reporting requirements of member states (e.g., Chile, Morocco, and Portugal), shows that rarely do these strategies refer specifically to WFPs or, if they do, are very vague in terms of the measures needed to protect them. Actions are mostly limited to ex situ conservation measures [46], while no concrete activities are put forward to support their conservation via sustainable use [45]. Furthermore, appropriate and effective governance mechanisms are seldom in place to safeguard the rights of indigenous people and local communities to sustainably manage and benefit from the use of WFPs (and prevent their over-exploitation by others) [119].

The use of wild species, however, is explicitly recognized as useful for improving food and nutrition security in several international agreements, strategies and action plans: in the 2030 Agenda for Sustainable Development (SDG2, Target 2.5), the International Treaty on Plant Genetic Resources for Food and Agriculture (International Treaty), the Second Global Plan of Action for Plant Genetic Resources for Food and Agriculture (Second GPA), and in the Global Strategy for Plant Conservation of the Convention on Biological Diversity (CBD). The CBD, the main international agreement aimed at conserving biological diversity, accords explicit recognition to sustainable use for the long-term conservation of ecosystems, species and genes, which must continue to be used, but "in a way and at a rate that does not lead to the long-term decline of biological diversity" [120]. Intrinsic in the term "sustainable use" is that it generates benefits (e.g., nutritional, cultural, and financial) for the custodians and users of these wild species. These benefits encourage people to continue conserving these biological resources and the habitats in which they grow or live. However, the real challenge is to ensure this sustainability is maintained given the rising demands on global resources imposed by population growth and economic development, combined with the uncertain effects of climate change mentioned above.

3. Barriers to the Greater Use of WFPs

The disregard of WFPs for food security and nutrition can be partly attributed to a lack of evidence and awareness among policymakers and other stakeholders of the importance of wild foods to diets, livelihoods, and food security, coupled with a number of market and non-market barriers limiting their untapped potential.

Underpinning the lack of recognition for WFPs is also limited or short-term research and extension funding to support the exploration of non-conventional, traditional and indigenous food resources. Many of these barriers were summarized by Heywood [4] and are still very much valid today:

- lack of information about the extent of their use and importance in rural economies;
- lack of information, especially statistics, concerning the economic value of WFPs;

- lack of reliable methods for measuring their contribution to farm households and the rural economy;
- lack of information on the sustainability of current harvest levels;
- poorly developed infrastructure and markets for WFPs, with the exception of small number of products (e.g., Açaí berries);
- unevenness of supply;
- lack of quality standards;
- general lack of storage and processing technology;
- availability of substitutes;
- policies and research mostly favoring commodity crops and commercial agriculture.

Like other neglected and underutilized species, additional barriers to the promotion of WFPs in food production and consumption patterns include: limited and fragmented data of the nutritional importance of these species; fragmented data on the quality and nutritional impacts of WFPs on household nutrition [121]; and knowledge gaps on the species' biology and ecology to develop domestication and management strategies [45,46].

Unfavorable and disabling national policies, coupled with the many stakeholders and interests involved, represent an additional obstacle to greater recognition for WFPs. The main policy barriers were identified and summarized by the Strategic Framework for Underutilized Plant Species [122], of which WFPs are part of. These are provided in Table 2 below.

Table 2. Barriers that hinder the improvement of national policy frameworks towards supporting WFPs.

Awareness	Focus	Financial Support	External Pressures
No adequate data	Mismatch with national priorities	No international financial or donor support	International trade favor R&D on conventional crops
Lack of priority in education and information systems	Limited capacity (institutional, research) to work with WFPs	Weak economies for investing in R&D for WFPs	International R&D priorities influence national priorities

Further contributing to the demise of WFPs, is the low recognition of value and perception of these foods as being "women's food" [66] "food for the poor" or "famine foods" to be harvested only when staple crops fail, as well as lack of institutional capacity to mainstream this diversity into national production and consumption patterns [28]. On the other hand, in some regions, such as West Sumatra, communities perceive WFPs positively, but the main barrier to their greater use is their reduced availability caused by land degradation and agriculture intensification [77]. In many places, traditional wild leafy vegetables are disappearing from local diets due to changing dietary patterns and preferences driven by globalization and increasing market integration [123]. Wild leafy vegetables (WLV) and wild food plants in general are undervalued and seen as "un-modern" in Morocco, Turkey [28,66], and many other parts of the world. This lack of value places the role of WFPs in the diet at risk, although it may ease pressures on overharvesting. In Brazil and Kenya, changing dietary patterns and lifestyles has reduced the diversity and availability of wild fruit and vegetables in market settings, which focus instead on a limited number of exotic crops [124]. This has led to people consuming sub-optimal diets that are increasingly unhealthy, unsustainable, and inequitable for many populations [125].

3.1. Contribution to Nutrition and Diets

The contribution of wild food biodiversity to diets and nutrition is simultaneously limited by a severe lack of food composition data for many neglected and underutilized cultivated and wild foods [126] as well as by a lack of accurate botanical identification for many foods recorded in dietary records or food composition tables [45,127,128]. Nutrient composition data indicates the presence and quantity of nutrients (e.g., energy, proteins, minerals, and vitamins) as well as the compounds that can impact the bioavailability of nutrients within a food. These data are combined with dietary records of the foods consumed to assess whether individuals or groups are meeting their dietary requirements [129]. Nutrient composition data do not exist for many WFPs, and when they do there may be high variation in nutrient composition for a given species across space and time [130]. The few WFPs that have nutrient composition data and that are included in local food composition tables are often identified by local names. This hinders the use of these data to fill nutrition gaps in other locations where the same species might be present and used but is identified by a different local name. Many data sets lump all wild foods into a single food group (e.g., wild greens). For example, in analyzing data on wild harvests in 24 developing countries across Africa, Asia, and Latin America, Hickey et al. [84] found that only a small percentage (0.9%) of the collected mushrooms were identified by species, the rest was reported nonspecifically as "mushrooms".

In some cases, when WFPs are lost from the diet they may be replaced by similar cultivated species, but in other cases they are not. Anecdotal evidence from Morocco suggests that when people stop or reduce the consumption of WLVs in their diet, these are not replaced with cultivated alternatives, leading to a reduced consumption of any leafy vegetable and fruit and vegetables in general. This is particularly worrying given global recommendations [131] to consume at least 5 servings of fresh fruit and vegetables (including berries, green leafy and cruciferous vegetables, and legumes) per day as a protective measure against cardiovascular diseases and type II diabetes [132–136].

Practical challenges also exist in measuring wild food consumption and contribution to the diet relative to other foods [5,137]. Although in recent years, several investigations have tried to assess the role of wild food biodiversity and the contribution of forests and agroforestry systems to human dietary intakes [13,14], the real dietary contribution of wild food plants, berries, fruit, nuts, and mushrooms harvested within and around people's homesteads and in forested areas remains poorly understood. Geographical variations exist regarding the proportion of WFPs consumed. While in in the global North WFPs mostly have cultural and recreational value [138], in some low-income countries they significantly enrich people's diets [119]. Rowland et al. [13] found that the collection of forest foods represents a regular livelihood strategy for many households and that forest dependent communities living in specific sites in Brazil, Cameroon, and Ethiopia derive as much as 80–96% of wild fruits and vegetables from the forest. In some areas, the nutritional contribution of fruits and vegetables is such to cover 50% and above the minimum dietary recommendation for these food groups [13]. Differences in consumption might also vary by ethnicity. For example, in documenting the traditional food systems of Western Sumatra, Pawera et al. [77] found that different ethnic communities living in the same environment have different knowledge and uses for the same WFPs. Seasonal fluctuations in WFP occurrence and therefore consumption by local communities might also not be adequately captured with a single survey [139]. Other challenges include cultural and language barriers and perceived power imbalances during questionnaire administration that can alter the surveys' accuracy and reliability [137]. There is a huge body of research that only lists the edible species known to community members but neglects to quantify the use of WFPs in local recipes nor is their use standardized in nutrition surveys [121].

3.2. Gathering Grounds, Collection Practices and Use

An additional knowledge gap is represented by the lack of information on traditional gathering grounds and the sustainability of collection practices. In the SOWBFA, the ecosystem origin reported for WFPs is either from forests (>25%) or unknown (>45%) [45]. An often-overlooked practice is urban and peri-urban foraging for WFPs. In their cross-continental study of urban foraging spanning India, South Africa, Sweden, and the US, Shackleton et al. [140] found that urban foraging is a widespread custom that is practiced independently of wealth and social status and is driven by different motivations varying in time and place. Wooded areas on public land, local lake beds, and other urban habitats harbor nutritionally rich greens and fruits. Even spontaneous vegetation growing in alleyways was reportedly used by Indian residents for food and culinary use [140]. Aside from direct consumption and small-scale trade, other benefits include "improved physical and psychological health, sense of place, increased ecological knowledge, stronger connections with nature, food, income or cash saving, and a source of pride" [140]. The important cultural ecosystem services offered by these plants are apparent in a study of WFP gathering and consumption trends across Spain [141]. The authors observe that WFPs continue to be used in areas with deep-rooted culinary traditions and in some instances have become gourmet ingredients for chefs. Schulp et al. [142] also suggest that the cultural benefits of wild foods in the European Union might exceed their income and food benefits and observe that wild mushroom and food plant collecting are generally highest in Southern European countries where gastronomic identity is strongest.

4. An Integrated Approach for Conserving and Sustainably Using WFPs

With the gradual disappearance of WFPs from nature and diets, the question is how to effectively promote their sustainable use and simultaneously conserve them for food security and nutrition. Because they exist on a continuum of human management, from truly wild to semi-domesticated [7], and because the germplasm and other plant material (e.g., tissue, embryos etc.) of some species may not be suitable for ex situ conservation [143], both in situ and ex situ conservation should be combined for optimal results [144–146] (Figure 2). In situ conservation strategies can complement ex situ conservation and allow WFPs to continue to evolve adaptive traits in their natural environments while benefiting those who need them most, particularly in areas where high diversity, rural poverty and malnutrition coexist.

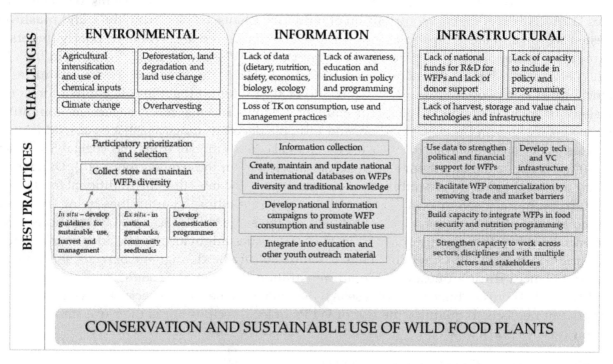

Figure 2. Proposed best practices for the long-term co-creation of conservation and sustainable use of WFPs help overcome many of the challenges identified.

Above, we have identified an array of threats to WFPs including: land use changes, deforestation and degradation; agricultural change, intensification and chemical input use; overharvest or unsustainable harvesting; loss of traditional management practices that communities used to promote the production of wild food plants (for example, pruning and burning); and climate change. We also identified a range of barriers that are contributing to the loss of use and value for WFPs, such as, lack of information (diet, nutrition, safety economics, and ecological); lack of harvest, storage and value chain tech and infrastructure; and lack of awareness, education and inclusion in policy and programming.

In the subsequent sections of this paper we propose a set of best practice actions that can be taken to support sustainable use and conservation of WFPs. This set of actions laid out in Figure 2 will act to overcome or mitigate against many of the threats and barriers identified.

The proposed set of best practice actions includes: the collection of information (identify the diversity of WFPs that are present in a given environment, information on nutrient composition and contribution to diet, economic importance, and ecological studies to determine sustainable offtake); (ii) prioritize the species with greatest potential to fill nutrition gaps, greatest need in terms of conservation, greatest cultural importance; (iii) protect species that are vulnerable through ex situ conservation; (iv) promote the use and management of WFPs in natural environments (in situ) (including sustainable management and collection guidelines where needed); (v) develop domestication programs where necessary and possible to avoid overexploitation in the wild; (vi) build local capacity to improve storage, processing, value chains, and markets (and all related technology and infrastructure); (vii) integrate WFP into programming and education and other youth outreach so as to raise awareness; (viii) develop and strengthen policies that support the conservation and sustainable use of WFPs; and (ix) and build donor commitment to funding efforts to support sustainable use and conservation of WFPs.

Each community and each WFP are unique, and will require a different set of actions, possibly occurring in a different order. Successful implementation of the set of best practice actions best suited to any given context will require working in a coordinated fashion across disciplines and sectors at the local, regional, and international level, and is largely dependent on the close and active participation of the national and local stakeholders. Due to the limits of time-bound projects (e.g., capacity, resources), it is rare for a single project or intervention to cover all elements or actions needed for a comprehensive and integrated approach. Below we present examples of best practice actions that we believe have successfully helped to further the conservation and sustainable use of WFPs.

4.1. Identify and Prioritize

The identification of WFPs to include in conservation and sustainable use strategies will almost invariably require close collaboration with indigenous and local communities who are the main users and custodians of this diversity. As opposed to extractive methods, participatory research approaches that integrate traditional and scientific knowledge are the most appropriate to collect information on WFPs while maximizing benefits for the communities involved [147]. Prior to the intervention, the community should be aware and agree on every aspect of the research process so that the methods, the analysis and the purposes of the data collection are clearly understood [148]. Ethnobotanical surveys and free-listing exercises are the most commonly used methods to complement scientific ecogeographic assessments. In the majority of the studies discussed in this paper, focus group discussions conducted with knowledgeable key informants were able to help fill knowledge gaps in WFP availability and use. Useful tools for assessing the potential of WFPs to fill seasonal food insecurity gaps, and low dietary diversity characterized by low fruit and vegetable consumption, are seasonal calendars, such as the one shown in Figure 3 developed by BFN Brazil to investigate flowering and fruiting seasons for wild fruit species. Data can then be transformed into an accessible and understandable tool to assist communities and decision makers adopt healthier diets based on local biodiversity [149].

Market surveys are also useful to understand what WFPs might be available for consumption within a community. A notable example is represented by BFN Turkey, which undertook market surveys and key informant interviews with 2334 local wild plant gatherers, sellers and consumers of WFPs to capture the diversity of WFPs still being used across three ecogeographic regions [28,150]. Documenting the use of wild plants in this participatory way has several benefits that include: (i) facilitating knowledge transmission from elders to younger generations and between community members; (ii) stimulating local innovation without undermining cultural traditions and local governance mechanisms, and (iii) ensuring that the community can use this diversity to address its own questions, challenges and needs [147]. In Western Kenya, for example, biodiversity surveys and dietary health assessments were followed by a series of participatory workshops that enabled five communities to gain and share knowledge on available wild and cultivated biodiversity, discuss options on ways to use this diversity to improve malnutrition within their communities, rank and prioritize the most suitable species and develop their own community action plans (CAP) towards this end. In collaboration with the ministries of Agriculture and Health, training was then provided to assist with the integration of the chosen species—mostly African leafy vegetables and legumes—into sustainable production systems and diets. One year into CAP implementation, mean dietary diversity scores and the percentage of children meeting minimum dietary diversity had significantly increased in all the households in the sublocation, irrespective of participation in the scheme, indicating the adoption of these best practices by neighboring households. The dietary diversity scores of women from participating households had also significantly increased [151].

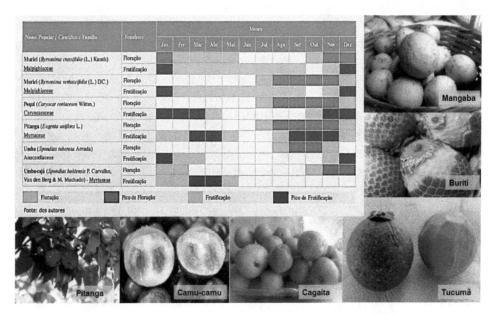

Figure 3. Research into the flowering and fruiting period of wild fruits and greens within a given geography can be used to develop an adaptable tool for informed decision making at both community and government level. Credit: BFN Brazil.

With all probability, surveys will reveal a long list of species that could be the focus of further research and promotion in food and nutrition strategies. Realistically, limited resources will often require a prioritization exercise that reduces the list to a manageable number. Since the intent is to ensure that WFPs are safeguarded and sustainably consumed, again community participation in the prioritization process is key, for example, to single out species that could be conserved in seed saving facilities, domesticated, or included in breeding programs, or to identify WFPs with the potential to contribute to nutrition, climate-change resilience and other aspects of community well-being. In the earlier example from Turkey, the BFN team developed an ad hoc sustainability index to reduce an initial sample size of 43 species, mostly WFPs, to three target species—foxtail lily (*Eremurus spectabilis*), golden thistle (*Scolymus hispanicus*), and einkorn wheat (*Triticum monococcum*)—which have since been the object of domestication research as well as post-harvest handling and value chain analysis [150].

4.2. The Nutritional Importance of WFPs and Associated Traditional Knowledge

Understanding the nutrient content and health properties of WFPs (e.g., compositional data) as well as their contribution to diets will also greatly assist in the prioritization process. Compositional data is key to national nutritional planning and for developing locally fitting dietary guidelines. Seldom, however, does nutrition information appear in national food composition tables and databases, and if data does exist it is either scattered across different sources in institutional databases, in academic journals and grey literature, or is outdated and/or incomplete making data compilation a daunting task [28,150]. An additional hurdle is the standardization of food composition values. Common component names are often expressed inaccurately (e.g., vitamin A: retinol activity equivalents vs. retinol equivalents) or differ in terms of units, denominators, significant figures, maximum decimal places, and conversion factors [152]. Of further importance, is the documentation and protection of traditional knowledge related to consumption and preparation of WFPs, available largely in the recollections of elderly users, i.e., rural, indigenous, and forest-dependent communities, including local farmers, and city migrants. Some information may be available in national floras, in herbaria and in ethnological studies of local human ethnical groups, but additional botanical, culinary, nutritional, cultural research is required to fill this knowledge gap. As explained in Section 4.1, to avoid issues of misuse and abuse of this information, it is important that respondents are always adequately informed about data use, that sources are acknowledged, and that the data is made available in public databases. Biological knowledge on individual species is also frequently lacking but particularly essential for both in situ and ex situ conservation.

One of the most recent and comprehensive attempts to fill the evidence gap in food composition data is provided by the GEF-supported Biodiversity for Food and Nutrition Project (BFN). Led by Brazil, Kenya, Sri Lanka, and Turkey, and implemented by Bioversity International with support from the UN Environment Programme (UNEP) and the Food and Agriculture Organization of the United Nations (FAO), the project has generated food composition data for 185 plant species, many of them wild, particularly in Brazil and Turkey [28,150,153]. Because of the high costs associated with food composition analysis, the four countries carried out literature reviews prior to the project to identify information gaps and narrow down the list of potentially interesting species to a practicable sample size for analysis and to select the species with the greatest potential for conservation, domestication/management, promotion and marketing. Following the literature review and identified data gaps, food composition analysis was carried out for those species and nutrients for which information was missing or incomplete. Examples of the high nutrient content of WFPs was demonstrated as part of the BFN project in Brazil and Turkey [28]. Similar results were obtained in Indonesia by reviewing the country's food composition data [114] in which wild leafy vegetables are reported to contain higher amounts of limiting micronutrients than more commonly consumed greens (Figure 4).

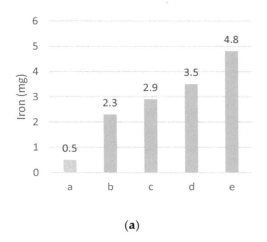
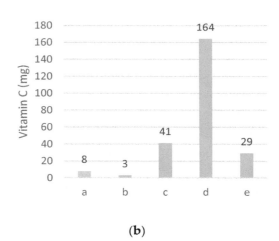

(a)   (b)

Figure 4. Four wild leafy vegetables from West Sumatra are compared to common lettuce (*Lactuca sativa*) in terms of (**a**) iron content (mg) and (**b**) vitamin C content (mg). In the graphs the letters stand for a lettuce; b vegetable fern "pakis" (*Diplazium esculentum*); c nightshade "leunca/ranti" (*Solanum americanum*), d sweet leaf "katuk/nasi-nasi" (*Sauropus androgynus*), and e water mimosa "komen" (*Neptunia prostrata*). Values are expressed per 100g of fresh, raw ingredient. *Source*: Indonesian Food Composition Data [114].

Species selection and prioritization, literature reviews, and generating food composition data is only the first step of a comprehensive and integrated conservation approach.

4.3. Collecting, Storing and Maintaining WFP Diversity

Once the species have been identified and prioritized, consideration will need to be given to safeguarding the species for future use, either through ex situ or in situ conservation strategies. Particularly for WFPs, ex situ measures are envisioned as a support to their propagation and reintroduction for habitat restoration [154]. In both cases, to be effective, conservation should involve a wide range of stakeholders working together both in the public and private sectors, across the agricultural and environmental domains [145].

In many cases, governments have established national plant genetic resources programs and seed saving facilities (e.g., gene banks) for ex situ conservation.

However, seed and planting material produced by these "formal" facilities are often inaccessible to smallholder farmers due to strict regulations limiting exchange, little involvement of community actors in the governance, and management of these services [146], as well as imbalances in seed availability, access, and quality for smallholders [155]. However, alternatives do exist. The MGU Useful Plants project, for example, worked closely with communities in Botswana, Kenya, Mali, South Africa, and Mexico to select useful indigenous plants for which high-quality seed collections were established. Seed lots were also banked in the five countries as well as being duplicated and tested at the Millennium Seed Bank in Kew [48,154,156]. Research on seed germination helped support plant propagation activities. The propagules were then planted in community gardens while facilities were established or improved at the local level to facilitate conservation of the prioritized species. Training and knowledge on seed conservation in seed conservation, plant propagation, and planting activities were also provided [49]. This form of conserving WFPs, which takes place in situ, either "on farm" or "in the wild" in natural habitats or protected areas, provides greater opportunity for the involvement of local communities. Once hotspots of WFP occurrence are identified, farmers and indigenous communities living within and around those habitats and protected areas should be involved in conservation activities with due recognition given to their roles and rights in managing WFPs. Further guidance on the establishment of sites for active in situ conservation (i.e., where populations are actively monitored and maintained) of WFPs can be found in the "Voluntary Guidelines on the Conservation and Sustainable Use of Crop Wild Relatives and Wild Food Plants" [145].

Midway between these two conservation approaches are community seed banks or gene banks, which are community-maintained facilities that preserve seeds and other planting materials for local use [146]. These are a collective forms of crop conservation that provide farmers with access to seed, planting material, and traditional knowledge that may otherwise be lost [147]. They also foster community engagement and strengthen the understanding of farmers' and community' intellectual property [157]. By documenting and storing biodiversity and associated traditional knowledge, the seed banks also raise awareness of unique biodiversity in a given area. The community-based organizations (CBO) operating in Vihiga County, Western Kenya, have now established their own community seed bank for African indigenous vegetables and legumes [158]. Creating markets for the seeds and planting material can create additional conservation incentives. Such is the case for the communities in Botswana engaged in the MGU UPP who collect the edible seeds of *Tylosema esculentum* (Burch.) A. Schreib (morama bean) for conservation and cultivation, consumption, sale, and processing into numerous marketable food products. Likewise, the Tsetseng community, through their community trust, have become leading innovators in marketable morama products [159].

4.4. Domestication Programmes and Guidelines for Sustainable Collection

Depending on conservation status and extent of utilization of WFPs, domestication programs may be required to facilitate cultivation of these wild species and thus to ease the pressure on wild populations and rebuild and restore the genetic diversity that has been lost. A successful example is provided by Turkey in its quest to reduce overexploitation of golden thistle (*Scolymus hispanicus* L.). Golden thistle is a flowering plant that is widely consumed across Turkey and is traditionally collected from the wild for its roots and immature leaves that are sold in local markets [62,160]. Selected by the BFN Project as one of the target species for potential commercialization, breeding, and domestication efforts were undertaken by the Aegean Agricultural Research Institute and the University of Anadolu in collaboration with 37 farmers to select, characterize, and evaluate the species [161]. Nurseries established following initial selection of the hardiest plants produced an average yield of 3.9 tons/ha and up to a maximum of 7 tons/ha. A cultivar called "Sari" was registered and seeds distributed to farmers in the İzmir province. Golden thistle is now cultivated on an area of 100 ha^{-1} [161]. To complement seed distribution, guidelines for the sustainable production of golden thistle were also produced to assist farmers in addressing critical aspects such as climate and soil conditions, plant management, harvest, and seed production (Figure 5).

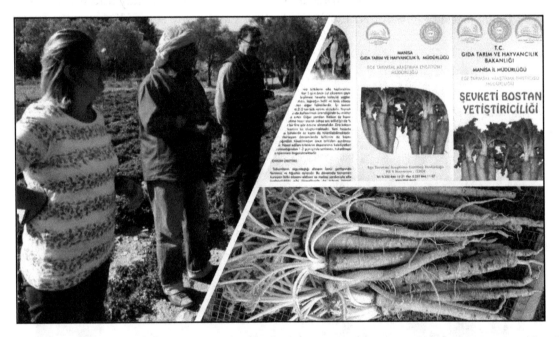

Figure 5. From left to right, top to bottom. BFN Turkey work with farmers to test domesticated golden thistle (*Scolymus hispanicus* L.); the sustainable production guidelines; and harvested golden thistle roots ready for sale Credit: BFN Turkey.

4.5. Strengthening Policies in Support of WFP Conservation and Sustainable Use

Once baseline data has been gathered, guidelines exist to assist countries in preparing a National Plan for the Conservation and Sustainable Use of Wild Food Plants and crop wild relatives, including setting up a monitoring plan for WFP diversity [145]. The scope of the action plan, its application and effectiveness will very much depend on the national context, the existing policy framework and institutional arrangements, the range of stakeholders involved and their interrelationships, as well as on the resources available. Guidelines are also provided for undertaking preparatory work towards this end [145]. Suggestions are made on how to promote wider use of crop wild relatives and WFPs, but few examples are given to show countries what is practical or actionable. One possibility, which has shown great promise in the BFN Project, is to link producers and collectors to institutional or private sector markets enabling them to benefit from the authorized trade of WFPs. Brazil has used its two largest public procurement programs, the Food Procurement Program (PAA) and the National School Feeding Program (PNAE), to stimulate engagement by family farmers and wild plant collectors (known as extractivists) in sustainable agriculture and the management of Brazilian food diversity, including many WFPs. Both PNAE and PAA are in fact obliged to buy a proportion of the food they distribute from family farmers and pay a 30% bonus for organic or agroecological produce, preferring suppliers from indigenous and traditional communities [162]. PAA also supports activities aimed at the conservation, production, storage, and distribution of local or traditional seed varieties (Beltrame et al., 2020) [28]. Working closely with government actors and using the nutritional data generated as part of the BFN project, BFN Brazil was also able to promote the publication of Ordinance N° 284/2018, which officially recognizes the nutritional and sociocultural value of over 100 plant species native to the Amazon, Caatinga, Atlantic Forest, and Cerrado biomes. This has boosted the market value of native biodiversity including WFPs, with ministries now referring to the list in the "Sociobiodiversity Ordinance" to purchase biodiversity and farmers and collectors eager to join the scheme. In order to do so, however, producers must adhere to procurement regulations, and follow training and guidelines for organic production and the sustainable management of these resources in the wild (Figure 6). Similar linkages were fostered in the other three BFN countries, increasing structured demand for African leafy vegetables in Kenya, for WFPs in Turkey and for native fruits such as wood apple (*Limonia acidissima*) in Sri Lanka including via private sector linkages (see next section).

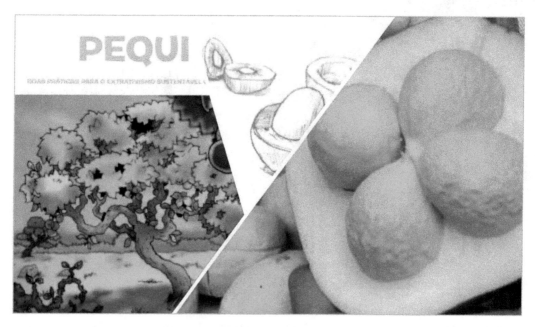

Figure 6. Best practices for the sustainable harvesting and management of pequi (*Caryocar brasiliense* Cambess), common to Brazil's Cerrado region. The guidelines are produced by the Ministry of Agriculture, Livestock and Supply (MAPA) in support of producers/extractivists intending to take part in the public procurement schemes.

4.6. Raising Public Awareness of the Importance of WFPs

Raising public awareness of the important contribution WFPs can make to diets and livelihoods is another effective way to secure research and policy investments targeting their conservation and use and creating a mutually reinforcing virtuous cycle [163]. This is probably the area in which countries invested in protecting WFPs let lose their creativity and excel in finding ingenious, innovative, and culturally acceptable ways of communicating the importance of WFPs to different target groups. Naturally, collaborating and partnering with the broadest range of stakeholders, e.g., farmer groups, NGOs, private sector enterprises, schools, the media, and ministries will ensure that there is clear and cohesive messaging that is able to reach the widest possible audience.

4.6.1. Youth

As future consumers and protectors of biodiversity, youth are an important target audience for WFP messaging. Awareness raising campaigns can take advantage of recurring activities such as biodiversity festivals or food fairs to organize nature walks or competitions for younger participants [28,150] or join forces with relevant ministries (e.g., Environment, Agriculture, and Education) to introduce messaging around WFP conservation and use in curricular activities and courses (Figure 7). For older students, WFPs offer an interesting opportunity for "greening" vocational training, particularly in the food and beverage sector. In Turkey, to raise the profile of WFPs, the BFN project partnered with the Halim Foçali Vocational School organizing a series of lectures and hands-on activities for 16 student chefs, who were trained to recognize and collect local edible species and use them in their cooking classes. Future plans for the institute include the establishment of an herb garden on the school premises where WFPs will be grown and harvested for use in cooking courses. Interest in the program from the National Education Directorate of Foça has led to plans for extending the training to other schools and officially include traditional WFPs in the school curriculum [150]. School gardens are also an effective way of promoting greater interest in biodiversity and can act as important conduit for improving nutrition, well-being and education of schoolchildren and their families [164], as well as acting as conservation networks for tree genetic resources [165] and reviving traditional food systems and culture [164].

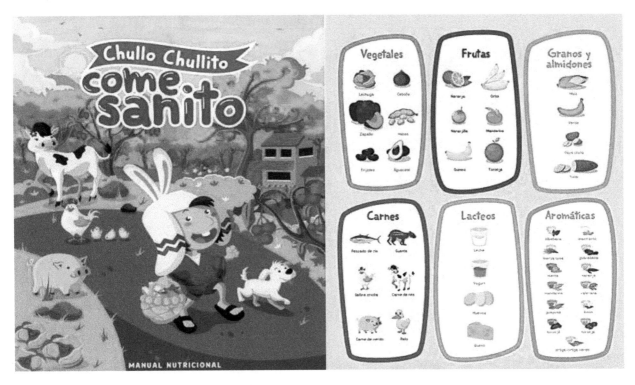

Figure 7. A nutrition education booklet from Ecuador that includes WFPs as a food group. On the left, the cover depicts the forest as an alternative source of foods, mainly fruits, while on the right, five food groups are shown along with a list of 13 WFPs (mostly aromatic plants) used for preparing hot beverages.

4.6.2. Communities and Households

As previously mentioned, it will be important to ensure that the main users of this diversity the communities that continue collecting and maintaining WFPs are aware of the species' nutritional and sociocultural importance. Seasonal food availability booklets and calendars, such as the one shown in Figure 5, and simple, locally appropriate picture posters (Figure 8) can serve the dual purpose of revitalizing the use of WFPs and imparting basic nutrition information derived from national nutrition guidelines. Translated into local languages, these tools can be used by government extension workers and NGO practitioners to offer an overview of local diet quality and consumption patterns derived from baseline assessments and provide recommendations on how WFPs and other local agrobiodiversity can fill existing nutrient gaps. To avoid issues of overharvesting, it will be important, that the above information is complemented by easy-to-understand guidelines on the sustainable collection and management of these species, as shown by the informative brochures that accompanied the revival of WFPs in Turkey (Figure 9).

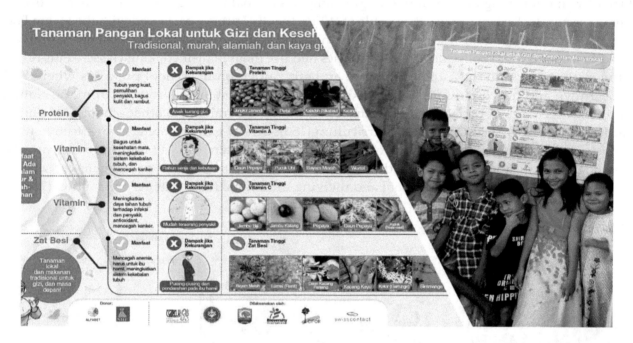

Figure 8. Community poster in local language developed in West Sumatra, Indonesia, as part of the "Food, Agrobiodiversity, and Diet project" explaining the health benefits of local food plants that are rich in protein, vitamin A, vitamin C, and iron, and Mandailing children learning about local foods. Credit: Lukas Pawera.

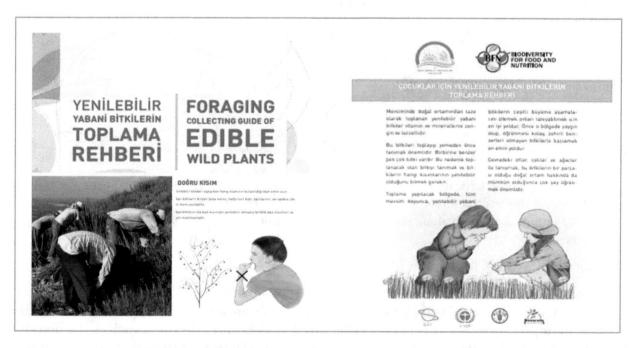

Figure 9. Foragers' guide to edible wild plants and illustrations taken from "A children's guide to the collection of wild edibles", produced by BFN Turkey to complement activities aimed at raising the profile of Turkish WFPs. Credit: BFN Turkey.

4.6.3. Policymakers

Policymakers and key change agents who can support the conservation and use of WFPs are to be found within the following sectors: nutrition, health, agriculture, forestry, education, environment, trade, planning, poverty reduction, food security, rural development, economy, and finance at national, regional, and international levels. Whatever their background, for effective decision-making to occur, policymakers need access to timely, independent and reliable information, in a simple and useful form, accompanied by the cost implications of the research, indicating whether it is feasible and affordable [166]. As demonstrated by the endorsement of the "Sociobiodiversity Ordinance" in Brazil, for example, nutrition evidence generated via food composition analysis was critical for expanding the list of sociobiodiversity species to include previously neglected WFPs, and for subsequent policy uptake by national programs dealing with food and nutrition security.

The recognition of WFPs as important elements of healthy diets and rural resilience has thus resulted in increased federal funding (approximately US$6 Million per year) for public procurement programs to purchase sociobiodiversity products directly from family farmers and provided an indication of the untapped market potential of WFPs in institutional markets [167]. The increased appreciation of the role WFPs play in rural diets is also leading to investigations into the affordability of diets that include WFPs [126]. As mentioned earlier, the study carried out in Eastern Baringo, Kenya, has shown that wild plant species, especially vegetables, are able to significantly reduce (by 30–70%) the cost of nutritious meal for vulnerable groups [54]. The tool, which provides an insight into the affordability of nutritious foods, offers a useful entry point for policy discussion around the types of commodities and delivery channels that are likely to achieve nutritional outcomes particularly for the most vulnerable segments of the population [168].

4.6.4. Broader Audiences

Recent interest in food and gastronomy programs worldwide has acted as the perfect jumping board for WFPs, particularly in developing countries. Many of the approaches adopted by BFN project countries have extensively been described [28,150,153], and broadly involve communities partnering with celebrity chefs, gastronomists, or taking advantage of existing food festivals to organize information and hands-on events on WFP collection, transformation, and cooking (Figure 10). Innovative approaches for reaching out to broader audiences are described in detail by Gee and Lee (2020) who look at emerging youth-led innovations that can be productively applied to the conservation and sustainable use of food biodiversity, including WFPs. The realms of social media and mobile technology are rapidly evolving, and via mobile apps consumers are now able to (i) find local crops in season and plan grocery purchases, (ii) identify plants through a global photo database, (iii) learn about wild edible plants (Wild Edibles and Foraging Flashcard Lite), (iv) and even trace fresh crops back to farms using blockchain technology. On the production side, a growing number of applications, including in developing countries, offer "smart phone farmers" unprecedented access to crop, field, and market information, which could easily be extended to incorporate WFPs. Gee and Lee [169] also explore the benefits of creating conservation networks for biodiversity through international movements such as via "Campesina" and Slow Food, which can connect different actors who are motivated to improve global and community-based food systems using food biodiversity.

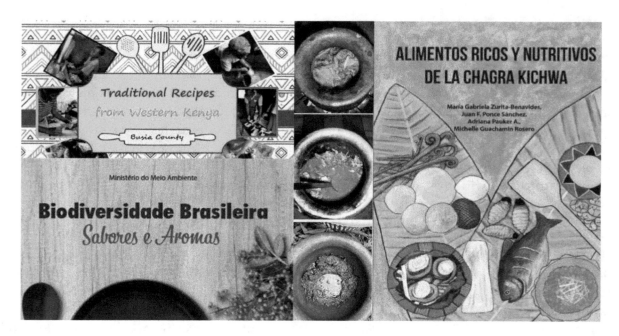

Figure 10. Front covers of recipe books developed as part of the WFP-focused projects in Brazil, Ecuador and Kenya. Credit: BFN Brazil, IKIAM and BFN Kenya.

5. Conclusions

While WFPs contribute to the diets and livelihoods of millions of people worldwide at the local level, there is still much that we do not yet fully understand about them and thus their role is not fully appreciated. This makes it a challenge when it comes to decisions and actions that might support more effective national and international conservation, sustainable management, and useful strategies for WFPs. Some of these actions are summarized in Table S2. While there are an increasing number of publications outlining the importance of WFPs, usually at a local level, there is largely a scarcity of data and information at a national level, and conservation assessments are still limited. This fails to convey the full contribution that WFPs make to food security and nutrition and the overall importance of these biological resources to national economies in many parts of the world. Furthermore, while we increasingly learn more about some of the threats which impact WFPs, we still know so little about their biology and ecology as well as the dynamics of their use and how climate change is impacting them now and in the future. The integrated conservation approach described in this paper is intended to guide stakeholders in creating plans and strategies to ensure that WFPs are used sustainably and are conserved for generations to come.

In this review we survey the contribution of WFPs to food security, nutrition, and livelihoods in a variety of geographical settings, many of which have benefited from the availability of donor-funded projects and therefore the dedicated attention of researchers and their organizations. It is by no means a comprehensive review. However, the limited cases and examples it highlights clearly demonstrate that the contribution of WFPs to food security, nutrition, and livelihoods is significant. With increased development attention and research investments, including a more effective enabling policy environment, the role of WFPs could be strengthened in the future.

A greater understanding and appreciation, especially by decision-makers, of the nutritional value of WFPs and their contribution to food security and nutrition could see the enhanced inclusion of WFPs in important national nutrition policy instruments such as dietary guidelines, development plans, or in nutrition education and school curricula. Greater use should also go hand in hand with increased research and investments targeting existing biological and ecological knowledge gaps on WFPs, such as plant demographic studies to calculate sustainable harvest levels in the wild or studies on seed biology and ecology to ensure they are adequately conserved ex situ. If WFPs were provided with greater policy recognition and support, especially through policy incentives and the development of innovative market-based demand approaches (with clear benefits arising to custodians), it would help create longer-term economic viability. This, in turn, could help greatly in better linking the conservation of WFPs and their sustainable traditional management and use, something which is currently missing in most national Plant Genetic Resources conservation strategies and action plans.

Supplementary Materials: Table S1: Plant families that include WFPs and semi-cultivated species that are known to contribute to food and nutrition security; Table S2: Summary of actions that can be undertaken across the four pillars by the main stakeholders involved in WFP conservation and use.

Author Contributions: Conceptualization, T.B. and D.H.; investigation, T.U., E.M., D.B., C.T., D.P., L.P., B.P., and A.T.; writing—original draft, T.B.; and writing—review and editing, T.B., B.P., T.U., E.M., D.H., D.B., C.T., D.P., L.P., A.T.; M.T., and J.E. All authors have read and agreed to the published version of the manuscript.

Funding: Overall support for the Biodiversity for Food and Nutrition (BFN) Project was provided by the Global Environment Facility (GEF Project ID 3808). Co-funding and implementation support were received from the UN Environment Programme; the Food and Agriculture Organization of the United Nations; Bioversity International and the governments of Brazil, Kenya, Sri Lanka, and Turkey. Additional funding was received by the Australian Centre for International Agriculture Research for work in Kenya (HORT2014/100, GP2017/007 and GP2018/101), as well as the CGIAR Research Program on Agriculture for Nutrition and Health (A4NH). For the Food, Agrobiodiversity, and Diet (FAD) Project in West Sumatra, Indonesia, the authors would like to thank the Neys-van Hoogstraten Foundation (Project IN305), and ALFABET mobility for supporting Lukas Pawera under the Erasmus Mundus Action 2 Programme. For work in Kenya, the support of Biovision Foundation Switzerland and A4NH CRP are gratefully acknowledged. The "MGU—Useful Plants Project" was funded by MGU, a kind and generous philanthropist based in Spain. E.M. is supported by the Kew Future Leaders Fellowship—Diversity and Livelihoods, of the Royal Botanic Gardens, Kew, UK.

Acknowledgments: The authors would also like to gratefully acknowledge the many colleagues and institutions in participating countries that contributed to the work described in this paper.

Abbreviations

BFN	Biodiversity for Food and Nutrition Project
CAP	Community action plans
CBD	Convention on Biological Diversity
CBO	Community-based organization
CIAT	International Center for Tropical Agriculture now part of the Alliance of Bioversity International and CIAT
EIARD	European Initiative for Agricultural Research for Development
FAD	Food, Agrobiodiversity and Diet Project
FAO	Food and Agriculture Organization of the United Nations
GEF	Global Environment Facility
GPA	Global Plan of Action for Plant Genetic Resources for Food and Agriculture of the FAO
IKIAM	Universidad Regional Amazónica - Amazon Regional University (Ecuador)
IUCN	International Union for Conservation of Nature
MAPA	Ministério da Agricultura, Pecuária e Abastecimento - Ministry of Agriculture, Livestock and Supply (Brazil)
NBSAPs	National Biodiversity Strategies and Action Plan (of the CBD)
NGO	Non-governmental organization
PAA	Programa de Aquisição de Alimentos - Food Procurement Program (Brazil)
PNAE	Programa nacional de alimentação escolar - National School Feeding Program (Brazil)
PNG	Papua New Guinea
PPF	Plantas Paro o Futuro (Plants for the Future Initiative – Brazil)
RAE	Retinol Activity Equivalents
R&D	Research and Development
SDG	Sustainable Development Goal

SOWBFA   State of the World's Biodiversity for Food and Agriculture of the FAO
UNEP   UN Environment Programme
UPP   Useful Plants Project, Kew
WFPs   Wild food plants
WLVs   Wild leafy vegetables

References

1.   Zohary, D.; Hopf, M.; Weiss, E. *Domestication of Plants in the Old World. The Origin and Spread of Domesticated Plants in South-West Asia, Europe, and the Mediterranean Basin*, 4th ed.; Oxford University Press: New York, NY, USA, 2012. [CrossRef]

2.   Sowunmi, M.A. The beginnings of agriculture in West Africa: Botanical evidence. *Curr. Anthropol.* **1985**, *26*, 127–129. [CrossRef]

3.   Johnson, A.; Behrens, C.A. Nutritional criteria in machiguenga food production decisions: A linear-programming analysis. *Hum. Ecol.* **1982**, *10*, 167–189. [CrossRef]

4.   Heywood, V.H. *Use and Potential of Wild Plants in Farm Households*; FAO Farm System Management Series; FAO: Rome, Italy, 1999; Volume 15.

5.   Bharucha, Z.; Pretty, J. The roles and values of wild foods in agricultural systems. *Philos. Trans. R. Soc. B Biol. Sci.* **2010**, *365*, 2913–2926. [CrossRef] [PubMed]

6.   Casas, A.; Otero-Arnaiz, A.; Perez-Negron, E.; Valiente-Banuet, A. In situ management and domestication of plants in Mesoamerica. *Ann. Bot.* **2007**, *100*, 1101–1115. [CrossRef]

7.   Cruz-Garcia, G.S. Management and motivations to manage "wild" food plants. A case study in a mestizo village in the amazon deforestation frontier. *Front. Ecol. Evol.* **2017**, *5*, 127. [CrossRef]

8.   Heywood, V.H. Overview of Agricultural Biodiversity and Its Contribution to Nutrition and Health. In *Diversifying Food and Diets: Using Agricultural Biodiversity to Improve Nutrition and Health*; Fanzo, J., Hunter, D., Borelli, T., Mattei, F., Eds.; Routledge: London, UK, 2013; pp. 35–67.

9.   Commission on Genetic Resources for Food and Agriculture—FAO. *Biodiversity for Food and Agriculture—Revised Draft—Needs and Possible Actions CGRFA/NFP-BFA-1/18/2*; FAO: Rome, Italy, 2018.

10.   Asprilla-Perea, J.; Díaz-Puente, J.M. Importance of wild foods to household food security in tropical forest areas. *Food Secur.* **2019**, *11*, 15–22. [CrossRef]

11.   Bioversity International. *Mainstreaming Agrobiodiversity in Sustainable Food Systems: Scientific Foundations for an Agrobiodiversity Index*, 1st ed.; Bioversity International: Rome, Italy, 2017.

12.   Broegaard, R.B.; Rasmussen, L.V.; Dawson, N.; Mertz, O.; Vongvisouk, T.; Grogan, K. Wild food collection and nutrition under commercial agriculture expansion in agriculture-forest landscapes. *For. Policy Econ.* **2017**. [CrossRef]

13.   Rowland, D.; Ickowitz, A.; Powell, B.; Nasi, R.; Sunderland, T. Forest foods and healthy diets: Quantifying the contributions. *Environ. Conserv.* **2017**, *44*, 102–114. [CrossRef]

14.   Ickowitz, A.; Powell, B.; Rowland, D.; Jones, A.; Sunderland, T. Agricultural intensification, dietary diversity, and markets in the global food security narrative. *Glob. Food Sec.* **2019**, *20*, 9–16. [CrossRef]

15.   Carvalho, A.M.; Barata, A.M. The Consumption of Wild Edible Plants. In *Wild Plants, Mushrooms and Nuts*; John Wiley & Sons, Ltd.: Chichester, UK, 2016; pp. 159–198. [CrossRef]

16.   Ojelel, S.; Mucunguzi, P.; Katuura, E.; Kakudidi, E.K.; Namaganda, M.; Kalema, J. Wild edible plants used by communities in and around selected forest reserves of Teso-Karamoja Region, Uganda. *J. Ethnobiol. Ethnomed.* **2019**, *15*, 3. [CrossRef]

17.   Kuhnlein, H.V.; Erasmus, B.; Spigelski, D. *Indigenous Peoples' Food Systems: The Many Dimensions of Culture, Diversity and Environment for Nutrition and Health*; Food and Agriculture Organization of the United Nations: Rome, Italy, 2009.

18.   Kuhnlein, H.V. Holding on to Agrobiodiversity: Human Nutrition and Health of Indigenous Peoples. In *Routledge Handbook of Agricultural Biodiversity*; Hunter, D., Guarino, L., Spillane, C., McKeown, P.C., Eds.; Routledge: London, UK, 2017; p. 692.

19.   United Nations. *State of the World's Indigenous Peoples*; United Nations: New York, NY, USA, 2009.

20.   Angelsen, A. Policies for reduced deforestation and their impact on agricultural production. *Proc. Natl. Acad. Sci. USA* **2010**, *107*, 19639–19644. [CrossRef] [PubMed]

21. Powell, B.; Thilsted, S.H.; Ickowitz, A.; Termote, C.; Sunderland, T.; Herforth, A. Improving diets with wild and cultivated biodiversity from across the landscape. *Food Secur.* **2015**, *7*, 535–554. [CrossRef]
22. Aryal, K.P.; Poudel, S.; Chaudhary, R.P.; Chettri, N.; Chaudhary, P.; Ning, W.; Kotru, R. Diversity and use of wild and non-cultivated edible plants in the western Himalaya. *J. Ethnobiol. Ethnomed.* **2018**, *14*, 10. [CrossRef] [PubMed]
23. Boedecker, J.; Termote, C.; Assogbadjo, A.E.; Van Damme, P.; Lachat, C. Dietary contribution of wild edible plants to women's diets in the buffer zone around the Lama forest, Benin—An underutilized potential. *Food Secur.* **2014**, *6*, 833–849. [CrossRef]
24. Ju, Y.; Zhuo, J.; Liu, B.; Long, C. Eating from the wild: Diversity of wild edible plants used by Tibetans in Shangri-La Region, Yunnan, China. *J. Ethnobiol. Ethnomed.* **2013**, *9*, 28. [CrossRef]
25. Shumsky, S.A.; Hickey, G.M.; Pelletier, B.; Johns, T. Understanding the contribution of wild edible plants to rural social-ecological resilience in Semi-Arid Kenya. *Ecol. Soc.* **2014**, *19*, art34. [CrossRef]
26. Smith, E.; Ahmed, S.; Dupuis, V.; Running Crane, M.; Eggers, M.; Pierre, M.; Flagg, K.; Byker Shanks, C. Contribution of wild foods to diet, food security, and cultural values amidst climate change. *J. Agric. Food Syst. Community Dev.* **2019**, 1–24. [CrossRef]
27. Fernández-Ruiz, V.; Morales, P.; Ruiz-Rodríguez, B.M.; Isasa, E.T. Nutrients and Bioactive Compounds in Wild Fruits Through Different Continents. In *Wild Plants, Mushrooms and Nuts*; John Wiley & Sons, Ltd.: Chichester, UK, 2016; pp. 263–314. [CrossRef]
28. Hunter, D.; Borelli, T.; Beltrame, D.M.O.; Oliveira, C.N.S.; Coradin, L.; Wasike, V.W.; Wasilwa, L.; Mwai, J.; Manjella, A.; Samarasinghe, G.W.L.; et al. The potential of neglected and underutilized species for improving diets and nutrition. *Planta* **2019**, *250*, 709–729. [CrossRef]
29. Morales, P.; Herrera, P.G.; González, M.C.M.; Hurtado, M.C.; de Cortes Sánchez Mata, M. Wild Greens As Source of Nutritive and Bioactive Compounds Over the World. In *Wild Plants, Mushrooms and Nuts*; John Wiley & Sons, Ltd.: Chichester, UK, 2016; pp. 199–261. [CrossRef]
30. Kinnunen, P.; Guillaume, J.H.A.; Taka, M.; D'Odorico, P.; Siebert, S.; Puma, M.J.; Jalava, M.; Kummu, M. Local food crop production can fulfil demand for less than one-third of the population. *Nat. Food* **2020**, *1*, 229–237. [CrossRef]
31. Padulosi, S.; Mal, B.; King, O.; Gotor, E. Minor millets as a central element for sustainably enhanced incomes, empowerment, and nutrition in rural India. *Sustainability* **2015**, *7*, 8904–8933. [CrossRef]
32. Shackleton, S.; Paumgarten, F.; Kassa, H.; Husselman, M.; Zida, M. Opportunities for enhancing poor women's socioeconomic empowerment in the value chains of three African Non-Timber Forest Products (NTFPs). *Int. For. Rev.* **2011**, *13*, 136–151. [CrossRef]
33. Torero, M. Without food, there can be no exit from the pandemic. *Nature* **2020**, *580*, 588–589. [CrossRef] [PubMed]
34. HLPE. *Food Security and Nutrition: Building a Global Narrative towards 2030*; HLPE: Rome, Italy, 2020.
35. Béné, C. Resilience of local food systems and links to food security—A review of some important concepts in the context of COVID-19 and other shocks. *Food Secur.* **2020**. [CrossRef] [PubMed]
36. Fernandes, N. Economic effects of coronavirus outbreak (COVID-19) on the world economy. *SSRN Electron. J.* **2020**. [CrossRef]
37. United Nations. *Policy Brief: The Impact of COVID-19 on Food Security and Nutrition*; United Nations: New York, NY, USA, 2020; p. 23.
38. Vandebroek, I.; Pieroni, A.; Stepp, J.R.; Hanazaki, N.; Ladio, A.; Alves, R.R.N.; Picking, D.; Delgoda, R.; Maroyi, A.; van Andel, T.; et al. Reshaping the future of ethnobiology research after the COVID-19 pandemic. *Nat. Plants* **2020**, *6*, 723–730. [CrossRef]
39. Cappelli, A.; Cini, E. Will the COVID-19 pandemic make us reconsider the relevance of short food supply chains and local productions? *Trends Food Sci. Technol.* **2020**, *99*, 566–567. [CrossRef]
40. IPES-Food. *COVID-19 and the Crisis in Food Systems: Symptoms, Causes, and Potential Solutions*; IPES-Food: Brussels, Belgium, 2020.
41. Poppick, L. The Effects of COVID-19 Will Ripple through Food Systems. Available online: https://www.scientificamerican.com/article/the-effects-of-covid-19-will-ripple-through-food-systems/ (accessed on 13 July 2020).

42. Mururia, D.; Mwale, A. Demand for Indigenous Vegetables Soar as Residents Grapple with COVID-19 Economic Shocks. Available online: https://www.kenyanews.go.ke/demand-for-indigenous-vegetables-soar-as-residents-grapple-with-covid-19-economic-shocks/ (accessed on 13 July 2020).

43. Giuliano, G. Coronavirus: From Wild Tobacco New Perspectives in the Treatment of COVID-19. Available online: https://www.enea.it/en/news-enea/news/coronavirus-from-wild-tobacco-new-perspectives-in-the-treatment-of-covid-19 (accessed on 13 July 2020).

44. Timoshyna, A.; Ling, X.; Zhang, K. COVID-19—The Role of Wild Plants in Health Treatment and Why Sustainability of Their Trade Matters. Available online: https://www.traffic.org/news/covid-19-the-role-of-wild-plants-in-health-treatment/ (accessed on 13 July 2020).

45. FAO. *The State of the World's Biodiversity for Food and Agriculture*; FAO: Rome, Italy, 2019. [CrossRef]

46. Ulian, T.; Diazgranados, M.; Pironon, S.; Padulosi, S.; Davies, L.; Howes, M.-J.; Borrell, J.; Ondo, I.; Perez Escobar, O.A.; Sharrock, S.; et al. Unlocking plant and fungal resources to support food security and promote sustainable agriculture. *Plants People Planet* **2020**. [CrossRef]

47. Zulu, D.; Ellis, R.H.; Culham, A. Collection, consumption, and sale of Lusala (*Dioscorea hirtiflora*)—A wild yam—By rural households in southern province, Zambia. *Econ. Bot.* **2019**, *73*, 47–63. [CrossRef]

48. Ulian, T.; Sacandé, M.; Hudson, A.; Mattana, E. Conservation of indigenous plants to support community livelihoods: The MGU—Useful plants project. *J. Environ. Plan. Manag.* **2017**, *60*, 668–683. [CrossRef]

49. Ulian, T.; Flores, C.; Lira, R.; Mamatsharaga, A.; Mogotsi, K.K. *Wild Plants for a Sustainable Future: 110 Multipurpose Species*, 1st ed.; Ulian, T., Flores, C., Lira, R., Mamatsharaga, A., Mogotsi, K.K., Muthoka, P., Ngwako, S., Nyamongo, D.O., Omondi, W., Sanogo, A.K., et al., Eds.; Kew Publishing: Kew, UK, 2019.

50. Maundu, P.M.; Njiro, E.I.; Chweya, J.A.; Imungi, J.K.; Seme, E.N. Kenya. In *The Biodiversity of Traditional Leafy Vegetables*; Chweya, J.A., Eyzaguirre, P.B., Eds.; International Plant Genetic Resources Institute: Rome, Italy, 1999; pp. 51–84.

51. Gotor, E.; Irungu, C. The impact of bioversity international's African leafy vegetables programme in Kenya. *Impact Assess. Proj. Apprais.* **2010**, *28*, 41–55. [CrossRef]

52. Bioversity International; European Initiative for Agricultural Research for Development. *African Leafy Vegetables Come out of the Shade*; Bioversity International: Rome, Italy, 2013; p. 6.

53. Borelli, T.; Gee, E.; Hunter, D. Neglected no more: Reframing the food systems narrative using agricultural biodiversity. In *Biodiversity, Food and Nutrition. A New Agenda for Sustainable Food Systems*; Hunter, D., Borelli, T., Gee, E., Eds.; Routledge: Oxford, UK, 2020.

54. Sarfo, J.; Keding, G.B.; Boedecker, J.; Pawelzik, E.; Termote, C. The impact of local agrobiodiversity and food interventions on cost, nutritional adequacy and affordability of women and children's diet in northern Kenya: A modeling exercise. *Front. Nutr.* **2020**. [CrossRef] [PubMed]

55. Penafiel, D.; Lachat, C.; Espinel, R.; Van Damme, P.; Kolsteren, P. A systematic review on the contributions of edible plant and animal biodiversity to human diets. *Ecohealth* **2011**, *8*, 381–399. [CrossRef] [PubMed]

56. Penafiel, D.; Vanhove, W.; Espinel, R.L.; Van Damme, P. Food biodiversity includes both locally cultivated and wild food species in Guasaganda, Central Ecuador. *J. Ethn. Foods* **2019**, *6*, 25. [CrossRef]

57. Jacob, M.C.M.; Araújo de Medeiros, M.F.; Albuquerque, U.P. Biodiverse food plants in the Semiarid Region of Brazil have unknown potential: A systematic review. *PLoS ONE* **2020**, *15*, e0230936. [CrossRef] [PubMed]

58. Baldermann, S.; Blagojević, L.; Frede, K.; Klopsch, R.; Neugart, S.; Neumann, A.; Ngwene, B.; Norkeweit, J.; Schröter, D.; Schröter, A.; et al. Are neglected plants the food for the future? *CRC Crit. Rev. Plant Sci.* **2016**, *35*, 106–119. [CrossRef]

59. Dogan, Y.; Baslar, S.; Ay, G.; Mert, H.H. The use of wild edible plants in western and central Anatolia (Turkey). *Econ. Bot.* **2004**, *58*, 684–690. [CrossRef]

60. Taylor, J.; Sarkis, L.; Hani, N.; Abulaila, K.; Ulian, T. Conservation and Sustainable Use of Wild Edible Plants in the Eastern Mediterranean Region. In *Role of Mediterranean Forests in the Paris Agreement, Proceedings of the Sixth Mediterranean Forest Week, Brummana, Lebanon, 1–5 April 2019*; Mohanna, C., Ed.; Forêt Méditerranéenne: Brummana, Lebanon, 2019; pp. 293–300.

61. Rivera, D.; Obón, C.; Heinrich, M.; Inocencio, C.; Verde, A.; Fajardo, J. Gathered Mediterranean Food Plants—Ethnobotanical Investigations and Historical Development. In *Local Mediterranean Food Plants and Nutraceuticals*; Heinrich, M., Müller, W.E., Galli, C., Eds.; KARGER: Basel, Switzerland, 2006; pp. 18–74. [CrossRef]

62. Dogan, Y. Traditionally Used Wild Edible Greens in the Aegean Region of Turkey. *Acta Soc. Bot. Pol.* **2012**, *81*, 329–342. [CrossRef]

63. Dogan, Y.; Ugulu, I.; Durkan, N. Wild edible plants sold in the local markets of Izmir, Turkey. *Pak. J. Bot.* **2013**, *45* (Suppl. 1), 177–184.

64. Nassif, F.; Tanji, A. Gathered food plants in Morocco: The long forgotten species in ethnobotanical research. *Life Sci. Leafl.* **2013**, *3*, 17–54.

65. Hadjichambis, A.C.; Paraskeva-Hadjichambi, D.; Della, A.; Elena Giusti, M.; De Pasquale, C.; Lenzarini, C.; Censorii, E.; Reyes Gonzales-Tejero, M.; Patricia Sanchez-Rojas, C.; Ramiro-Gutierrez, J.M.; et al. Wild and semi-domesticated food plant consumption in seven Circum-Mediterranean areas. *Int. J. Food Sci. Nutr.* **2008**, *59*, 383–414. [CrossRef] [PubMed]

66. Powell, B.; Ouarghidi, A.; Johns, T.; Ibn Tattou, M.; Eyzaguirre, P. Wild leafy vegetable use and knowledge across multiple sites in Morocco: A case study for transmission of local knowledge? *J. Ethnobiol. Ethnomed.* **2014**, *10*. [CrossRef] [PubMed]

67. Ellatifi, M. The situation of non-wood forest products in Morocco. In *Proceedings of the Joint FAO/ECE/ILO Committee on Forest Technology, Management and Training Seminar Proceedings on Harvesting of Non-Wood Forest Products, Menemen-Izmir, Turkey, 2–8 October 2000*; Food and Agricultural Organization of The United Nations: Menemen, Turkey, 2000.

68. Thomson, L.; Doran, J.; Clarke, B. *Trees for Life in Oceania: Conservation and Utilisation of Genetic Diversity*; ACIAR Mono.; Australian Centre for International Agricultural Research: Canberra, Australia, 2018.

69. French, B. *Food Plants of Papua New Guinea*; Australia and Pacific Science Foundation: Sheffield, Tasmania, 1986.

70. Powell, J.M. Ethnobotany. In *New Guinea Vegetation*; Paijmans, K., Ed.; Elsevier Scientific Publishing: Amsterdam, The Netherlands, 1976; pp. 106–183.

71. Bourke, M.R.; Allen, B. Nuts. In *Food and Agriculture in Papua New Guinea*; Bourke, M., Harwood, T., Eds.; ANU E Press: Canberra, Australia; The Australian National University: Canberra, Australia, 2009; pp. 215–222.

72. Townsend, P.K. Sago production in a New Guinea economy. *Hum. Ecol.* **1974**, *2*, 217–236. [CrossRef]

73. Roscoe, P. The hunters and gatherers of New Guinea. *Curr. Anthropol.* **2002**, *43*, 153–162. [CrossRef]

74. Government of Niue. *The State of Niue's Biodiversity for Food and Agriculture*; Niue Country Report; FAO: Rome, Italy, 2019.

75. Thaman, R.R. The Evolution of the Fiji Food System. In *Food and Nutrition in Fiji: A Historical View*; Jansen, A.A.J., Parkinson, S., Robertson, A.F.S., Eds.; University of the South Pacific: Suva, Fiji, 1990; pp. 23–109.

76. Novaczek, I. *A Guide to the Common and Edible Medicinal Sea Plants of the Pacific Islands*; Secretariat of the Pacific Community: Suva, Fiji, 2001.

77. Pawera, L.; Khomsan, A.; Zuhud, E.A.M.; Hunter, D.; Ickowitz, A.; Polesny, Z. Wild food plants and trends in their use: From knowledge and perceptions to drivers of change in West Sumatra, Indonesia. *Foods* **2020**, *9*, 1240. [CrossRef] [PubMed]

78. Pawera, L.; Lipoeto, N.I.; Khomsan, A.; Zuhud, E.A.D. *Food Plants of Minang and Mandailing Communities in Pasaman District, West Sumatra. A Community Guidebook on Biodiversity for Nutrition and Health*; Swisscontact: Jakarta, Indonesia, 2018.

79. Sen, A. *Poverty and Famines: An Essay on Entitlement and Deprivation*; Clarendon Press: Oxford, UK, 1981.

80. Shackleton, S.; Cocks, M.; Dold, T.; Kaschula, S.; Mbata, K.; Mickels-Kokwe, G.; von Maltitz, G. Contribution of Non-Wood Forest Products to Livelihoods and Poverty Alleviation. In *The Dry Forests and Woodlands of Africa. Managing for Products and Services*; Chidumayo, E.N., Gumbo, D.J., Eds.; Routledge: Abingdon, UK, 2010; pp. 93–129.

81. FAO. *The State of the World's Forests. Forest Pathways to Sustainable Development*; Food and Agriculture Organization of the United Nations: Rome, Italy, 2018. [CrossRef]

82. Petersen, L.M.; Moll, E.J.; Collins, R.; Hockings, M.T. Development of a compendium of local, wild-harvested species used in the informal economy trade, Cape Town, South Africa. *Ecol. Soc.* **2012**, *17*. [CrossRef]

83. Hudson, A.; Milliken, W.; Timberlake, J.; Giovannini, P.; Fijamo, V.; Massunde, J.; Chipanga, H.; Nivunga, M.; Ulian, T. Natural plant resources for sustainable development: Insights from community use in the Chimanimani trans-frontier conservation area, Mozambique. *Hum. Ecol.* **2020**, *48*, 55–67. [CrossRef]

84. Hickey, G.M.; Pouliot, M.; Smith-Hall, C.; Wunder, S.; Nielsen, M.R. Quantifying the economic contribution of wild food harvests to rural livelihoods: A global-comparative analysis. *Food Policy* **2016**, *62*, 122–132. [CrossRef]

85. Karabak, S. Economic and socio-cultural importance of edible wild species. *ANADOLU J. AARI* **2017**, *27*, 26–38.

86. Morris, C.; Bala, S.; South, G.R.; Lako, J.; Lober, M.; Simos, T. Supply chain and marketing of sea grapes, *Caulerpa racemosa* (Forsskål) J. Agardh (Chlorophyta: Caulerpaceae) in Fiji, Samoa and Tonga. *J. Appl. Phycol.* **2014**, *26*, 783–789. [CrossRef]

87. Lovrić, M.; Da Re, R.; Vidale, E.; Prokofieva, I.; Wong, J.; Pettenella, D.; Verkerk, P.J.; Mavsar, R. Non-wood forest products in Europe—A quantitative overview. *For. Policy Econ.* **2020**, *116*, 102175. [CrossRef]

88. Díaz, S.; Settele, J.; Eduardo, B.; Ngo, H.T.; Guèze, M.; Agard, J.; Arneth, A.; Balvanera, P.; Brauman, K.; Butchart, S.; et al. *The Global Assessment Report on Report on Biodiversity and Ecosystem Services. Summary for Policymakers*; IPBES: Bonn, Germany, 2019. [CrossRef]

89. Masson-Delmotte, V.; Zhai, P.; Pörtner, H.-O.; Roberts, D.; Skea, J.; Calvo, E.; Priyadarshi, B.; Shukla, R.; Ferrat, M.; Haughey, E.; et al. *Climate Change and Land: IPCC Report*; IPCC: Geneva, Switzerland, 2019.

90. Royal Botanic Gardens, Kew. *State of the World's Plants*; Royal Botanic Gardens, Kew: London, UK, 2016.

91. Sunderland, T.C.H. Food Security: Why Is Biodiversity Important? *Int. For. Rev.* **2011**, *13*, 265–274. [CrossRef]

92. Kew. *Plants under Pressure—A Global Assessment*; Royal Botanic Gardens: Kew, UK; Natural History Museum: London, UK, 2016.

93. Khoury, C.K.; Amariles, D.; Soto, J.S.; Diaz, M.V.; Sotelo, S.; Sosa, C.C.; Ramírez-Villegas, J.; Achicanoy, H.A.; Velásquez-Tibatá, J.; Guarino, L.; et al. Comprehensiveness of conservation of useful wild plants: An operational indicator for biodiversity and sustainable development targets. *Ecol. Indic.* **2019**, *98*, 420–429. [CrossRef]

94. Jarvis, A.; Upadhyaya, H.; Gowda, C.; Aggarwal, P.K.; Fugisaka, S.; Anderson, B. *Climate Change and Its Effect on Conservation and Use of Plant Genetic Resources for Food and Agriculture and Associated Biodiversity for Food Security*; Thematic Study SoW Report PGRFA; FAO: Rome Italy, 2008; p. 26.

95. Cooper, M.; Zvoleff, A.; Gonzalez-Roglich, M.; Tusiime, F.; Musumba, M.; Noon, M.; Alele, P.; Nyiratuza, M. Geographic factors predict wild food and nonfood NTFP collection by households across four African countries. *For. Policy Econ.* **2018**, *96*, 38–53. [CrossRef] [PubMed]

96. Willett, W.; Rockström, J.; Loken, B.; Springmann, M.; Lang, T.; Vermeulen, S.; Garnett, T.; Tilman, D.; DeClerck, F.; Wood, A.; et al. Food in the anthropocene: The EAT–Lancet Commission on healthy diets from sustainable food systems. *Lancet* **2019**, *393*, 447–492. [CrossRef]

97. Belcher, B.; Ruíz-Pérez, M.; Achdiawan, R. Global patterns and trends in the use and management of commercial NTFPs: Implications for livelihoods and conservation. *World Dev.* **2005**, *33*, 1435–1452. [CrossRef]

98. Lamrani-Alaoui, M.; Hassikou, R. Rapid risk assessment to harvesting of wild medicinal and aromatic plant species in Morocco for conservation and sustainable management purposes. *Biodivers. Conserv.* **2018**, *27*, 2729–2745. [CrossRef]

99. Government of Brazil; BFN Project. SiBBr—Information Platform on Brazilian Biodiversity. Available online: https://ferramentas.sibbr.gov.br/ficha/bin/view/FN/ (accessed on 29 July 2020).

100. Martinelli, G.; Moraes, M.A. *Livro Vermelho da Flora do Brasil*, 1st ed.; Instituto de Pesquisas Jardim Botânico do Rio de Janeiro: Rio de Janeiro, Brazil, 2013.

101. Kim, D.-S.; Joo, N. Nutritional composition of *Sacha inchi* (*Plukenetia volubilis* L.) as affected by different cooking methods. *Int. J. Food Prop.* **2019**, *22*, 1235–1241. [CrossRef]

102. de Gaillande, C.; Payri, C.; Remoissenet, G.; Zubia, M. Caulerpa consumption, nutritional value and farming in the Indo-Pacific Region. *J. Appl. Phycol.* **2017**, *29*, 2249–2266. [CrossRef]

103. Chweya, J.A.; Mnzava, N.A. *Cat's Whiskers. Cleome Gynandra L. Promoting the Conservation and Use of Underutilized and Neglected Crops*; International Plant Genetic Resources Institute: Rome, Italy, 1997.

104. FAO/Government of Kenya. *Kenya Food Composition Tables*; Food and Agricultural Organization of the United Nations: Nairobi, Kenya, 2018.

105. BFN Project. BFN Species Database. Available online: http://www.b4fn.org/resources/species-database/ (accessed on 29 July 2020).

Aquatic Foods and Nutrition in the Pacific

Anna K. Farmery [1,*](ID), Jessica M. Scott [1], Tom D. Brewer [1], Hampus Eriksson [1,2],
Dirk J. Steenbergen [1], Joelle Albert [3], Jacob Raubani [4], Jillian Tutuo [2], Michael K. Sharp [5]
and Neil L. Andrew [1]

[1]   Australian National Centre for Ocean Resource and Security, Faculty of Business and Law,
University of Wollongong, Wollongong 2522, Australia; scottj@uow.edu.au (J.M.S.);
tbrewer@uow.edu.au (T.D.B.); H.Eriksson@cgiar.org (H.E.); dirks@uow.edu.au (D.J.S.);
nandrew@uow.edu.au (N.L.A.)

[2]   WorldFish, Honiara, Faculty of Agriculture, Fisheries and Forestry,
C/O Solomon Islands National University, Ranadi, Solomon Islands; J.Wate@cgiar.org

[3]   Island Elements, Brisbane 4069, Australia; joellealbert099@gmail.com

[4]   Fisheries, Aquaculture and Marine Ecosystems Division, The Pacific Community,
Noumea Cedex 98849, New Caledonia; jasonr@spc.int

[5]   Statistics for Development Division, The Pacific Community, Noumea Cedex 98849, New Caledonia;
michaels@spc.int

*   Correspondence: afarmery@uow.edu.au

Abstract: National rates of aquatic food consumption in Pacific Island Countries and Territories are among the highest in the world, yet the region is suffering from extensive levels of diet-related ill health. The aim of this paper is to examine the variation in consumption patterns and in nutrient composition of aquatic foods in the Pacific, to help improve understanding of their contribution to food and nutrition security. For this examination we analysed nutrient composition data and trade data from two novel region-specific databases, as well as consumption data from national and village level surveys for two Melanesian case studies, Vanuatu and Solomon Islands. Results demonstrated that consumption depends on availability and the amount and type of aquatic food consumed, and its contribution to nutrition security varies within different geographic and socio-demographic contexts. More data is needed on locally relevant species and consumption patterns, to better inform dietary guidelines and improve public health both now and into the future. Advice on aquatic food consumption must consider the nutrient composition and quantity of products consumed, as well as accessibility through local food systems, to ensure they contribute to diverse and healthy diets.

Keywords: fish consumption; malnutrition; Melanesia; dietary diversity; healthy diets; food systems; seafood trade

1. Introduction

Consumption rates of aquatic food(aquatic animals and plants grown in, or wild-harvested from, water and used for food or feed) in Pacific Island Countries and Territories (PICTs) are among the highest in the world [1]. Annual average consumption by coastal rural populations ranges from 30–118 kg per person in Melanesia, 62–115 kg in Micronesia, and 50–146 kg in Polynesia [2]. Aquatic food provides 50–90% of the dietary animal protein in rural areas [1]. While consumption in urban centres is lower than in rural areas, it usually still exceeds the global average of around 20 kg per person per year [3]. Aquatic foods are highly nutritious [4], however, despite the high rate of aquatic food consumption, many PICTs experience extensive levels of diet-related ill health [5].

Malnutrition, as distinct from food insecurity, is a persistent challenge in the Pacific Island region. While micronutrient deficiencies and undernutrition are major problems [6–8], many PICTs (PICTs include: Commonwealth of the Northern Mariana Islands *, Guam *, Palau, the Federated States of Micronesia, Marshall Islands, Papua New Guinea *, Solomon Islands, Vanuatu, New Caledonia, Fiji, Nauru, Tuvalu, Kiribati, Tonga, Samoa, American Samoa *, Wallis and Futuna, French Polynesia, Niue, Cook Islands, Tokelau and Pitcairn Island *. * not included in our analysis) are experiencing the triple burden of malnutrition—the coexistence of under-nutrition, over-nutrition and micronutrient deficiencies [9–11]. Eight of the world's ten most obese nations are PICTs and the prevalence of diet-related non-communicable diseases (NCDs) is particularly high [12]. NCDs are responsible for around 70% of all deaths in PICTs and have resulted in falling life expectancy in some countries [13].

In most Melanesian and Polynesian countries, rates of urban population growth are much higher than in rural areas and some countries now have a large percentage of their population living in urban areas [14]. As a result of urbanization and the growth of food imports, dietary patterns have shifted from traditional diets comprising a variety of fresh fish, tubers and local vegetables toward diets high in fat and sugar [12,15]. These dietary changes have been influenced by multiple drivers including limited access to land within urban centres, low household incomes and the availability of cheaper and convenient, imported and processed foods such as noodles, white rice, and canned fish and meats [12,16]. This ongoing dietary transition, combined with the resulting over-reliance on commercially sourced foods and consumption of a poor variety of foods, has led to the subsequent rise in food and nutrition insecurity and non-communicable diseases [15–17]. However, dietary transitions and their impacts unfold differently at local scales and are not adequately captured in national data.

Although aquatic foods play an important role in the diets of Pacific Island people, there are many gaps in the evidence needed to understand the broader contribution to nutritional adequacy and health status in PICT populations [18]. Previous studies have reported consumption of "fish", but do not provide further detail on species, or on other types of aquatic food consumed. For example, "fish" consumption has been recorded, noting if it was fresh or canned, in Vanuatu [19–21] and Solomon Islands [22–24]. In one study investigating the percentage of women and young children consuming fresh fish, canned fish, and other seafood, it was noted that a small percentage of women (4%) reported consuming other seafood, principally shellfish [25].

Reporting consumption under the broad category of "fish" belies the great diversity of fish and invertebrates, especially coral reef species, that support coastal fisheries in the region [26]. More than 300 species of finfish are harvested by small-scale fisheries as well as a range of invertebrate species [27], although relatively few species dominate small-scale, commercial reef fisheries in the western and central areas of the region. While invertebrates such as trochus and sea cucumber are commonly harvested for export, many invertebrates including molluscs, crustaceans and cephalopods may be as critically important in the Pacific as in other subsistence fisheries and local markets [28], but there are limited catch statistics available [29,30]. The volume of production from coastal subsistence fisheries is generally greater than that from coastal commercial fishing, and involves hundreds of different taxa, including fish, molluscs, crustaceans, algae and other groups [31]. The potential for aquaculture to contribute to food and nutrition security in the Pacific has been recognised, in particular for pond aquaculture enterprises in peri-urban areas [32]. However, much of the investment made in establishing animal aquaculture has targeted export commodity markets with limited scope for food security [33]. Investments have also been made in diversifying seaweed industries in Pacific island countries with the aim of improving marine-based livelihoods through food and health applications [34]. The variation in aquatic food types, their nutrient composition and patterns of consumption is important from a health and nutrition perspective and represents a significant data gap.

Although subsistence fishing is important for coastal rural populations, the amount of aquatic food being traded for cash is growing as rural economies become increasingly monetized. The result has been a gradual shift away from fishing for home consumption, or to meet social obligations, towards fishing to generate income [31]. Some of this income is used to purchase other food, including imported processed foods such as canned fish.

While consumption of aquatic food, both fresh and canned, remains high, public health in the Pacific is not improving. Increasing aquatic food consumption is promoted in many countries for public health benefits, particularly where current consumption rates are low [35]. However, broad promotion of aquatic food consumption on its own is unlikely to result in improved health outcomes in the Pacific Island context. Filling data gaps on the contribution of aquatic food to Pacific diets, based on the availability of different aquatic food types and their nutrient composition, is essential for addressing food and nutrition security. In addition, developing a better understanding of the variation in consumption among countries, across urban and rural divides, and within intra-household distribution of food is critical to improving public health interventions. In particular, understanding consumption of aquatic foods in the context of broader dietary diversity in nutritionally vulnerable groups, particularly women and children, will be key to leveraging aquatic foods to address intergenerational malnutrition [36]. This study contributes to the development of a more holistic understanding of why NCDs and malnutrition remain prevalent amidst such high rates of national aquatic food consumption.

Recent work has shown there is considerable potential for marine fisheries to help address deficiencies globally through the supply of essential micronutrients [37]. If Pacific countries are to harness the potential of aquatic food to help address the triple burden of malnutrition, developing a better understanding of consumption patterns, and the influence of access to a diverse range of healthy food through local food systems, are critical next steps. The aim of this paper is to examine the variation in consumption patterns and nutrient composition of aquatic foods in the Pacific, to help improve understanding of their contribution to food and nutrition security. For this examination we analysed nutrient composition data and trade data from two novel region-specific databases, as well as consumption data from national and village level surveys for two Melanesian case studies, Vanuatu and Solomon Islands.

2. Materials and Methods

A mixed method approach was used to incorporate data from different sources, including: nutrient composition data from the newly created Pacific Nutrient Database; national level data on aquatic food consumption from Household Income Expenditure Surveys; village-level data on women's food consumption collected as part of an ongoing diet diversity study in Solomon Islands and Vanuatu; and trade data from the newly developed Pacific Food Trade Database. These diverse datasets are analysed jointly here and methods for each analysis are described below.

2.1. The Pacific Island Region and Case Study Countries

The Pacific Island region consists of fourteen independent countries and eight territories located in the western and central Pacific Ocean, made up of thousands of high islands, low islands and atolls [3]. Depending on the type of island, Pacific populations have access to varied local environments that support different types of domestic food production; their geography influences productivity for example [38]. The region experienced a rapid 30% drop in domestic crop production during the 1980s which has not been recovered–these declining trends in domestic food production have happened concurrently with the doubling of food net-imports [39]. The variation in local environments, combined with factors such as distance to markets, can influence diets and nutrient intake. Most of the population is rural but movement from outer islands and rural areas to urban centres is increasing. Many urban centres are coastal with an estimated 95% people living within 5 km of the coast [40].

The diversity in fishing practices, marine resource consumption and dependency on the sea across PICTs is rooted in the various social and physical factors shaping island lives. Early human migration into the region by different ethnic groups from South East Asia and Australasia has formed three distinct ethnographic regions; including Melanesia spanning the western islands to the north and northeast of Australia, and Micronesia and Polynesia spanning the islands respectively north of New Guinea and east into the central Pacific Ocean. In geophysical terms, the Andesite line forms a geological divide that traces a deep ocean trench along the western tectonic shelf and separates the continental islands to its west from the oceanic islands to its east (Figure 1). As such, Melanesia's large and high-elevation continental islands provide better agriculture conditions, and thus over time have come to support larger, culturally and linguistically diverse populations that maintain a more landward livelihood orientation. The land area and population of Melanesia account for about 98% and 90% of the regions' total [41], harbouring around 1500 indigenous languages [42]. The smaller more dispersed oceanic islands of Micronesia and Polynesia on the other hand, include low-lying coral atolls with poor soils and volcanic islands that have extreme topography. These islands over time have come to support smaller populations that have settled along coastlines, and exhibit a stronger seaward orientation in their culture and livelihood. Living in a maritime region where, if excluding Papua New Guinea, less than 0.5% (about 88,600 km^2 of the estimated total 27 million km^2) of the combined area of the 22 PICTs' jurisdictions is land [43], rural Pacific islander life reflects an existence characterized by limited social and economic connectivity due to relative isolation of its many islands. (Due to its size, Papua New Guinea skews the region's population and land area statistics, hiding the region's predominant island environment. When including Papua New Guinea, about 1.8% of total jurisdiction is land (about 550,000 km^2 of the approximate 30 million km^2 total area). Papua New Guinea and New Zealand are not included in this analysis.)

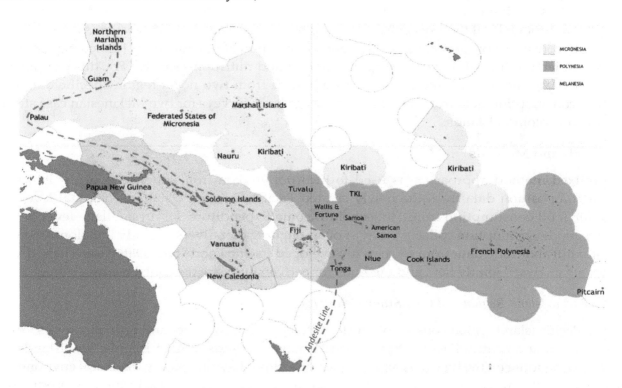

Figure 1. Map of Pacific Islands' countries and territories.

2.2. Vanuatu

Three quarters of Vanuatu's 292,675 population [44] live in rural areas, across an archipelago of 80 islands. Vanuatu is ranked amongst the most natural disaster prone countries in the world, primarily due to frequency of seasonal cyclone events and volcanic activity [45]. Most land is forested, or of extreme topography, and only 12% is estimated to be cultivated. The agriculture sector, including fishing, makes up 26% of the gross domestic product (US$ 802 million) [46]. Major urban populations center around Luganville, on the island of Espiritu Santo, and the country's capital Port Vila on the island of Efate. Growth of these urban populations is significant, with an estimated 2.9% annual growth [47], putting increased pressure on domestic food production systems to meet demand for food. In rural areas, households derive most of their income and consumption needs from agriculture-based activities, with 32% from sales of agriculture and home-made products at local markets and 39% from subsistence production [48]. On average, over half (56%) of household annual expenditure is on food

(62% and 42% respectively for rural and urban populations) [48]. In 2013, the government of Vanuatu set out a policy direction to address food and nutrition security challenges in the country. Therein it "outlines a holistic approach to address all key elements of food security along the food chain from farm to fork, i.e., from primary production, processing, trading, marketing, preparation and consumption", with emphasis put on "investing in improving and increasing production and productivity of the agricultural and fisheries sectors" [49] (p. 12).

2.3. Solomon Islands

Solomon Islands is an archipelago of more than 1000 islands in the south-west Pacific Ocean with a population of 652 856 [44]. The country experienced a period of civil conflict that was brought to an end through international intervention in 2003. Since then the country's economy has grown at an average annual rate of 5.5 percent [50]. However, this metric masks a development struggle. The country is ranked 152nd on the human development index and is among the least developed countries in the world [51]; approximately 13% of the population is classified as poor [52] and this is projected to rise anywhere from 2–12 percent due to the most recent external shock—COVID-19 [53].

Most economic activities in the country takes place in the informal sector, which includes small-scale agriculture and fisheries [54]. Most Solomon Islanders live in rural, coastal communities where fish is the primary animal-source food and gardens provide root crops and vegetables for household needs and income generation [12].Growing conditions are favorable for a range of crops, and the majority of the population is engaged in agriculture in some way on the 1.1 million ha of agricultural land in use [55]. Fishing is widespread and productive, with 68% of households in rural areas reporting catching fish or shellfish, and one-third of all households in urban areas engaged in fishing activity [56]. Despite this largely subsistence mode of living, rapid population growth, shortages of arable land in urban environs, declining fish stocks and cheap, low-quality food imports create challenges for nutrition security [16].

2.4. Nutrient Composition

The Pacific Nutrient Database (PNDB) [57] is a new database developed to address the need for a standardised method for linking data between the Household Income Expenditure Surveys (HIES) and nutrient composition data for foods consumed in the region. The PNDB matched 822 food items from the HIES with their respective macro- and micro-nutrient composition available from the literature. The PNDB presents values per 100 g edible portions for total energy, all macronutrients, fibre, and 17 micronutrients. The PNDB authors' process was limited by the availability of secondary data, where items were matched to their closest taxa or description; not all micronutrients are represented in the PNDB for this reason. For example, while aquatic food is a rich source of marine long chain omega -3 fatty acids, iodine and selenium [58,59], these nutrients are absent from the current iteration of the PNDB. Other key nutrients relevant to aquatic food as a source are included, such as protein, calcium, iron, zinc, vitamin A and vitamin B12. As such, nine nutrients are displayed within this paper based on their inclusion in the PNDB, their relevance to aquatic food and the purpose of the study.

At present there are 42 individual aquatic food items, or species, included in the PNDB. These individual species were aggregated into taxonomic groupings and the mean value was presented to demonstrate the nutritional composition of different aquatic food groups. The range between highest and lowest value was also determined for each aggregate group containing three or more species. The range was included, rather than standard deviation, as the number of individual species within aggregated groups were too small to apply standard deviations. Further information on grouping of species is available in the supplementary material (Table S1).

2.5. Consumption Data

Consumption of aquatic foods was explored at different scales using two data sources. National level data on consumption of different aquatic food groups was quantified using HIES data (Section 2.5.1), and village-level data on the number of food groups consumed by women was sourced through dietary diversity surveys (Section 2.5.2).

2.5.1. National Consumption of Aquatic Foods

Mean annual per capita apparent consumption of a range of aquatic foods was calculated from HIES data for Vanuatu and Solomon Islands, at a national level, as well as by urban and rural settings. The 2012–13 Solomon Islands HIES was implemented over the course of 12 months from October 2012 and was stratified by urban and rural areas in all 10 provinces, except for the province of Rennell and Bellona, which has only rural clusters, and Honiara, which has only urban clusters. The 2010 Vanuatu HIES was implemented in all provinces over the course of four months from October 2009 (See also http://www.statistics.gov.sb/statistics/demographic-statistics/household-income-and-expenditure-surveys, https://microdata.pacificdata.org/index.php/catalog/731 and https://microdata.pacificdata.org/index.php/catalog/727/ for further detail on design and implementation of the surveys.).

As with other HIES analyses at the national level, we used income and expenditure on specific food groups as proxies for acquisition and consumption. Apparent consumption data (hereafter more simply consumption) from the HIES were converted to per capita edible portions for analysis using the conversion factors from the PNDB. We recognize the limitations of using HIES to generate proxies of per capita consumption but in the data sparse landscape of the Pacific region they provide an important and under-utilized source of evidence [60,61].

2.5.2. Village-Level Food Consumption

Data on food consumption, including aquatic food, was collected as part of an ongoing diet diversity study in Solomon Islands and Vanuatu [25]. The study applied the internationally validated tool, the Minimum Dietary Diversity for Women of Reproductive Age (MDD-W) [62], as an indicator of the micronutrient adequacy of the diets of women of reproductive age (15–49 years). The MDD-W is a categorical indicator of the proportion of women who consumed at least five out of ten food groups within the past 24 h recall period. The tool does not quantify amounts of the reported food group consumed or quantify intakes of processed/excess non-nutritious foods. Instead, it is a measure of the number of different food groups consumed, as recalled by respondents in the 24 h recall period. The MDD-W tool and study method detailed by Albert et al. [25] was further applied in an extended study in seven rural sites in 2018 and 2019. This previously unpublished data on diet diversity scores based on food group recall of the second study are presented within this paper.

The 24 h recall method for MDD-W was carried out with women aged 15–49. The survey team convened a community meeting to introduce the survey and its objectives to understand dietary patterns in the village. Eligible and consenting respondents were then randomly recruited for the survey, representing at least 50% of households in each village surveyed ($n = 260$). The total sample across sites was 260 women of reproductive age. Data were collected at different times of the year (Site A and B in September and November respectively, Sites C and D in March, Sites E, F and G were sampled on two occasions in February/March and in April). Seasonality is a major feature in rural growing practices and food production. The north-western trade winds, *koburu*, extends from January to March, which is generally the lean period in many of the sampled sites [63]. Our sampling of consumption patterns is therefore likely influenced by season.

Within this study, we have modified the presentation of the ten MDD-W food groups [62] by separating aquatic foods from the meat, poultry, fish group. However, the total diversity score out of ten is calculated per the original MDD-W method as a combined fish and meat group.

2.6. Trade of Aquatic Foods

PICT import and export of aquatic foods is limited, in terms of quantity, primarily due to the significant domestic harvest. However, two aquatic food groups do comprise substantial trade quantities; tuna and canned fish. The dominant fishery in the Pacific, in terms of total catch volume is the oceanic tuna fishery. A large portion of the fishery occurs within PICT national waters, with harvesting conducted predominantly by foreign-flagged vessels and transhipped to countries outside the region. Only a small portion is harvested by domestic vessels. These fisheries provide significant benefit to PICTs, including foreign fleet revenues and contributions of landed catch to GDP [64]. We present existing tuna harvest data (Pacific Islands Forum Fisheries Agency (https://www.ffa.int/catch_value), in terms of potentially available grams per capita per day to consider the potential role of commercial tuna in Pacific diets. Papua New Guinea was excluded from analysis because it is more agriculture focused and has a human population size which exceeds all other PICTs combined, and would, therefore, skew interpretation. Canned fish, including tuna, mackerel, sardines and pilchards comprise an increasing portion of Pacific diets [65]. Here we assess apparent consumption of canned fish import data using the new Pacific Food Trade Database (PFTD) [66]. The PFTD was developed to better understand international trade in food and beverages in the region. The database is based on data from BACI international trade database, which amends Comtrade data [67], including the use of mirror data to fill gaps. Development of the PFTD included significant expert input to identify categorical errors (e.g., commodity, exporter, and importer) and imputation to address quantity errors. The resulting database, covering all food and beverage trade for 18 PICTs for the years 1995–2018, addresses substantial error in global data and delivers the benchmark in reliable food and beverage trade data for the region.

3. Results

3.1. Nutrient Composition of Aquatic Foods in the Pacific

The available nutrient composition data in Table 1 represents only a small proportion of the thousands of aquatic foods available in the Pacific, yet it demonstrates that large variation exists in the nutrient composition of aquatic foods commonly consumed in the region. The results also highlight consistency in valuing aquatic foods as a nutrient dense food group with large variation across specific micronutrients.

Aquatic food is an important source of quality protein; however, it is also rich in a variety of highly bioavailable micronutrients, of which several are of public health concern in the Pacific Island region. Small pelagics, crabs and crayfish, turtle and canned fish, for example, are good sources of calcium, containing 725, 143, 100, 154 mg/100 g respectively. Small fish that can be consumed whole including the bones, such as sardines, and those softened in canned fish are especially rich in calcium. Some aquatic groups examined showed substantial range in nutrient content between species, for example, bivalves, such as oysters contain high amounts of calcium, while others such as sici-shells contain very little (see Table S1).

Bivalves and gastropods, seaweed and small pelagics are important sources of iron. Small pelagics, bivalves and gastropods contain similar amounts of iron (4 mg/100 g), which is almost seven times higher than the amount contained in demersal and reef fish. Seaweed contains 8 mg/100 g which is double the amount contained by pelagics, bivalves and gastropods. Cephalopods, bivalves and gastropods, and small pelagics are very rich in vitamin B12 (10.2, 9.4, 8.3 µg/100 g respectively), in comparison to other groups, for example, tuna (1.1 µg/100 g) and prawns (1.5 µg/100 g). Small pelagics (consumed whole) also provide more vitamin A (106 µg RAE/100 g) than all other aquatic groups examined (Table 1). All groups examined, except sea urchin and seaweed, contained a meaningful contribution to daily requirements per 100 g portions important for cognitive function and development.

Large nutrient variations are seen within the different types of canned fish. This is due to the varied species types and species-specific nutrients, as well as variance in ingredients such as oil, brine, salt, or tomato and the recipe of the final product. The higher mean value for fat in canned fish is from the oil added to some canned varieties.

Table 1. Nutritional composition of aggregated aquatic food groups consumed in the Pacific (Nutrient values are based on 100 g edible portions; nutrient composition data adapted from the Pacific Nutrient Database).*

Aquatic Food Group	Energy (kcal)	Protein (g)	Fat (g)	Sodium (mg)	Calcium (mg)	Iron (mg)	Zinc (mg)	Vitamin A (μg RAE)	Vitamin B12 (μg)
Tuna (n= 4)	164 (77)	25 (3)	5.4 (8)	38.3 (14)	5.5 (6)	1.2 (0.9)	0.5 (0.23)	54.8 (58)	1.1 (1.4)
Small pelagic fish (n = 1)	105	19.7	2.9	665	725	4	3.1	106	8.3
Large pelagic fish (n = 2)	132	21	5.2	110	14	0.8	0.7	31	0.9
Demersal/reef fish (n = 3)	101 (28)	19.8 (0.3)	2.2 (3.1)	78.3 (11)	25.3 (21)	0.6 (0.3)	0.6 (0.1)	30.3 (2)	1.7 (1.6)
Elasmobranchs (n = 2)	97.5	22.6	0.8	97.5	11.0	1.0	0.5	12.0	1.1
Prawn/shrimp (n = 2)	92	20.4	1.2	249	89	1.6	1.31	27	1.5
Crabs/crayfish (n = 5)	76 (18)	15.7 (5.2)	1.4 (0.8)	279 (244)	143 (139)	1.3 (1.1)	3.5 (0.6)	16.2 (21)	2.9 (3.9)
Bivalves, gastropods (n = 6)	104 (98)	19.1 (16)	1.9 (3)	437 (464)	77.5 (227)	4.0 (8)	4.4 (17)	56.3 (180)	9.4 (15)
Cephalopods (n = 2)	78.5	17.2	1.1	285	14.5	0.8	1.4	21.5	10.2
Echinoids (n = 1)	91.0	8.2	6.5	147	50.0	0.9	0.4	tr	0.0
Sea cucumber (n = 1)	52.0	12.8	0.1	716	87.0	1.2	0.2	tr	2.3
Turtle (n = 2)	73	16	1.0	129	100	1	1.3	5	1.1
Seaweed (n = 2)	9	0.6	0.3	810	56	8	tr	50	0
Canned Fish (mixed fish, oil, brine, other) (n = 12)	177 (139)	21.8 (14.7)	9.5 (11.1)	937 (5310)	154 (399)	1.5 (1.7)	1.2 (2.4)	16.8 (37)	3.3 (7.6)

* 'n' represents number of species within an aggregated group; mean group values are displayed—the range between the minimum and maximum values in parentheses for groups with three or more species; see supplementary material Table S1 for individual species within groups; 'tr' indicates trace amounts detected.

Aquatic food can also contain high levels of sodium, particularly processed and canned fish. The high sodium content, and variation of recipes of processed products, must be taken into consideration in recommendations to increase aquatic food intake from processed forms.

3.2. National Consumption of Aqautic Foods

Apparent consumption of aquatic foods is high in PICTs, however, consumption trends are not homogenous and the volume and type of aquatic food consumed varies among sub-regions, countries and within countries. For example, variation exists between rural and urban consumers (Table 2) and between communities, partially as a result of availability. Solomon Islanders each consume, on average, 73 kg of aquatic food (all types) per year. In contrast, 14 kg of aquatic food is consumed per person per year in Vanuatu, which is less than the global average of 20 kg/p.c./year [68]. Within Solomon Islands, rural consumption of pelagic fish alone is equivalent to the global average consumption of aquatic food, with an additional 63 kg/p.c./year of other fish and seafood consumed. Urban consumption of 48 kg/year of aquatic food is still high in terms of the global average, but is much lower than rural consumption of 83 kg/yr. Different types of aquatic food make different contributions to consumption, for example, shellfish account for over 15% of total consumption in Solomon Islands and 4% in Vanuatu. Within Solomon Islands, shellfish account for 17% or rural aquatic food consumption and 7% of urban consumption (Table 2). Canned fish is consumed more by urban than rural consumers in both Vanuatu and Solomon Islands. Urban and rural consumers typically have different access to healthy and nutritious food, as well as differing dietary gaps. As demonstrated by this variance in volumes and types of aquatic foods consumed, further food and nutrition requirements must be considered within a localized context to inform relevant and appropriate interventions to address dietary gaps.

Table 2. Mean daily per capita apparent consumption of aquatic foods (edible portion in grams ± standard error) in Vanuatu (2010) and Solomon Islands (2011–12), by national, rural and urban.

Aquatic Food Group	Solomon Islands			Vanuatu		
	National	Rural	Urban	National	Rural	Urban
Pelagic fish	53.2 (1.51)	56.1 (1.92)	45.8 (2.08)	14.4 (0.63)	18.0 (0.82)	4.4 (0.49)
Reef fish	97.5 (2.33)	116.1 (3.07)	50.9 (2.30)	7.2 (0.49)	7.6 (0.58)	6.1 (0.88)
Canned fish	13.5 (0.22)	9.2 (0.19)	24.3 (0.49)	14.1 (0.30)	13.3 (0.30)	16.3 (0.68)
Shellfish	30.7 (1.26)	39.0 (1.67)	9.7 (1.04)	1.6 (0.08)	2.0 (0.11)	0.44 (0.05)
Mixed fresh/frozen fish	6.3 (0.60)	8.3 (0.82)	1.2 (0.38)	1.4 (0.11)	1.7 (0.14)	0.58 (0.16)
Aquatic food (total)	201.2 (3.45)	228.8 (4.52)	131.8 (3.70)	38.8 (0.99)	42.6 (1.23)	27.9 (1.40)

3.3. Individual Consumption

The majority of Pacific Islanders live in rural settings where food access and availability vary according to factors such as the amount of arable land, distance from nearest market, population size and coastal habitat. The result is substantial variation at village and household level in the diversity of foods consumed, as well as the species of aquatic food types consumed.

Women's dietary diversity was low with 14–42% meeting the minimum dietary diversity score of five across the seven rural sites in Melanesia included in our study (Figure 2A). Some similarities between women's diets were evident across sites. Grains, tubers and plantains were consumed by virtually all respondents (96%) (Figure 2B). Products in this group include food such as locally grown tubers as well as imported rice. Dark leafy greens, Vitamin A rich foods, and other fruits were consumed by over 50% of respondents at all sites. Consumption of other vegetables was generally low. The three major food groups with low consumption included pulses, nuts seeds, milk/dairy and eggs.

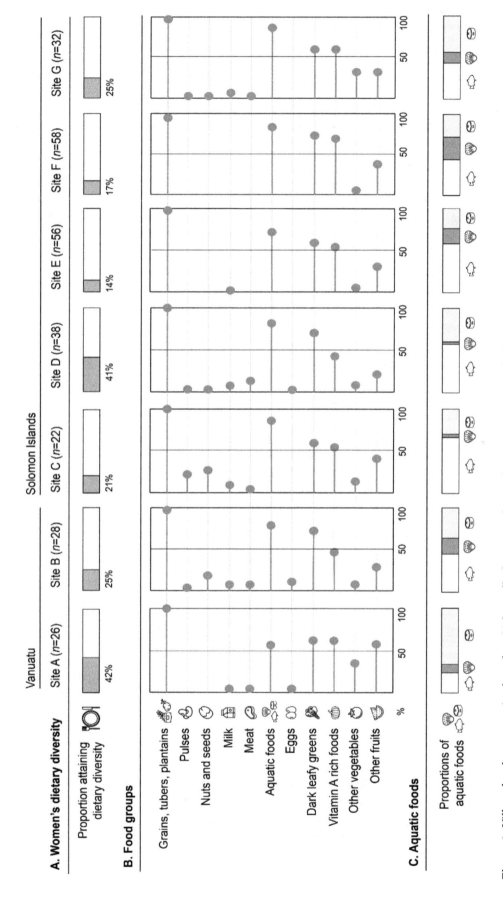

Figure 2. Village-level consumption based on 24-h recall of women of reproductive age (*n* = 260) [25]. (**A**). Proportion of women attaining minimum dietary diversity (five or more food groups); (**B**). Frequency of food group consumption in 24-h recall; (**C**). Proportion of three categories of aquatic foods (finfish, invertebrates, canned tuna) reported in 24-h recall. Foods are grouped based on their nutritional content as defined in the MDD-W index method [62]. The group 'Vitamin A rich foods' includes other Vitamin A rich fruit and vegetables not included in other groups. 'Aquatic foods' includes animal sourced aquatic foods only. Together, meat and aquatic foods (separated for this figure) contribute as an aggregate score out of one in calculating total diet diversity scores.

Of the respondents that reported consuming meat, poultry, and fish, the majority (78%) of this consumption was from aquatic foods. While finfish, including reef, mangrove and pelagic species, were important for consumption across all sites (Figure 2C), the type of aquatic food consumed varied between sites. For example, canned tuna was the main source of aquatic food at site A in Vanuatu, where there are few lagoons to harvest aquatic food from and limited arable land. However, fishers have access to deep oceanic high-value fisheries and fishing activity in this site is predominantly commercially-oriented, where aquatic food is caught to generate income rather than for local consumption.

In contrast, invertebrates, including shellfish and crabs, were an important source of aquatic food at sites B, E, F. These sites are complex habitats where fishers have access to shallow reef, lagoon and/or mangrove habitats to harvest food for local consumption. They are also located far from provincial market centres and so exhibit a dietary composition largely reflecting the growing and fishing conditions at their location, with addition of long shelf-life foods bought at rural stores (e.g., rice, biscuits and canned tuna).

3.4. Movement of Nutrients from Aquatic Foods through Imports and Exports

3.4.1. Canned Fish

The majority of aquatic food consumed in PICTs is caught domestically, however, aquatic food imports play an increasingly prominent role in the diets of Pacific Island people [65] (Figure 3). Canned mackerel, tuna, pilchards and sardines comprise the bulk of consumed canned fish. These fish species have different nutrient compositions, and further variance from ingredients within the final canned product (Table 1).

There has been a significant increase in imports of canned fish to the region over the last two decades, with a rapid increase from 1999 to 2007 and a subsequent plateau, mostly imported from China and Thailand [66]. Total regional consumption of canned fish increased from 3.6 to 14.8 g per capita per day, between 1995 and 2018 (Figure 3). Regional import of canned mackerel (grams per capita per day) has increased from 1.8 in 1995 to 4.9 in 2018, with a peak of 8.3 in 2008. Import of canned tuna (grams per capita per day) increased nearly 6-fold, from 0.8 in 1995 to 4.7 kg in 2018. In consumption terms, this is an underestimate as it excludes tuna canned in Fiji and Solomon Islands, and sold domestically, which contributes substantially to total consumption [65]. Across the region, canned sardine and pilchard imports increased from 1 in 1995 to 5.2 g/capita/day in 2018. Importantly, there are significant differences in per capita imports between sub-regions (Melanesia, Micronesia, and Polynesia) (Figure 3).

3.4.2. Oceanic Tuna Fishery

Between 1997 and 2018 over 17.5 million metric tonnes of the four dominant species of tuna (Albacore, Bigeye, Skipjack and Yellowfin) were harvested from national waters of the 17 PICTs included here, with Skipjack accounting for the majority of the harvest (Figure 4). There are, however, drastic differences in harvest, on a per capita basis, between Pacific sub-regions. In 2018, total catch in grams per capita per day, was 80, 440, and 4630 in Melanesia, Polynesia, and Micronesia respectively. While there are large differences in per capita harvest rates among sub-regions and individual PICTs, in edible portion terms (0.58 * total weight) [53], the catch harvested has risen from around 250,000 metric tonnes in 1997 to 700,000 metric tonnes in 2018. These quantities relative to PICT populations and economies represent a profound asset in terms of revenue, although in terms of food and nutrition security, the majority of this nutritional value is exported from the region. The estimated need for tuna for good nutrition across the region by 2035 is estimated to be 87,500 tonnes [69].

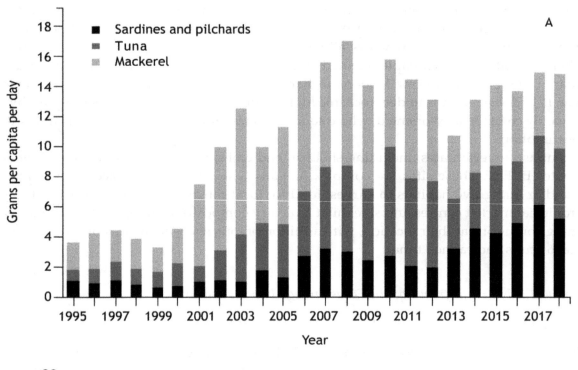

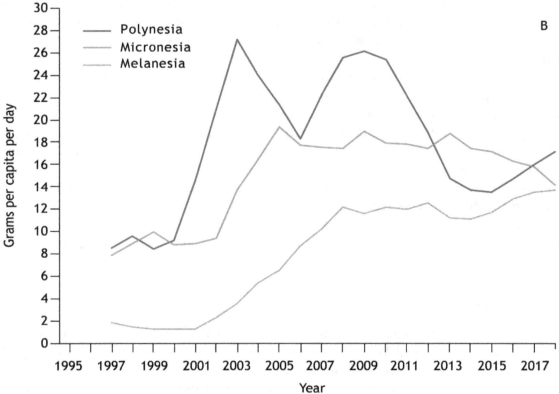

Figure 3. Per capita import (apparent consumption) of canned fish to 17 Pacific Island Countries and Territories (full list available in supplementary information, Papua New Guinea excluded because of its relative dominance in the data set) ncluding (**A**) regional trend by fish types and (**B**) total import by sub-region. Estimates exclude other minor quantities of canned fish including salmon and herring. Sub-regional trends are a 3-year moving average and include all canned fish types included in the regional estimate. Edible portions are likely to be 0.7 to 0.85 of the estimates shown due to inedible portions (e.g., brine, oil and cans) and variation in proportion of fish by total weight across different fish types and processing methods (see Table 1). Canned fish data from the Pacific Food Trade Database [66]. Human population data from UN Population division (https://www.un.org/development/desa/pd/).

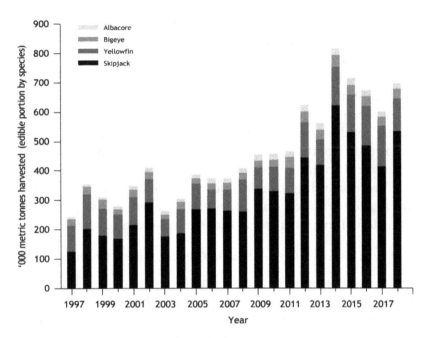

Figure 4. Temporal trend in total edible portion of registered catch (1997–2018) within PICT (same PICTs as Figure 3) national waters. Total catch was calculated as the total catch of Albacore, Bigeye, Skipjack and Yellowfin tuna by domestic and foreign-flagged vessels multiplied by 0.58 [53] to derive a measure of edible harvest. Tuna data from Pacific Islands Forum Fisheries Agency (https://www.ffa.int/catch_value). Human population data from UN Population division (https://www.un.org/development/desa/pd/).

4. Discussion

Aquatic foods play an essential role in food and nutrition security in the Pacific region, however, they are not a homogenous food group in terms of nutrient composition. The variation in nutrient composition indicates that some groups may be more suited to addressing specific health issues in the Pacific region than others. Consumption of aquatic foods is highly variable among sub-regions, countries and within countries, with people consuming what they can access. The majority of aquatic food consumed in PICTs is caught domestically, however, aquatic food imports play an increasingly prominent role in the diets of Pacific Island people. Fisheries, such as the oceanic tuna fishery, represent a profound asset in terms of revenue, although in terms of food and nutrition security, the majority of this nutritional value is exported from the region. While most Pacific Islanders consume large amounts of aquatic food, this consumption is part of a diet that does not meet the recommended dietary diversity. More data is needed on the micronutrient content of locally relevant aquatic foods, as well as on whole diet consumption at regional, national, household and individual levels, to improve public health, particularly in regions where aquatic food consumption is already high, yet overall dietary diversity remains low.

4.1. Aquatic Food Is Not a Homogenous Group

Unlike the term "chicken" or "pig", which denotes an animal from a single genus (*Gallus* and *Sus* respectively) [70], "aquatic food" and "seafood" include multiple taxa of biologically divergent animals, and often plants, from freshwater and marine habitats. As a result, the nutrient composition of different aquatic foods varies considerably and the nutritional value of aquatic food far exceeds its common description as a quality protein source. Aquatic food is an important source of micronutrients, of which several are of public health concern in the Pacific Island region. Sardine, crabs, crayfish, turtle and canned fish, for example, are good sources of calcium, highlighting these alternate calcium sources of importance as compared to the negligible dairy intake reported by the diet diversity respondents in this, and other, research [25]. Iron rich species such as bivalves and gastropods, seaweed and sardines, are important sources of iron which can contribute to meeting iron requirements in Pacific populations suffering diet and parasitic related anemia [7]. Aquatic foods have also been identified for provision of high biological vitamin A, as well as calcium, iron and zinc and as a target food for combating these micronutrient deficiencies in S/SE Asia [59,71].

Our results, based on what is currently available in the PNDB, support current evidence that there is considerable variation in the nutrient composition of different aquatic food groups [37,72]. This variation is of importance in nutrition sensitive food systems and food-based dietary guidelines, whereby specific aquatic food sources can be targeted to fill particular nutrient gaps. However, the ability to identify aquatic foods to target nutrient gaps is limited by the lack of data on the concentration of nutrients and contaminants in aquatic foods, especially in low- and middle-income countries [73]. Greater understanding of micronutrient content of locally relevant aquatic foods is critical to formulating advice around consumption and harness the potential of aquatic foods in addressing the triple burden of malnutrition in the Pacific, and elsewhere.

4.2. Integrating Nutrient Compostion Information with Consumption Patterns

Combined with the need for greater understanding of nutrient composition, is the need for information on quantified consumption at regional, national, household and individual levels, and the factors that drive differences in consumption patterns. In particular, better understanding of the needs, access and modes of acquisition of rural and urban consumers and vulnerable groups is required. Local environments and cultural contexts have a major influence over the types of aquatic foods that can be accessed and consumed. For example, our results identified that in areas where there are few lagoons to harvest aquatic food from and limited arable land, canned tuna is an important source of aquatic food. In contrast, invertebrates, including shellfish and crabs, were an important source in areas located far from provincial market centres, where fishers can harvest aquatic food from shallow reef, lagoon and/or mangrove habitats.

Aquatic food consumption is strongly influenced by local environments, as well as local customs, which can determine whether the aquatic foods are consumed or sold. For example, some diet data analysed as part of this study were collected during a "kustom" or traditional fishing season, which may have influenced results. In addition, for some PICTs, religious dietary proscriptions limit consumption of different types of animal source food (e.g., the Seventh Day Adventist church, a major faith in Solomon Islands, prohibits consumption of shellfish).

The Pacific Community (SPC) Public Health Division advises that, on average, each person in the region should eat about 35 kg of fish per year. This value reflects aquatic food contributing up to 50% of the daily protein intake recommended by the World Health Organization for good nutrition [74]. National consumption in some PICTs already exceeds of this amount, yet major health problems continue to plague a large proportion of the Pacific population [9,75,76]. While most Pacific Islanders consume large amounts of aquatic food, this consumption is part of a diet that does not meet the recommended dietary diversity. With exceptions, such as Vanuatu and Papua New Guinea, recommendations to increase "fish" consumption at national levels are unlikely to benefit the health of the population. Contemporary national level recommendations around "fish" or "seafood" now need to take in to account the varied needs of different population groups, the food groups that are absent from their diets and the relative nutritional benefits of different aquatic foods. For example, the village site in Solomon Islands with the lowest dietary diversity score showed almost all people ate aquatic foods including fish, shellfish and canned tuna. In this situation, health advice should be to maintain consumption of aquatic foods in conjunction with messages to increase the diversity of other foods consumed. In contrast, where dietary diversity is higher, but consumption of aquatic foods is lower and less diverse, health messages should focus on increasing diversity of aquatic food consumption for improved nutrition rather than increasing consumption per se. Achieving Recommended Dietary Intakes (RDIs) for specific nutrients through one source of aquatic food, for example a species group such as tuna, is unrealistic. RDIs should instead be reached through a combination of different food groups, including a diverse range of aquatic food.

4.3. Aquatic Food as Part of the Pacific Food System

Advice to increase consumption of aquatic foods will also need to be considerate of the broader transition in diets occurring in Pacific countries, including consumption of less healthy foods. Progress in shifting dietary and health trajectories toward better outcomes will require nutrition-sensitive interventions aimed at the structural drivers of national food systems and the external food environment [25,77].

Broader development (e.g., infrastructure, communication, banking, public services) is lacking, so the transportation and distribution of highly perishable fresh foods from the garden or sea to the urban market place are difficult and expensive. This is a driving factor to the influx and acceptance of refined foods like rice and flour or long shelf-life convenience foods, all of which paradoxically tend to outcompete domestic grown crops and fish in price, access and availability in urban settings [78]. Enhancing storage, processing, and distribution of food commodities is vital in mitigating food and nutrition security impacts from changing food production patterns and during the current COVID-19 crisis [39].

Aquatic foods also play a key role in disaster recovery in the Pacific, where terrestrial-based food and income generation capacity has been reduced. The capacity for marine resources to support recovery, however, is dependent on factors such as market access, as well as fishing skills and technology in many sectors of the community [79–81].

4.4. Effects of Aquatic Food Trade on Nutrition

4.4.1. Imports

Most of the aquatic food consumed in the Pacific is caught domestically, however, consumption of imported aquatic food is increasing, particularly canned fish. Paradoxically, although there are major canneries in Solomon Islands, Fiji and Papua New Guinea, much of the tuna caught in the EEZs of PICTs is transshipped to Asia for processing [65]. The contribution of canned fish to national security in the region is mixed, and in need of more research to better place it within national and local dietary patterns. Canning an otherwise highly perishable food greatly increases access to aquatic food for people that do not have reliable access to fresh fish or refrigeration, but canned fish can be high in salt and consuming high amounts can lead to negative health implications [82]. However, unlike other processed foods high in sodium, which can be of overall low nutritional value, aquatic food also contains other nutrients. An opportunity exists to revisit sodium guidelines to ensure that canned fished does not contribute excess sodium.

Identifying differences in per capita aquatic food imports among sub-regions (Melanesia, Micronesia, and Polynesia) and individual PICTs, is important for understanding trade-derived nutrition at the community and urban/rural scale. Reviewing population-level trade in food through a nutrition lens deepens the understanding of potential micronutrient sources. If a population were deficient in calcium intake, for example, canned fish such as mackerel and other small pelagic species with bones, could be promoted. If canned fish is not disaggregated by species and recipe type, the nutritional value could be largely over- or under-estimated. Future studies examining food availability of specific canned fish types from trade data, converted to respective micronutrient composition, can help to ensure appropriate estimation of trade derived nutrition.

4.4.2. Exports

Unlike other aquatic foods, the majority of tuna caught in Pacific waters is currently exported. There has been considerable debate over the food security costs and benefits for developing countries engaging in aquatic food trade [83,84]. Hicks et al. [37] identified the need for more research on the relationship between potential nutrient supply from fisheries and international trade and foreign fishing in countries with populations at risk of dietary deficiency. Nash et al. [85] examined the impact of growing global redistribution of fish products on current and future supply of fishery-derived nutrients.

They found that international trade contributes to inequities when considering micronutrient supply and that countries currently benefiting from trade and foreign fishing tend to be more vulnerable to future changes in nutrient supplies. An important part of the aquatic food and nutrition story in many PICTs is understanding the quantity of nutrients leaving the region without being landed, in particular the micronutrients needed to overcome stunting, or other deficiencies. Determining the right balance between efforts to divert aquatic food from export markets for domestic consumption, and income generation from international fleets, is an area requiring further investigation [80]. The cost-benefit of such comparisons will need to be measured in terms of public health outcomes.

4.5. Future Opportunities and Constraints for Aquatic Foods and Nutrition

4.5.1. Data Gaps

There remains a paucity of nutrient composition data for the Pacific. While the PNDB makes an important contribution to improving data availability, many of the species included in the PNDB are not Pacific species or local samples. Several key nutrients are absent from the current iteration of the PNDB. Our finding that there are large variations in the composition of different species and aquatic food groups highlights that this is an important gap in the literature. The integration of local catch data (that can be disaggregated by species) is much needed to provide a more accurate picture of catch composition and the macro/micronutrients sourced through the consumption of aquatic food. Further sampling of species from both wild capture fisheries and aquaculture is also needed to strengthen the empirical nutrition composition data for aquatic foods in the Pacific region.

4.5.2. Addressing the Predicted Supply Gap from Coastal Fisheries

Coastal habitats that have traditionally provided most of the aquatic foods caught by small-scale fishers are predicted to be progressively degraded by ocean warming and acidification, leading to declines in catch potential [86,87]. These impacts are predicted to occur alongside existing pressures, such as overfishing, erosion and siltation of coastal ecosystems from logging, and mangrove clearing [88] as well as increased coastal urban development, population growth and coastal pollution [86,89]. For many PICTs, the gap between the aquatic foods required for food and the amount of aquatic foods that can be harvested sustainably from reefs will increase considerably [1,69]. The reduced availability of aquatic food from coastal fisheries may be exacerbated by trade disruptions to imports, as evidenced by the Covid-19 pandemic [39]. Proposed solutions to address this supply gap include increasing consumption of canned fish and landing more tuna and bycatch in PICTs from off-shore fisheries [69].

In terms of volume and calories, based on the data presented here, all Pacific sub-regions could increase the availability of aquatic food based solely by landing, rather than exporting, more of the tuna harvested in national waters by registered vessels. While landing more tuna may help contribute to filling the supply gap from declines in coastal fisheries, it may not have the same nutrient densities as the aquatic foods it replaces. Higher quantities of tuna may need to be consumed to get the same amount of a micronutrient and eating this volume of tuna may be unrealistic. A large volume of tuna is already consumed domestically, from a number of sources including domestically produced and imported canned tuna, products entering the region from foreign-flagged tuna vessels, catch from domestic commercial fleets, and coastal artisanal capture from various methods including the use of fish aggregation devices (FADS). However, the total quantity of tuna consumed across PICTs, or for individual PICTs is not accurately known. Such information is essential for measuring the success of the food security goal of the Regional Roadmap for Sustainable Pacific Fisheries [90], which aims to increase access to tuna for domestic consumption by 40,000 tonnes between 2015 and 2024.

Increasing the availability of tuna for Pacific consumers may be an important option for overcoming undernutrition where access is prioritized for vulnerable groups. Given the large differences in per capita harvest rates between Pacific sub-regions and individual PICTs, an understanding of the geopolitical heterogeneity of harvestable tuna will be essential for understanding the potential role of the fishery in meeting future dietary requirements in the region [64]. Other fisheries including inshore finfish and invertebrates, which already contribute to local livelihoods and food security, can potentially play a greater role in food and nutrition security in the Pacific. Inshore species have a varied nutrient composition and together with tuna present a nutrition sensitive approach to increase the supply of aquatic foods. In addition, invertebrates are predicted to be impacted by climate change to a lesser degree than other aquatic foods [26], and future dietary advice will need to consider these eventualities. Where consumption of these species is currently low, efforts to promote consumption may be needed, particularly to target nutrient deficiency in vulnerable groups. Developing messaging around "culturally significant local aquatic foods" may help promote consumption via targeting foods significant to a local environment that may not currently have a place on the "daily plate" for various reasons. Linking these foods with their high nutritional value could potentially increase their consumption. For example, the small mud whelk found in mangroves is often considered a "poor persons food" i.e., people collect it when they have nothing else. If this food source was celebrated for its nutritional value, it may help increase its consumption. Care would also need to be taken to ensure overexploitation did not occur.

Aquatic foods may be substituted with other animal source foods if supply of aquatic foods is reduced. Understanding consumption patterns and the nutrient composition of aquatic foods will provide an evidence base for national context food group substitutions, such as aquatic food portion within respective animal source foods portions and providing alternate non-diary calcium sources. These data will also inform culturally appropriate food-based dietary guidelines (FBDGs). Customizing FBDGs to local food practices, preferences, availability and access, with consideration of the local food system and health education, will be necessary to best support healthy diets.

4.5.3. Addressing Contaminants

As well as being an important source of micronutrients, aquatic food is a source of contaminates, including metals, persistent organic pollutants (POPs), and plastics accumulated from the marine environment [73]. Developing a better picture of variability in aquatic foods is also important for understanding the effects of these contaminants, as well as toxins which cause poisoning such as ciguatera. Mercury levels are typically low in fast growing species but are much higher in larger fish, such as some tunas [91]. Excess consumption of fish with high mercury levels, particularly by pregnant women and children, is harmful [92]. Understanding mercury contamination and safe levels of consumption for each species and size of tuna in PICTs will become increasingly important from a public health perspective if more tuna is landed nationally, rather than exported [93].

Understanding the temporal and spatial variation in Ciguatera Fish Poisoning (CFP) cases will be important in predicting the future role of coral reef fish in local diets. CFP, the most frequently reported seafood toxin illness in the world, can produce a diverse array of complex and debilitating symptoms [94]. CFP is caused by consumption of coral reef associated fish contaminated by ciguatoxin and related toxins from dinoflagellates (microalgae) and cyanobacteria. The toxin bioaccumulates up the food web, with particular fish species being more prone to having higher levels of ciguatoxin [94]. Presence of ciguatoxic fish not only causes ill-health but can alter fishing practices and overall fishing effort which reduces local fish consumption. Public health challenges, in terms of both CFP symptoms and nutrition have worsened over the past 35 years, and are expected to continue to do so as the coastal habitats continue to degrade [95]. In addition to CFP, scrombroid syndrome can result from eating "spoiled fish", particularly tuna and other, mostly pelagic species, in the family Scombridae. While the syndrome has been reported in local hospitals in Solomon Islands, it is generally considered an underreported form of food poisoning [90]. Improving fish hygiene and ensuring food safety and quality along supply chains will be essential components of improving the contribution of aquatic foods to nutrition.

5. Conclusions

General messages to increase consumption of "aquatic food" will not be adequate to improve nutrition and health in the Pacific region. For aquatic foods to best contribute to food and nutrition security in the Pacific region, and more broadly, consumption advice needs to be shaped to match the type of aquatic food already being consumed, its nutritional composition, and its place in contributing to dietary diversity with other foods, both domestically produced and imported.

Author Contributions: Conceptualization, A.K.F., J.M.S., T.D.B., H.E., D.S. and N.A.; methodology, J.M.S., T.D.B., H.E., J.W., M.S. and J.A.; formal analysis, A.K.F., J.M.S., T.D.B., H.E., M.S. and D.J.S.; data curation, A.K.F., J.M.S., T.D.B., J.T., M.S. and H.E.; Writing—Original draft preparation, A.K.F., J.M.S., T.D.B., H.E., D.J.S., M.S.; Writing—review and editing, A.K.F., J.M.S., T.D.B., H.E., D.J.S., J.A., J.T., J.R. and N.A.; funding acquisition, N.A., M.S. and H.E. All authors have read and agreed to the published version of the manuscript.

Acknowledgments: We are grateful to Elle McNeill for graphics and Johann Bell for comments on the manuscript. This work contributes to the CGIAR research program on Fish Agri-Food Systems (FISH) led by WorldFish. We acknowledge the original sources of the HIES data: Solomon Islands National Statistics Office and Vanuatu National Statistics Office.

References

1. Bell, J.D.; Kronen, M.; Vunisea, A.; Nash, W.J.; Keeble, G.; Demmke, A.; Pontifex, S.; Andréfouët, S. Planning the use of fish for food security in the Pacific. *Mar. Policy* **2009**, *33*, 64–76. [CrossRef]
2. FAO. *Global Blue Growth Initiative and Small Island Developing States*; Food and Agriculture Organization of the United Nations: Rome, Italy, 2014.
3. Gillet, R. *Fisheries in the Economies of Pacifi Island Countries and Territories*; Pacific Community: Noumea, New Caledonia, 2016.
4. Thilsted, S.H.; Thorne-Lyman, A.; Webb, P.; Bogard, J.R.; Subasinghe, R.; Phillips, M.J.; Allison, E.H. Sustaining healthy diets: The role of capture fisheries and aquaculture for improving nutrition in the post-2015 era. *Food Policy* **2016**, *61*, 126–131. [CrossRef]
5. WHO. *Global Status Report on Noncommunicable Diseases 2014*; World Health Organization: Geneva, Switzerland, 2014.
6. Haddad, L.; Cameron, L.; Barnett, I. The double burden of malnutrition in SE Asia and the Pacific: Priorities, policies and politics. *Health Policy Plan.* **2015**, *30*, 1193–1206. [CrossRef] [PubMed]
7. WHO. *The Global Prevalence of Anaemia in 2011*; World Health Organization: Geneva, Switzerland, 2015.
8. United Nations Children's Fund. *Situation Analysis of Children in the Pacific Island Countries*; UNICEF: Suva, Fiji, 2017.
9. Sievert, K.; Lawrence, M.; Naika, A.; Baker, P. Processed foods and nutrition transition in the Pacific: Regional trends, patterns and food system drivers. *Nutrients* **2019**, *11*, 1328. [CrossRef]
10. Fanzo, J.; Hawkes, C.; Udomkesmalee, E.; Afshin, A.; Allemandi, L.; Assery, O.; Baker, P.; Battersby, J.; Bhutta, Z.; Chen, K. *2018 Global Nutrition Report: Shining a Light to Spur Action on Nutrition*; Development Initiatives: Bristol, UK, 2018.
11. Hughes, R.G.; Lawrence, M. Globalisation, food and health in Pacific Island countries. *Asia Pacific J. Clin. Nutr.* **2005**, *14*, 298–305.
12. Andersen, A.B.; Thilsted, S.H.; Schwarz, A.M. *Food and Nutrition Security in Solomon Islands*; Working Paper, AAS-2013-06; WorldFish: Penang, Malaysia, 2013; p. 15.
13. Hawley, N.L.; McGarvey, S.T. Obesity and diabetes in Pacific Islanders: The current burden and the need for urgent action. *Curr. Diabetes Rep.* **2015**, *15*, 29. [CrossRef]

14. United Nations Population Fund. *Population and Development Profiles: Pacific Island Countries*; UNFPA Pacific Sub-Regional Office: Suva, Fiji, 2014.
15. Thow, A.M.; Snowdon, W. The effect of trade and trade policy on diet and health in the Pacific Islands. *Trade Food Diet Health Perspect. Policy Options* **2010**, *147*, 168.
16. Horsey, B.; Swanepoel, L.; Underhill, S.; Aliakbari, J.; Burkhart, S. Dietary diversity of an adult Solomon Islands population. *Nutrients* **2019**, *11*, 1622. [CrossRef]
17. Popkin, B.M.; Horton, S.; Kim, S. The nutrition Transition and Prevention of Diet-Related Chronic Diseases in Asia and the Pacific. *Food Nutr. Bull.* **2012**, *22*, 1–58.
18. Charlton, K.E.; Russell, J.; Gorman, E.; Hanich, Q.; Delisle, A.; Campbell, B.; Bell, J. Fish, food security and health in Pacific Island countries and territories: A systematic literature review. *BMC Public Health* **2016**, *16*, 285. [CrossRef]
19. Li, M.; McKelleher, N.; Moses, T.; Mark, J.; Byth, K.; Ma, G.; Eastman, C.J. Iodine nutritional status of children on the island of Tanna, Republic of Vanuatu. *Public Health Nutr.* **2009**, *12*, 1512–1518. [CrossRef] [PubMed]
20. Dancause, K.N.; Dehuff, C.; Soloway, L.E.; Vilar, M.; Chan, C.; Wilson, M.; Tarivonda, L.; Regenvanu, R.; Kaneko, A.; Garruto, R.M. Behavioral changes associated with economic development in the South Pacific: Health transition in Vanuatu. *Am. J. Hum. Biol.* **2011**, *23*, 366–376. [CrossRef] [PubMed]
21. Dancause, K.N.; Vilar, M.; Wilson, M.; Soloway, L.E.; DeHuff, C.; Chan, C.; Tarivonda, L.; Regenvanu, R.; Kaneko, A.; Lum, J.K. Behavioral risk factors for obesity during health transition in Vanuatu, South Pacific. *Obesity* **2013**, *21*, E98–E104. [CrossRef] [PubMed]
22. Mertz, O.; Bruun, T.B.; Fog, B.; Rasmussen, K.; Agergaard, J. Sustainable land use in Tikopia: Food production and consumption in an isolated agricultural system. *Singap. J. Trop. Geogr.* **2010**, *31*, 10–26. [CrossRef]
23. Aswani, S.; Furusawa, T. Do marine protected areas affect human nutrition and health? A comparison between villages in Roviana, Solomon Islands. *Coast. Manag.* **2007**, *35*, 545–565. [CrossRef]
24. Albert, J.A.; Beare, D.; Schwarz, A.M.; Albert, S.; Warren, R.; Teri, J.; Siota, F.; Andrew, N.L. The contribution of nearshore fish aggregating devices (FADs) to food security and livelihoods in Solomon Islands. *PLoS ONE* **2014**, *9*, e115386. [CrossRef]
25. Albert, J.; Bogard, J.; Siota, F.; McCarter, J.; Diatalau, S.; Maelaua, J.; Brewer, T.; Andrew, N. Malnutrition in rural Solomon Islands: An analysis of the problem and its drivers. *Matern. Child Nutr.* **2020**, *16*, e12921. [CrossRef]
26. Bell, J.D.; Ganachaud, A.; Gehrke, P.C.; Griffiths, S.P.; Hobday, A.J.; Hoegh-Guldberg, O.; Johnson, J.E.; le Borgne, R.; Lehodey, P.; Lough, J.M. Mixed responses of tropical Pacific fisheries and aquaculture to climate change. *Nat. Clim. Chang.* **2013**, *3*, 591–599. [CrossRef]
27. Andrew, N.; Campbell, B.; Delisle, A.; Li, O.; Neihapi, P.; Nikiara, B.; Sami, A.; Steenbergen, D.; Urium, T. *Developing Participatory Monitoring of Community Fisheries in Kiribati and Vanuatu*; SPC Fisheries Newsletter #162: Noumea, New Caledonia, 2020.
28. Tilley, A.; Burgos, A.; Duarte, A.; dos Reis Lopes, J.; Eriksson, H.; Mills, D. Contribution of women's fisheries substantial, but overlooked, in Timor-Leste. *Ambio* **2020**. [CrossRef]
29. SPC. *Status Report: Pacific Islands Reef and Nearshore Fisheries and Aquaculture*; SPC: Noumea, New Caledonia, 2013.
30. Pratchett, M.S.; Munday, P.L.; Graham, N.A.; Kronen, M.; Pinca, S.; Friedman, K.; Brewer, T.D.; Bell, J.D.; Wilson, S.K.; Cinner, J.E.; et al. Vulnerability of coastal fisheries. In *Vulnerability of Tropical Pacific Fisheries and Aquaculture to Climate Change*; Bell, J.D., Johnson, J.E., Hobday, A.J., Eds.; Secretariat of the Pacific Community: Noumea, New Caledonia, 2011; pp. 167–185.
31. Gillett, R.; Tauati, M.I. *Fisheries of the Pacific Islands: Regional and National Information*; Fisheries and Aquaculture Technical Paper; FAO: Rome, Italy, 2018; pp. 1–47.
32. Pickering, T.D.; Ponia, B.; Hair, C.A.; Southgate, P.C.; Poloczanska, E.; Patrona, L.; Teitelbaum, A.; Mohan, C.V.; Phillips, M.J.; Bell, J.D. *Vulnerability of Aquaculture in the Tropical Pacific to Climate Change*; Secretariat of the Pacific Community: Noumea, New Caledonia, 2011.
33. Hambrey, J.; Govan, H.; Carleton, C. Opportunities for the development of the Pacific islands' mariculture sector. In *Report to the Secretariat of the Pacific Community by Hambrey Consulting*; SPC: Noumea, New Caledonia, 2012; ISBN 978-982-00-0529-7.
34. Paul, N. *Diversification of Seaweed Industries in Pacific Island Countries: Final Report FIS/2010/098*; Australian Centre for International Agricultural Research: Canberra, Australia, 2020.

35. Farmery, A.K.; O'Kane, G.; McManus, A.; Green, B.S. Consuming sustainable seafood: Guidelines, recommendations and realities. *Public Health Nutr.* **2018**, *21*, 1503–1514. [CrossRef]

36. Black, R.E.; Victora, C.G.; Walker, S.P.; Bhutta, Z.A.; Christian, P.; de Onis, M.; Ezzati, M.; Grantham-McGregor, S.; Katz, J.; Martorell, R. Maternal and child undernutrition and overweight in low-income and middle-income countries. *Lancet* **2013**, *382*, 427–451. [CrossRef]

37. Hicks, C.C.; Cohen, P.J.; Graham, N.A.; Nash, K.L.; Allison, E.H.; D'Lima, C.; Mills, D.J.; Roscher, M.; Thilsted, S.H.; Thorne-Lyman, A.L. Harnessing global fisheries to tackle micronutrient deficiencies. *Nature* **2019**, *574*, 95–98. [CrossRef]

38. Eriksson, H.; Friedman, K.; Amos, M.; Bertram, I.; Pakoa, K.; Fisher, R.; Andrew, N. Geography limits island small-scale fishery production. *Fish Fish.* **2018**, *19*, 308–320. [CrossRef]

39. Farrell, P.; Thow, A.M.; Wate, J.T.; Nonga, N.; Vatucawaqa, P.; Brewer, T.; Sharp, M.K.; Farmery, A.; Trevena, H.; Reeve, E. COVID-19 and Pacific food system resilience: Opportunities to build a robust response. *Food Secur.* **2020**, *12*, 783–791. [CrossRef] [PubMed]

40. Andrew, N.L.; Bright, P.; de la Rua, L.; Teoh, S.J.; Vickers, M. Coastal proximity of populations in 22 Pacific Island Countries and Territories. *PLoS ONE* **2019**, *14*, e0223249. [CrossRef]

41. SPC. *Pacific Island Populations (Les Populations du Pacifique) 2020*; The Pacific Community (SPC): Noumea, New Caledonia, 2020.

42. Schapper, A. Linguistic Melanesia. In *The Routledge Handbook of Language Contact*; Matras, A.A.Y., Ed.; Routledge: New York, NY, USA, 2020.

43. Govan, H.; Tawake, A.; Tabunakawai, K.; Jenkins, A.; Lasgorceix, A.; Techera, E.; Tafea, H.; Kinch, J.; Feehely, J.; Ifopo, P. Community Conserved Areas: A review of status & needs in Melanesia and Polynesia. In *ICCA Regional Review for CENESTA/TILCEPA/TGER/IUCN/GEF—SGP*; IUCN: Gland, Switzerland, 2009; 66p.

44. DESA. World Population Prospects 2019. Available online: https://population.un.org/wpp/Download/Standard/Population/ (accessed on 17 November 2020).

45. Day, J.; Forster, T.; Himmelsbach, J.; Korte, L.; Mucke, P.; Radtke, K.; Thielbörger, P.; Weller, D. *World Risk Report 2019*; Bündnis Entwicklung Hilft and Ruhr University Bochum–Institute for International Law of Peace and Armed Conflict (IFHV): Berlin, Germany, 2019.

46. FAO. *AQUASTAT Country Profile–Vanuatu*; Food and Agriculture Organization of the United Nations FAO: Rome, Italy, 2016.

47. World Bank. Country Profile Vanuatu. In *World Development Indicators Database*; World Bank: Washington, DC, USA, 2019.

48. VNSO. *Vanuatu Household Income and Expenditure Survey 2010*; Vanuatu National Statistics Office: Port Vila, Vanuatu, 2012.

49. Government of Vanuatu. *Vanuatu National Plan of Action on Food and Nutrition Security*; National Advosry Board on Climate Change and Disaster Risk Reduction: Port Vila, Vanuatu, 2013.

50. Bank, W. *Solomon Islands Systematic Country Diagnostic: Priorities for Supporting Poverty Reduction and Promoting Shared Prosperity*; World Bank: Washington, DC, USA, 2017.

51. UNDP. *Human Development Indices and Indicators: 2018 Statisticalupdate*; United Nations Development Program: New York, NY, USA, 2018.

52. SIG. *Solomon Islands Poverty Profile Based on the 2012/13 Household Income and Expenditure Survey*; Solomon Islands Government: Honiara, Solomon Islands, 2015.

53. Hoy, C. Poverty and the pandemic in the Pacific. In *Devpolicy Blog*; Betteridge, S.H.A.A., Ed.; The Australian National University: Canberra, Australia, 2020; Volume 2020.

54. Woo, S.; Perera Mubarak, K.N.; Mahmood, N.L.; Ride, A.K.; Naidoo, D.; Ki'l, M.; Resture, M.; Aluta, R.; Funa, J. *Enhancing the Economic Participation of Vulnerable Young Women in Solomon Islands*; The World Bank: Washington, DC, USA, 2019.

55. SIG. *Report on National Agricultural Survey 2017*; Solomon Islands Government, National Statistics Office: Honiara, Solomon Islands, 2019.

56. SINSO. *Solomon Islands 2012–2013 Household Income and Expenditure Survey: National Report*; Solomon Islands National Statistics Office: Honiara, Solomon Islands, 2013.

57. SPC; UOW; FAO. *The Pacific Nutrient Database User Guide: A Tool to Facilitate the Analysis of Poverty, Nutrition and Food Security in the Pacific Region*; Pacific Community, University of Wollongong and the Food and Agriculture Organization of the United Nations: Noumea, New Caledonia, 2020; p. 15.

58. Aakre, I.; Næss, S.; Kjellevold, M.; Markhus, M.W.; Alvheim, A.R.; Dalane, J.Ø.; Kielland, E.; Dahl, L. New data on nutrient composition in large selection of commercially available seafood products and its impact on micronutrient intake. *Food Nutr. Res.* **2019**, *63*. [CrossRef]

59. Nordhagen, A.; Rizwan, A.A.M.; Aakre, I.; Moxness Reksten, A.; Pincus, L.M.; Bøkevoll, A.; Mamun, A.; Haraksingh Thilsted, S.; Htut, T.; Somasundaram, T. Nutrient Composition of Demersal, Pelagic, and Mesopelagic Fish Species Sampled Off the Coast of Bangladesh and Their Potential Contribution to Food and Nutrition Security—The EAF-Nansen Programme. *Foods* **2020**, *9*, 730. [CrossRef]

60. Fiedler, J.L.; Lividini, K.; Bermudez, O.I.; Smitz, M.F. Household Consumption and Expenditures Surveys (HCES): A primer for food and nutrition analysts in low-and middle-income countries. *Food Nutr. Bull.* **2012**, *33*, S170–S184. [CrossRef]

61. Fiedler, J.L.; Carletto, C.; Dupriez, O. Still waiting for Godot? Improving Household Consumption and Expenditures Surveys (HCES) to enable more evidence-based nutrition policies. *Food Nutr. Bull.* **2012**, *33*, S242–S251. [CrossRef]

62. FAO. *Minimum Dietary Diversity for Women: A Guide for Measurement*; FAO: Rome, Italy, 2016; p. 82.

63. Kastom Garden Association. *People on the Edge. A Report of the 2005 Kastom Gaden Association Assessment of the Food Security, Livelihoods Potential and Energy Resources of the Guadalcanal Weather Coast, Solomon Islands*; Kastom Garden Association: Rockdale, Australia, 2005.

64. Bell, J.D.; Reid, C.; Batty, M.J.; Lehodey, P.; Rodwell, L.; Hobday, A.J.; Johnson, J.E.; Demmke, A. Effects of climate change on oceanic fisheries in the tropical Pacific: Implications for economic development and food security. *Clim. Chang.* **2013**, *119*, 199–212. [CrossRef]

65. Bell, J.D.; Sharp, M.K.; Havice, E.; Batty, M.; Charlton, K.E.; Russell, J.; Adams, W.; Azmi, K.; Romeo, A.; Wabnitz, C.C. Realising the food security benefits of canned fish for Pacific Island countries. *Mar. Policy* **2019**, *100*, 183–191. [CrossRef]

66. Brewer, T.D.; Andrew, N.L.; Sharp, M.K.; Thow, A.; Kottage, H.; Jones, S. *A Method for Cleaning Trade Data for Regional Analysis: The Pacific Food Trade Database (Version 2, 1995–2018)*; Pacific Community Working Paper; SPC: Noumea, New Caledonia, 2020.

67. Gaulier, G.; Zignago, S. Baci: International Trade Database at the Product-Level (The 1994–2007 Version). Paris, France; 2010. Available online: https://ssrn.com/abstract=1994500 (accessed on 26 November 2020).

68. FAO. *The State of World Fisheries and Aquaculture 2020. Sustainability in Action*; Food and Agriculture Organization of the United Nations: Rome, Italy, 2020.

69. Bell, J.D.; Allain, V.; Allison, E.H.; Andréfouët, S.; Andrew, N.L.; Batty, M.J.; Blanc, M.; Dambacher, J.M.; Hampton, J.; Hanich, Q. Diversifying the use of tuna to improve food security and public health in Pacific Island countries and territories. *Mar. Policy* **2015**, *51*, 584–591. [CrossRef]

70. Scherf, B.D. *World Watch List for Domestic Animal Diversity*; Food and Agriculture Organization (FAO): Rome, Italy, 2000.

71. Roos, N.; Wahab, M.A.; Hossain, M.A.R.; Thilsted, S.H. Linking human nutrition and fisheries: Incorporating micronutrient-dense, small indigenous fish species in carp polyculture production in Bangladesh. *Food Nutr. Bull.* **2007**, *28*, S280–S293. [CrossRef] [PubMed]

72. Farmery, A.K.; Hendrie, G.; O'Kane, G.; McManus, A.; Green, B. Sociodemographic variation in consumption patterns of sustainable and nutritious seafood in Australia. *Front. Nutr.* **2018**, *5*, 118. [CrossRef]

73. Moxness Reksten, A.; Bøkevoll, A.; Frantzen, S.; Lundebye, A.K.; Kögel, T.; Kolås, K.; Aakre, I.; Kjellevold, M. Sampling protocol for the determination of nutrients and contaminants in fish and other seafood–The EAF-Nansen Programme. *Methods X* **2020**, *7*, 101063. [CrossRef]

74. SPC. *Fish and Food Security*; Secretariat of the Pacific Community: Noumea, New Caledonia, 2008.

75. Cheng, M.H. Asia-Pacific faces diabetes challenge. *Lancet* **2010**, *375*, 2207–2210. [CrossRef]

76. Cassels, S. Overweight in the Pacific: Links between foreign dependence, global food trade, and obesity in the Federated States of Micronesia. *Glob. Health* **2006**, *2*, 10. [CrossRef]

77. HLPE. *Nutrition and Food Systems*; High Level Panel of Experts on Food Security and Nutrition of the Committee on World Food Security: Rome, Italy, 2017.

78. Coyne, T.; Hughes, R.; Langi, S. *Lifestyle Diseases in Pacific Communities*; Secretariat of the Pacific Community: Noumea, New Caledonia, 2000.

79. Eriksson, H.; Ride, A.; Notere Boso, D.; Sukulu, M.; Batalofo, M.; Siota, F.; Gomese, C. *Changes and Adaptations in Village Food Systems in Solomon Islands: A Rapid Appraisal during the Early Stages of the COVID-19 Pandemic;* WorldFish: Honiara, Solomon Isalnds, 2020.

80. Steenbergen, D.; Neihapi, P.; Koran, D.; Sami, A.; Malverus, V.; Ephraim, R.; Andrew, N. COVID-19 restrictions amidst cyclones and volcanoes: A rapid assessment of early impacts on livelihoods and food security in coastal communities in Vanuatu. *Mar. Policy* **2020**, *121*, 104199. [CrossRef]

81. Eriksson, H.; Albert, J.; Albert, S.; Warren, R.; Pakoa, K.; Andrew, N. The role of fish and fisheries in recovering from natural hazards: Lessons learned from Vanuatu. *Environ. Sci. Policy* **2017**, *76*, 50–58. [CrossRef]

82. Christoforou, A.; Snowdon, W.; Laesango, N.; Vatucawaqa, S.; Lamar, D.; Alam, L.; Lippwe, K.; Havea, I.L.; Tairea, K.; Hoejskov, P.; et al. Progress on Salt Reduction in the Pacific Islands: From Strategies to Action. *Heart Lung Circ.* **2015**, *24*, 503–509. [CrossRef]

83. Asche, F.; Bellemare, M.; Roheim, C.; Smith, M.; Tveterås, S. Fair Enough? Food Security and the International Seafood Trade. *World Dev.* **2015**, *67*, 151–160. [CrossRef]

84. Béné, C.; Lawton, R.; Allison, E.H. "Trade Matters in the Fight Against Poverty": Narratives, Perceptions, and (Lack of) Evidence in the Case of Fish Trade in Africa. *World Dev.* **2010**, *38*, 933–954. [CrossRef]

85. Nash, K.L.; MacNeil, M.A.; Blanchard, J.L.; Cohen, P.J.; Farmery, A.; Graham, N.A.J.; Thorne-Lyman, A.; Watson, R.; Hicks, C. Foreign fishing and trade mediate nutrient supply from fisheries. *Nature*. in review.

86. Bell, J.D.; Cisneros-Montemayor, A.; Hanich, Q.; Johnson, J.E.; Lehodey, P.; Moore, B.R.; Pratchett, M.S.; Reygondeau, G.; Senina, I.; Virdin, J.; et al. Adaptations to maintain the contributions of small-scale fisheries to food security in the Pacific Islands. *Mar. Policy* **2018**, *88*, 303–314. [CrossRef]

87. Asch, R.G.; Cheung, W.W.; Reygondeau, G. Future marine ecosystem drivers, biodiversity, and fisheries maximum catch potential in Pacific Island countries and territories under climate change. *Mar. Policy* **2018**, *88*, 285–294. [CrossRef]

88. van der Ploeg, J.; Sukulu, M.; Govan, H.; Minter, T.; Eriksson, H. Sinking Islands, Drowned Logic; Climate Change and Community-Based Adaptation Discourses in Solomon Islands. *Sustainability* **2020**, *12*, 7225. [CrossRef]

89. Hernández-Delgado, E.A. The emerging threats of climate change on tropical coastal ecosystem services, public health, local economies and livelihood sustainability of small islands: Cumulative impacts and synergies. *Mar. Pollut. Bull.* **2015**, *101*, 5–28. [CrossRef]

90. FFA. A Regional Roadmap for Sustainable Pacific Fisheries. Available online: https://www.ffa.int/system/files/Roadmap_web_0.pdf (accessed on 21 May 2020).

91. Houssard, P.; Point, D.; Tremblay-Boyer, L.; Allain, V.; Pethybridge, H.; Masbou, J.; Ferriss, B.E.; Baya, P.A.; Lagane, C.; Menkes, C.E. A model of mercury distribution in tuna from the western and central Pacific Ocean: Influence of physiology, ecology and environmental factors. *Environ. Sci. Technol.* **2019**, *53*, 1422–1431. [CrossRef]

92. FSANZ. Advice on Fish Consumption: Mercury in Fish. Availabe online:. Available online: http://www.foodstandards.gov.au/consumer/chemicals/mercury/Pages/default.aspx (accessed on 25 February 2020).

93. Médieu, A.; Point, D.; Receveur, A.; Gauthier, O.; Allain, V.; Pethybridge, H.; Menkes, C.E.; Gillikin, D.P.; Revill, A.T.; Somes, C.J. Stable mercury concentrations of tropical tuna in the south western Pacific ocean: An 18-year monitoring study. *Chemosphere* **2020**, *263*, 128024. [CrossRef]

94. Friedman, M.A.; Fernandez, M.; Backer, L.C.; Dickey, R.W.; Bernstein, J.; Schrank, K.; Kibler, S.; Stephan, W.; Gribble, M.O.; Bienfang, P. An updated review of ciguatera fish poisoning: Clinical, epidemiological, environmental, and public health management. *Mar. Drugs* **2017**, *15*, 72. [CrossRef]

95. Skinner, M.P.; Brewer, T.D.; Johnstone, R.; Fleming, L.E.; Lewis, R.J. Ciguatera fish poisoning in the Pacific Islands (1998 to 2008). *PLoS Negl. Trop Dis.* **2011**, *5*, e1416. [CrossRef] [PubMed]

3

'Sustainable' Rather than 'Subsistence' Food Assistance Solutions to Food Insecurity: South Australian Recipients' Perspectives on Traditional and Social Enterprise Models

Sue Booth [1],*, Christina Pollard [2]🆔, John Coveney [3] and Ian Goodwin-Smith [4]

[1] College of Medicine and Public Health, Flinders University, Adelaide 5000, Australia
[2] Faculty of Health Sciences, School of Public Health, Curtin University, Perth 6102, Australia; C.Pollard@curtin.edu.au
[3] College of Nursing & Health Sciences, Flinders University, Adelaide 5000, Australia; john.coveney@flinders.edu.au
[4] College of Business, Government and Law, Flinders University, Adelaide 5000, Australia; ian.goodwinsmith@flinder.edu.au
* Correspondence: sue.booth@flinders.edu.au

Abstract: South Australian (SA) food charity recipients' perspectives were sought on existing services and ideas for improvement of food assistance models to address food insecurity. Seven focus groups were conducted between October and November 2017 with 54 adults. Thematically analysed data revealed five themes: (1) Emotional cost and consequences of seeking food relief; (2) Dissatisfaction with inaccessible services and inappropriate food; (3) Returning the favour—a desire for reciprocity; (4) Desiring help beyond food; and, (5) "It's a social thing", the desire for social interaction and connection. Findings revealed that some aspects of the SA food assistance services were disempowering for recipients. Recipients desired more empowering forms of food assistance that humanise their experience and shift the locus of control and place power back into their hands. Some traditional models, such as provision of supermarket vouchers, empower individuals by fostering autonomy and enabling food choice in socially acceptable ways. Improvement in the quality of existing food assistance models, should focus on recipient informed models which re-dress existing power relations. Services which are more strongly aligned with typical features of social enterprise models were generally favoured over traditional models. Services which are recipient-centred, strive to empower recipients and provide opportunities for active involvement, social connection and broader support were preferred.

Keywords: food assistance; food insecurity; food charity; food service; social enterprise models

1. Introduction

Despite comprehensive social welfare provisions in Australia, such as unemployment benefits and universal health care, increasing neoliberalism and economic pressures have resulted in insufficient and inadequate levels of income support for vulnerable groups [1]. The United Nations Committee on the Rights of the Child recommended that Australia improve its social services (for education, health, income support, disability services and employment to strengthen their responsiveness for those at risk) [1]. Liberal state welfare models increase reliance on markets, individual responsibility and charitable responses rather than the state acting to universally respect, protect and fulfil the needs of vulnerable citizens [2]. As a consequence of the liberal model of welfare capitalism [3], more Australians are experiencing poverty, leading to food inequality [4] and a reliance on food assistance. In countries without robust, adequate welfare safety nets, people rely on food relief provided by charitable organisations such as foodbanks, faith-based groups and non-government organisations [5,6].

South Australia has experienced an economic downturn due in part to key industries relocating, resulting in unemployment and population subgroups at increasing risk of food insecurity [7,8]. In 2015, approximately 75,000 South Australians (4.2% of the population) were classified as food insecure, with higher prevalence among: women (4.9% compared to 4.1% of men); the unemployed (12.3% compared to 2.2% of full-time employed); households with an income of less than AUD$20,000 (12.1% compared to 1.2% of income over AUD$80,000); and Aboriginal and Torres Strait Islander people (16% compared to 4.4% non-Indigenous) [9]. The demand for food relief has increased, with recipients described as socially isolated, homeless, unemployed, financially struggling and marginalised [10]. Complex client needs, intergenerational poverty, limited education and employment opportunities contribute to the demand [11]. There is also evidence of food insecurity and reliance on food charity among middle-income Australian families [12]. The growing number of 'working poor' may reflect the unaffordability of household utility costs [13].

Australian food relief is predominantly provided by charitable food services [6,14]. In 2015, the Federal government provided ~AUD$64 million to support the provision of emergency relief, which was estimated to provide food assistance for up to eight percent of the population [14]. State governments assist in managing the distribution of funds and may allocate additional grant funding for targeted programs, for example, school breakfast programs. Between 3000 and 4000 emergency relief services provided short-term, immediate food assistance to eligible recipients in 2015 [14]. Seventy percent of emergency relief agencies reported increasing demand for food assistance in 2016, up by eight percent since 2015 [15].

The effectiveness and appropriateness of the traditional charitable food assistance model, has been questioned by government and academics, in light of the increasing demand for food assistance and an emerging interest in social enterprise models [16]. The South Australian Government's former Department of Communities and Social Inclusion (DCSI) (now Human Services) and SA Health commissioned research to explore recipients' experience of charitable food services and their recommendations for service improvements.

Traditional food assistance models are delivered via partnerships between the non-profit sector and supermarket chains—often with some government funding—with the aim of redistributing food waste to those living below the poverty line [17]. Food services are diverse and include mobile soup vans, food parcels, supermarket vouchers, pantries, seated meal services, food hubs and food banks [6,14]. The food provided is usually donated by supermarkets to food banks, where it is collected by direct services or "rescued" and delivered by food rescue organisations and faith-based groups, or purchased directly from supermarkets. Food is usually provided to recipients free or at a minimal cost. There is limited information on the types of foods provided in Australia; however, internationally, the types of food provided by these types of services have been found likely to exacerbate recipients' diet-related chronic disease conditions [6,18,19].

There are consistent reports from other jurisdictions of the recipients of traditional charitable food assistance being dissatisfied with the quality and quantity of food provided [20–22]. In addition to negative experiences due to limited food choice and poor food quality, recipients report feelings of shame, and describe the stigma and embarrassment associated with using food banks [23–25]. In Australia similar results are reported particularly concerning gratitude and shame: dissatisfaction with the variety, quality and types of food offered [26–28].

Social enterprise food assistance models, such as community or social supermarkets, social cafes, buying groups, and co-operatives, are uncommon in Australia, but are emerging as alternatives to the traditional charitable model [16]. Social enterprise broadly means 'trading for a social purpose', that is to say not for profit and for public benefit. However, there is little uniformity on what they are or do [29,30]. In other words, social enterprises are diverse, heterogeneous types of organisations using multiple activities to address the social needs of different client groups [31,32]. They vary in approach, but include: nonprofits' income earning strategies; voluntary organisations contracted to deliver public services; democratically controlled organisations primarily aiming to benefit the community with limited profits for external investors; commercial businesses operating in public welfare fields or with a social conscience; and, locally driven community enterprises combatting a shared problem [29,30].

Market, government and voluntary sector failures have been identified as the reason for the lack of uptake of social enterprise models in Australia, even though social enterprise models have the potential to address all three failures [16]. When reviewing these models in Australia, Wills (2017) found that resistance to them may be a consequence of commercial stakeholders fearing devaluation of their product range, lack of government legislative support, and/or current legislation undermining practices that social entrepreneurs wish to take [16].

There is no research on Australian food assistance recipients' perspectives on the likely benefits and limitations of social enterprise models to address food insecurity. Yet, the views of current food assistance recipients bring the lived experience perspective on receiving food assistance as well as helping to identify the elements of service delivery that are important to better meet needs. This study aimed to investigate recipients' views on both of these approaches (traditional and social enterprise), compare food relief models and their perspectives on each model's potential to meet the needs of food insecure people.

2. Materials and Methods

This study used a qualitative focus group methodology. Ethical approval was granted by the Flinders University Social and Behavioural Research Ethics Committee (Project No. 7770).

2.1. Recruitment and Data Collection

The DCSI provided researchers with an email contact list of South Australian emergency food relief services which they fund. Purposive sampling was used to capture inner metropolitan, outer metropolitan and country areas, as well as a diversity of service types. This enabled researchers to capture multiple and different perspectives. An email was sent to the CEO or similar explaining the study. Of the twelve organisations invited, seven (2 inner city, 3 outer metropolitan and 2 country) were agreeable and provided the name and contact details of their service manager to assist with focus group recruitment. The researchers were in regular contact with service managers regarding the most convenient day, and time to run the focus group. During times of food relief operations, the service manager and researchers would randomly approach recipients, advise them of the study and invite them to participate. All service managers were invited to attend the focus groups which were run in conjunction with a scheduled food relief session. Three experienced researchers (SB, JC and I G-S) conducted the focus groups in pairs. Service staff approached food relief participants and invited them to participate using a standard verbal script outlining the time and location of the focus group. The focus groups were held on site in a private room approximately an hour later. Invitees were provided with a study information sheet and consent form and a verbal explanation was given and written consent was obtained before the focus group commenced.

Each group was digitally recorded, field notes were written up afterwards and a commercial service transcribed each group. Participants were given a AUD$30 supermarket gift card as a token of appreciation for their time and contribution.

2.2. Focus Group Guide

A semi-structured guide was developed by the research team to direct the discussion while allowing for diversions reflective of participants' statements. Participants were asked to describe the type of charitable services they had used in the last year and the appropriateness and effectiveness of these services. A set of visual prompts were then used to assist participants to consider the pros and cons of traditional charitable and emerging social enterprise food relief service models. Finally, the group was asked to describe their ideal service for food relief provision.

2.3. Visual Prompts and Ranking of Preferences

A set of eight pictorial flash-cards was developed by the researchers. Each card had a short description of the type of service on the back to assist participants in considering the pros and cons of a variety of different food assistance models. The cards were used to stimulate focus group discussion and for an assessment of overall preference for services (Figure 1). The cards were divided into 2 groups based on availability. The first five cards showed and described traditional charitable food relief options commonly available in South Australia: (i) Food parcels, (ii) Food pantries, (iii) Gift cards/vouchers, (iv) Seated meal services, and (v) and Foodbank Food hubs. The remaining three cards showed social enterprise models of food relief which were not available in South Australia, but examples existing interstate or internationally. These were (vi) Social café program, (vii) Food co-operatives, and (viii) Social supermarkets. Each Group was asked to place the cards in rank order, starting with the service type they would be least likely to use. In each focus group, discussion continued until consensus was reached on the preferential ranking of cards. The discussions during the group ranking exercise highlighted some of the potential positive and negative attributions of services.

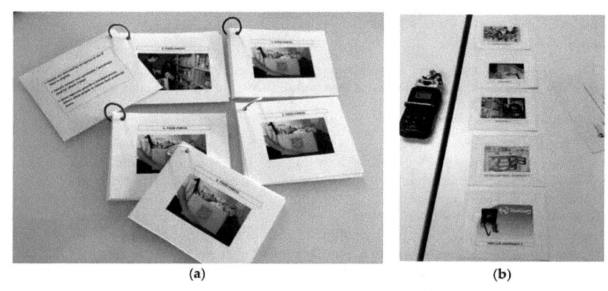

(a)   **(b)**

Figure 1. (**a**) The visual flash cards; (**b**) Visual flash cards in ranked order of preference during a focus group.

2.4. Data Analysis

Focus group recordings and notes were transcribed and de-identified. CMP and SB read and re-read all the transcripts and a sub-sample were read by the remaining researchers. The data was then analysed using the qualitative software program QSR NVivo (version 11.4.3, QSR International, Doncaster, Victoria, Australia). Deductive codes were initially developed from the focus group schedule as well as from the researchers' knowledge of the literature on experiences of charitable food service users. Inductive codes were developed from the focus group participant responses and discussed with the team to ensure rigour [33]. A thematic analysis was conducted by CMP with the codes and emergent themes cross-checked with the other members of the team until consensus was reached. SB double-coded three of the seven focus group transcript and any disagreements with the coding structure were discussed and the codes subsequently revised. Throughout the analysis, the data was further tested with the literature and subsequent focus groups in an iterative process. Data on the preferential ranking of service models across all focus group was tabulated. Verbal comments on the reasons for the ranking, pros, cons and recommendations to improve models were included in the thematic analysis.

3. Results

Fifty-four adults, 34 males and 20 females, who were recipients of food relief, participated in seven focus groups. Table 1 provides details of focus group location, service types from which participants were recruited and their gender.

Table 1. Location of focus group services, brief description, date and number of participants.

Group	Location	Service Description	Participants (*n*) Gender Split
1	Inner city	Seated breakfast program and emergency food relief appointments (Voucher)	(10) 7 men, 3 women
2	Inner city	Emergency food relief appointments (Food pantry access), free bread service	(7) 6 men, 1 woman
3	Country	Emergency food relief appointments (Food hub)	(7) 5 men, 2 women
4	Country	Emergency food relief appointments (Food parcels)	(4) 2 men, 2 women
5	Outer metropolitan	Volunteer run food hub—free food plus access to some items at reduced prices	(9) 2 men, 7 women
6	Outer metropolitan	Emergency food relief appointments (Food pantry access)	(7) 5 men, 2 women
7	Outer metropolitan	Food pantry, free bread, fruit and vegetables	(10) 3 men and 7 women

Overall, participants had used nine different food relief models, often accessing multiple services to overcome service food restrictions on frequency and amount. Several vulnerabilities led participants to use charitable food services, these included: homelessness; precarious employment; low income due to insufficient welfare payments; relationship breakdown; gambling addiction; and rises in the cost of living. The long-term nature of the need for food relief was evident, for example the chronicity recorded in the field note of SB,

"A woman on the far side of the table from me is of medium-thick build with shoulder-length strawberry blonde hair. She has broad facial features and makes intermittent eye contact. She tells the group she has been on the streets since she was 11 and she's now about 41. She looks much older. She has diabetes and food allergies. After the focus group she says I look familiar to her. We work out that I interviewed her for my PhD on homeless youth and food insecurity in 2000. She is terribly excited by this and tells everyone in the vicinity . . . She shouts she can't believe it and tells the people she is sitting with the story." Field note extract, SB Focus Group 1.

Participants' views on the pros, cons, and recommendations for improvement for the five traditional and three social enterprise food service models were varied and to some extent dependent on their current circumstances, as shown in Table 2.

Table 2. Participants' perspectives on the pros and cons of food service models and their recommendations to improve them.

Model	Pros	Cons	Recommendation
Food Parcel	• Commonly available • Grateful for parcels when have nothing	• 'Harsh' eligibility criteria • Inappropriate amount of food for family, types of food for special diets • Inadequate nutritious foods • No choice • Short term (1–3 day) solution • Food expires if you get more • Incomplete meals—no meat • Homeless people cannot carry	• Respectful and dignifying eligibility processes • Appropriate amounts and type of food to suit nutrition needs (e.g., meat, recipes, full meals, nutritious foods, length of time to cover) • Ability to choose items
Food Pantry	• Allows choice • Other items available (toiletries, washing powder etc.) • Fresh produce • Suitable if have access to cooking facilities	• Limits to number of items • Close to expired food • Limited types of foods, e.g., meat • Can only use twice a year • Must prove need • Difficulty securing an assessment appointment • Insufficient daily appointments • Have to waiting for appointment despite immediate need • Not suitable if no cooking facilities	• Respectful and dignifying eligibility processes • Reduce appointments waiting time, e.g., free calls or 1800 number • Appropriate amounts and type of food to suit nutritional needs (meat, recipes, full meals, nutritious foods) • Align food quantity with need • Increase access during holidays and weekends
Supermarket gift card	• Allows choice • Can buy other essential items • Easy to carry • Dignifying and 'normal' way to acquire food	• 'Harsh' eligibility criteria • Amount ($20) is inadequate • Only allowed to spend at major supermarket chains where food is expensive	• Increase supermarket voucher card value • Relax eligibility criteria • Cash for purchases from alternative food businesses
Seated meal services	• Best for people without dwelling, social isolated or cooking facilities • Able to combine with other services (e.g., shower, phone charging) • Social engagement with volunteers	• Families with young children too noisy • Sometimes unpleasant environment/people • Do not want children to experience the stigma • Cost to recipient • Can miss out on food because there is not enough and waiting time is too long • No-one sits down to and talks to you • Agency referral needed	• Combine with other services • Maintain pleasant, quiet, dignified atmosphere • Tailor food service to client needs • Universal eligibility • Socially connect with recipients
Foodbank Food Hubs	• Membership-based • Reward/incentive program • Discounts towards end of year, pre-saving for Christmas hampers • Free bread, fruit and vegetables	• Agency-issued vouchers require assessment appointments. Viewed as judgemental, embarrassing and undignified • Food that is unsaleable or approaching its use by date or expired.	• Universal eligibility or respectful and dignifying eligibility processes • Membership includes rewards scheme for every dollar spent • Food is purchased using own money • Blended model—free food and some discounted for purchase • Increase access during holidays and weekends

Table 2. *Cont.*

Model	Pros	Cons	Recommendation
Co-operative	• Dignifying • Dietitian assessed low-cost food packs with recipes for preparing at home • Offer toiletries, toys etc. • Best with other services including seated meals	• Membership fee • Having to pay for food if no income	• Include other services, e.g., seated meals or cafes • Make it more accessible to people e.g., transport • Increase access—Open during school holidays, weekends and major holidays
Social cafe	• Allows access to mainstream café—normalising experience • Helps isolated individuals • An outing for a special occasion	• Agency eligibility and assessment • Meal subsidy is time limited • Does not allow for family members and children • Dependent on participating café in local area	• Universal eligibility or respectful and dignifying eligibility processes • Incorporate access for children and family members • Free community barbecues to reduce social isolation and provide a treat/family outing
Social supermarket	• Opportunity for capacity building and volunteerism • Associated café providing cheap meals • Membership and discounted food • Supermarket style format, can exercise individual food choice • Other services can be accessed via the social supermarket—the idea of linked service valued • One-stop shop • Opportunity for socialisation, community connection	• Stocked with food that may be expired or close to use by date. Purchased food may have a shorter life span?	• Increased access—Open during school holidays, weekends and major holidays

Consensus on the preferential ranking of the five existing food service models varied across focus groups, depending on participants' social circumstances. Preference also varied for the three new models presented; however, social supermarkets were ranked highest by half of the groups, see Table 3.

Table 3. Focus group consensus ranking scores for participants' preference for five traditional models and three social enterprise food service models.

Ranking *	Traditional Models					Social Enterprise Models		
Focus group	Hub	Voucher	Pantry	Seated Meal	Parcel	Social Supermarket	Co-op	Social Café
1	5	2	3	1	4	2	3	1
2	5	4	3	2	1	2	1	3
3	1	2	3	5	4	1	3	2
4	2	1	3	5	4	1	3	2
5	1	4	3	2	5	1	2	3
6	2	1	3	5	5	2	1	3
7	1	3	2	5	4	1	2	3
Total	17	17	20	25	27	10	15	17

* Traditional models ranked from 1 most preferred to 5 least preferred (total possible 35) and social enterprise models from 1 most preferred to 3 the least preferred (total possible = 21).

When participants ranked the traditional food assistance service models, the hub, supermarket voucher and pantry were the most preferred. Discussions of the pros and cons revealed that these models enabled choice and allowed recipients to behave as mainstream consumers, that is, to engage in socially acceptable methods of food procurement. These types of food service models were the most likely to create a sense of empowerment for those who used them. Participants' recommendations to improve the traditional models generally focussed on universal eligibility or, if not possible, timely, dignified and respectful eligibility assessment processes. Traditional food assistance services also need to be re-engineered to provide the appropriate types and amounts of food to meet recipient's physical needs, specifically for: family composition, nutrition requirements, duration of food insecurity; and availability of food preparation facilities. They believed that services should also be re-engineered to provide opportunities reduce social isolation and foster social connection over a meal, for example, to incorporate seated meal services including cafes.

When participants ranked the three social enterprise food assistance service models, the social supermarket was first, co-operatives second and social cafe third. Again, the preference was to engage in socially acceptable models of food procurement. When informed about these models, participants viewed them favourability, particularly the normalising of food procurement processes, and the opportunity for neighbourhood and community connection. Social supermarkets and co-operatives were viewed as offering a dignified eligibility process, as a member rather than a recipient, and the opportunity to access additional services to assist recipients out of food insecurity. The opportunity to visit a café was viewed as highly desirable but out of reach for most participants. The main barriers to the social café model were the short-term nature, agency eligibility assessment, and the fact that recipients could not bring along their family members.

Five key themes emerged from all of the focus group and model ranking discussions (Figure 2). These were: (1) Emotional cost and consequences of seeking food relief; (2) Dissatisfaction with inaccessible services and inappropriate food; (3) Returning the favour—a desire for reciprocity; (4) Desiring help beyond food; and (5) "It's a social thing", the desire for social interaction and connection.

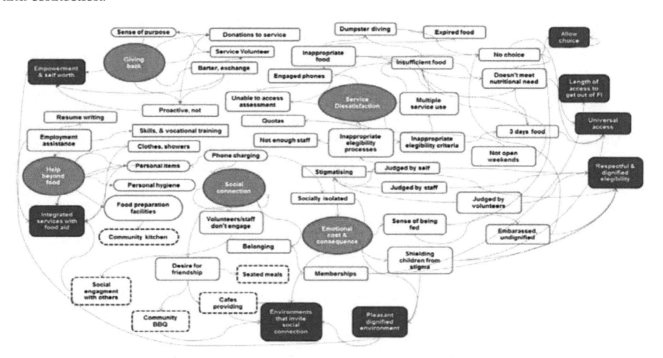

Figure 2. The thematic of food charity recipient perspectives on existing services and ideas for improvement—major themes (solid green), sub-themes (green outline), recipient recommendations (red outline), and final recommendations (solid red).

Each theme is described below.

3.1. Theme One: Emotional Cost and Consequences of Seeking Food Relief

Feelings of stigma, embarrassment, being judged or patronised as a result of many of the food service procedures or eligibility requirements. As one male said, *"I think the stigma should be the highlight I think and you shouldn't be made to feel embarrassed because, you know, you're sort of in need"*.

Negative comments regarding strict eligibility criteria for food relief were made in most groups and the notion of being referred by an agency to a particular service was seen as degrading and embarrassing,

> *"Yeah, if you have more than two visits you've got to take all these documents and you asked all the questions 'what do you do with the money, with the pension?' They say 'I get the same. How come I can do it and you can't do it?"* Male, Focus Group 1.

> *"See, the problem with most of those is that, like you said, you have to go to an agency where they make you feel so degraded. They're like 'how much do you earn? What do you do with that money? Why don't you have any money to buy food?' and it is embarrassing whereas here you don't have to explain yourself and the food co-op you don't have to explain yourself, you go in, buy what you want or get what you want and you walk out the door. They're not looking at you like 'oh my God what.'"* Female, Focus Group 2.

Operational inefficiencies had an emotional impact on recipients, contributing to their frustration and despair, for example, constantly engaged telephone lines that limited the opportunity for appointments to assess food assistance eligibility (Focus Group 6). One female participant showed the group her mobile telephone record of 39 calls logged trying to get an assessment appointment the morning of the interview. Delays in food eligibility assessments meant no food, and participants sometimes waited without food for up to three days for an appointment.

The impact of experiencing humiliation, judgment, embarrassment, or indignity during the food assistance process had some recipients stating they would not return to specific services, *"They make me feel this small. I never went there again."* Male, Focus Group 1.

Participants wanted services that were accepting and non-judgmental, *"If I could go somewhere that did not make me feel degraded to ask for help, that'd be awesome."* Female, Focus Group 5.

Some types of food relief models were seen as less stigmatising, for example, supermarket gift cards,

> *"Well, the card system is okay because there's no sort of stigma, is not it? Some people feel sort of embarrassed or ashamed in entering places like these and if you go in a place like this and, you know, if a card is given to you, I mean you're free to go and buy without no sort of stigma attached because nobody knows."* Male, Focus Group 2.

3.2. Theme Two: Inaccessible Services with Inappropriate Food

Food services were appreciated, but this was tempered by dissatisfaction due to problems related to food services, including: access, food types, the amount, and quality. Several participants mentioned that services were only available Monday to Friday and this made their life difficult, especially for those experiencing acute food shortages and needing emergency help.

> *"Yeah I think just even general —like in general, not just food or whatever, for the homeless, for the shutting down on the weekend, you know, people have crises on weekends, people have crises—you know, it is a real business structure and does not conform to business hours."* Female, Focus Group 2.

Supermarket vouchers and gift cards usually had a AUD$20 value. The amount was considered meagre and, although possibly suitable to pay for an individual's food for one day, the amount was viewed as insufficient for a family,

"They [cards] are very useful but realistically what can you get out of them, $20? I have a family of eight." Female, Focus Group 4.

Some participants said that the food offered was generally poor or may have exacerbated their existing health conditions, for example, diabetes, eating disorders, irritable bowel, allergies or mental health issues.

"I'm allergic to tomatoes and things like that so literally for myself, like trying to find—something like macaroni and cheese for me would be all right but I'm not supposed to eat too much pasta because of my diabetes so I'd have to actually find a way of being able to split that into two because two nights of—that whole meal would put me in hospital because of how much gluten's in it so I'm probably queen of the fuss but I'd just still rather be healthy by what I'm eating as well." Female, Focus Group 1.

"Pies are bad for diabetics because of the pastry. Pastry is really bad." Female, Focus Group 1.

Ready-made emergency food parcels also caused concern for people with existing health conditions because participants said they may contain food they were unable to eat. Negotiating to change the parcel contents or asking for a supermarket voucher instead caused some participant to experience guilt,

" … if I was to say 'look, I've got food issues and the food parcel that you've just given me, I really can't eat anything out of that' I would feel really—I feel guilty getting a [supermarket voucher/ gift] card." Female, Focus Group 2.

Supermarket vouchers and food pantries were preferred over ready-made food parcels because they afforded the opportunity for individuals to choose their own food items, with the statements below being typical:

"if you've got the card (supermarket gift card), you feel free to pick up what you want … " Male, Focus Group 2.

I like the … *"Food pantry because then you get to choose it."* Female, Focus Group 1.

Some service aspects and management strategies seemed to work better for recipients,

" … we paid $2. You get a little card. For every dollar you spend it gets accumulated up and at a Christmas time that amount would come off a Christmas hamper that they'd do, which I thought was absolutely fantastic. Go in there if you've made anything. If you've grown veggies or fruit you could take it in there and they give back to you. Like you give them that, you can get a couple of meals." Female, Focus Group 4.

To enable individuals to better manage their food insecurity, rather than seek help from food relief agencies, one Focus Group suggested a person's entire welfare payment should be directly deposited into supermarkets. They said this would avoid the money for food not being available if individually managed,

"You give it to—whatever shopping centre you use, you give it to them, the whole cheque, and so, okay, you can spend this much every week or every fortnight. You can't spend the whole lot in one hit. That will allow people to go there when they need something for tea or breakfast or whatever. They can grab the specific items and then go home 'oh well, I can make a meal and everything now' and then tomorrow comes 'well, I need this. I need onions and I need carrots and stuff'. Go in and buy them because if you gave someone a cheque they'd just go in and blow the whole lot." Male, Focus Group 1.

3.3. Theme Three: Returning the Favour—Reciprocity

Some participants engaged with services as both volunteers and recipients of food relief. Others desired to volunteer at services; however, the degree to which both men and women wanted to reciprocate at a 'pop up' service was sometimes unable to be accommodated. One comment indicated that children had also offered to volunteer at this same service. The quotes below are illustrative,

"We have on average maybe seven requests to volunteer every week. Well we don't [take more volunteers on]—I mean we're not ungrateful but we don't need them ... " Female, Focus Group 6.

"I volunteer and then sort of just pick some bits and pieces during my shift to take home to help out the family. I also am on a single parent pension so coming here for food relief by the volunteering ... " Female, Focus Group 7.

For some, the volunteering at a food relief service was driven by a desire to reciprocate for the assistance they had received.

"(I was) one of the people that lined up every week and then I started volunteering and I actually like returned the favour, giving back to the community." Female, Focus, Group 5.

Duties included staffing the café, preparing and/or re-packaging food items for distribution, or chatting to people lining up. Volunteers empathised with the circumstances and feelings of those seeking food relief variously commenting,

"We're not judging them", and *"we don't hold ourselves higher than what they are. We're one of them."* Female, Focus group 5.

Potential volunteer duties at food relief services were variable with garden maintenance on the premises suggested. Others suggested donating fresh home grown produce to food relief services as an acknowledgement of previous help or using produce to barter for pre-prepared meals or other food items,

" ... people could be working on an idea of providing food for—and people could contribute to that facility, if you know what I mean, and providing food for people on a regular basis, so people would be going there for meals and working in the garden and socialising ... " Male, Focus Group 2.

"'oh the lemon tree is nearly ready for picking' and then they go 'oh we'll bring lemons'. You know, big boxes like this that they've walked down the street with in wheelbarrow ... things or oranges, mandarins. If people have got trees they bring in the stuff to share back, like to say thank you to us." Female, Focus Group 5.

"Go in there if you've made anything. If you've grown veggies or fruit you could take it in there and they give back to you. Like you give them that, you can get a couple of meals." Female, Focus Group 4.

3.4. Theme Four: Help Beyond Food

Many participants described a need for help with other parts of their lives. For example, there was a need for items like nappies and toiletries, homeless people needed access to showers, laundry facilities and phone charging, domiciled people needed white goods (fridges, washing machines). Phone charging was important to keep people connected and the removal of free power points in the city mall was noted. Alternative charging stations were used including at McDonald's restaurants, suburban train carriages, some street locations, and libraries. Existing shower services were sometimes described as "hopeless" and the lack of showers in places like parklands were noted, prompting suggestions for alternative showers,

"Most people will pay . . . $20 and go to the bus terminal, give $20 over because it is a $20 deposit for the key and get the key and you can have a shower as long as you like. Then you go hand your key back and get your $20 back. That is how a lot of people get their showers . . . . And sometimes they let you put your phone [in] and go in the shower." Male, Focus Group 1.

"Can I just say something about the showers? I was talking to Orange Sky* not long ago because Orange Sky showers are going to be hopefully starting in January." Male, Focus Group 1 (Orange Sky is free of charge mobile laundry service).

Some participants wanted financial assistance and management, others were interested in support to increase the likelihood of employment such as resume development or assistance from a social worker.

" . . . you go to Centrelink and they go 'oh, it is nice if you start looking for work'—like before I had the babies—and it is like well, how do you put a resume together?" Female, Focus Group 4.

" . . . there needs to be like a social worker or someone that can be there to listen . . . " Female, Focus Group 4.

There were positive comments on the social supermarket model, centred around learning and training opportunities, which offered pathways out of poverty and a reliance on food relief.

"I really like the fact that with that one you're actually doing something as well. I just think that anything where people can learn to become better . . . . I would see it as a building and a stepping stone even more so because you get training . . . . They're the sort of things and for me that gives a person hope. That builds hope that I can get out of this position and get a bit better in life. You know, that I love." Female, Focus Group 7.

These suggestions, along with giving back, indicate a desire to gain skills and resources to seek financial independence or employment and get out of poverty.

3.5. Theme Five: "It's a Social Thing"—Desire for Social Interaction and Connection

In seeking food assistance, participants simultaneously sought meaningful social interaction and connection in a friendly atmosphere. They described how they wanted opportunities to engage with other regulars and volunteers, laugh, converse over coffee, or a meal or engage in fun activities.

"I'd rather the person that is handing the meal out, when you've finished handing the meals out sit down and talk to us, spend time with us. Don't just hand the meal out and go 'zoom' and take off and go somewhere else." Male, Focus Group 4.

"I'd rather go to [Service] because they sit down and talk and laugh and have fun and everything like that." Male, Focus Group 5.

Participants who had used food relief and who now volunteered their time registered the importance of providing social support for recipients,

"We get a lot of people that don't come here for the food; they come here because they know they can have a chat. Sometimes we're the only people in the whole entire week that they've spoken to . . . " Female, Focus group 5.

An outcome of social connection at food relief services included the development of friendships, and in one case marriage and cohabitation,

"Those people that are getting married, be it that they're elderly but they were facing nursing homes because they had no-one to look after them. They were living on their own and they met here. They've now moved in together. They don't have to move into nursing homes." Female, Focus Group 8.

4. Discussion

The aim of this study was to investigate food assistance recipients' views on both existing services in South Australia and on examples of social enterprise models. We also sought to understand how food assistance might be improved more broadly to better meet the needs of food insecure people. Five themes emerged from the discussions: (i) considerable emotional costs and consequences in receiving food assistance, (ii) dissatisfaction with inaccessible services and inappropriate food, (iii) desire to reciprocate for food assistance by volunteering at services, (iv) the need for help goes beyond food, and (v) a strong desire for social connection.

Participants desired food assistance models that afforded some of the features characteristic of social enterprise models, particularly the opportunity to exercise food choice, meet their desire for social connection and commensality, and provide access to other services such as training or skills development. Social supermarkets offer an innovative model of food assistance which could address some of these points, but are unavailable in Australia [34]. Internationally, there are a variety of novel food assistance practices that have the potential to transform incrementally and interact with other food systems to deliver pathways out of food poverty [35]. Our work suggests that recipients support the re-making of traditional food relief models as a way to support individual empowerment and pathways out of food insecurity.

The findings highlighted the power imbalances inherent in the provision of food assistance and suggests that they are deeply embedded at an operational level in existing South Australian services. The intrinsic design and delivery of charitable food assistance can be either disempowering or empowering. Forms of assistance which are empowering help vulnerable people climb out of their neediness and offers real pathways out of food insecurity. In contrast, disempowering assistance traps clients in a continuous, chronic food assistance cycle.

This study found evidence of disempowerment within traditional South Australian food charity models such as stigma or embarrassment, having to prove their eligibility, need or worthiness for assistance. Empowering options aligned more strongly with social enterprise models.

4.1. Disempowering Food Assistance

Although recipients were grateful for food assistance, there were several aspects of the system that were experienced as disempowering, which contributed to the emotional costs and consequences in receiving food relief including loss of power, similar to those described by van der Horst et al. (2014) [36]. Aspects of traditional food assistance models inadvertently impact the emotional wellbeing of recipients by fostering negative feelings such as judgment, embarrassment and stigma. The emotional consequences of having to ask for food assistance in the first place speaks to an admission of failure that one cannot provide food for oneself. This can be so overwhelming for some people that they would rather avoid seeking food assistance [36]. These findings are consistent with evidence from other wealthy industrial countries for recipients of food bank users and other types of food charities [25].

The power imbalance is also evidenced by the dissatisfaction with inaccessible and inappropriate food services, particularly recipient's inability to enforce their right to food, their freedom to choose food the food they want in socially acceptable ways, or eat in dignified settings. Riches (2018) asserts that it is "the universal right of vulnerable individuals and families to be able to feed themselves with choice and human dignity" (p. 3) [37]. Recipients were frustrated with the lack of choice in the current system and desired the dignity of being able to choose their own food, recommending models that were considered empowering and less stigmatising, such as supermarket gift cards. These finding were consistent with those of recipients in Perth, Western Australia [27].

4.2. Empowering Food Assistance

Study participants expressed a desire to receive flexible, recipient-oriented services that were empowering, encouraged independence and autonomy. They had a strong desire for giving back—that is, wanting to 'return the favour'—for example, by volunteering at services when their circumstances allowed them to. Applying Mauss's 1925 framework of gift exchange, food [charity] is this context is essentially a gift which cannot be reciprocated and may render the recipient powerless [38]. Inherent in Mauss's theory of gift giving is the obligation to reciprocate. This may explain the strong desire of participants to 'return the favour', namely, to regain a modicum of situational power by donating fruit or volunteer labour.

Recipients described the need for 'Help beyond food'. Their desire for empowerment went beyond food. Participants spoke positively of food assistance models that extended to the social purpose of tackling food insecurity and offered a viable pathway out of chronic reliance on food assistance. The current findings align with the UK's All-Party Parliamentary Group (AAPG) recommendations on the Hunger and Food Poverty inquiry into foodbanks in the UK [39]. The AAPG called for models to end food poverty which were 'sustainable' rather than offering 'subsistence' and recommended a 'food bank plus model', as described by Paget et al. (2015) [40]. The nature of the 'food plus model' included multiple services, all of which should be considered when reviewing funding to food assistance services in South Australia.

In Australia, charitable food assistance services rely on foodbanks and food rescue organisations to redistribute retail food waste. The participants in this current study, although grateful, were dissatisfied with the food provided by services, describing issues with the appropriateness and quality of food and the reliance on charity, and ultimately their inability to attain a varied and healthy diet in an autonomous way. The conversations rang true to the sentiment of 'Left over food for left over people' previously described by Dowler [41]. Participants wanted to 'fit in' and to shop at supermarkets and eat at cafes like 'normal people', and they did not want their children to know they were struggling. The findings suggest the retail sector reconsider their moral and social obligation in light of the right to food for the most vulnerable citizens residing in countries where they operate. For example, as part of their retail practice they could directly provide dignified access to appropriate food by assisting people during times of economic hardship to access their goods in socially acceptable ways.

The current study findings also highlight the acceptability of some of the aspects of social enterprise models to address food insecurity among recipients. A well-developed example of a social enterprise model to food insecurity are social supermarkets (SSMs). SSMs are a retail formula where the outlet receives free surplus food and consumer goods from partner companies and sells them at symbolic prices to people who are at risk of, or living in poverty (Holweg and Lienbaucher 2010) [34]. They may also operate as retail training grounds to assist people who are long term unemployed or disabled re-integrate into society. In doing so, SSMs provide opportunities for work and immediate positive fulfilment and feedback; they provide a wage rather than government handouts and subsidies, and they build individual confidence and resilience [42]. SSMs are widespread in continental Europe, with more than 1000 in operation in 2013 [43], but few, if any, examples exist in Australia. Despite being widespread, however, there is no available literature evaluating the effectiveness of social supermarkets.

Successful programs for food assistance and other support pathways are likely to be ones that are co-produced with recipients [39] and the current findings highlight the value in obtaining recipient reviews on current and future service options. Co-production has become synonymous with innovative approaches to service delivery and been defined as "A meeting of minds coming together to find a shared solution. It involves people who use services being consulted, included and working together from the start to the end of any project that affects them" (p.7) [44].

4.3. The Desire for Social Interaction and Connection

Participants desired meaningful social interaction and connection, recognition and acknowledgement, and friendship networks. The sense of isolation and loneliness experienced by homeless people or those living in poverty is well documented and may constitute a risk to survival [45]. Loneliness is adversely associated with physical and mental health and lifestyle factors [46]. The experience of social pain, defined as the unpleasantness that is associated with actual or potential damage to one's sense of social connection or social value (owing to social rejection, exclusion, negative social evaluation or loss) may involve an overlap of the neural circuitry underpinning physical pain (defined as the unpleasant experience that is associated with actual or potential tissue damage) [47].

High levels of concern about the consequences of loneliness experienced by all ages has prompted calls for it to be considered a public health issue [48]. The strong preference for seated shared meal services, commensality and connection with others in the current study suggest that social enterprise models integrated with cafes and restaurant dining are an option [49,50].

The study has several strengths and limitations. A strength of this study is that the 54 participants were recipients of food assistance from different geographic locations (metropolitan, regional and country areas) in South Australia. They provided a real-life perspective on the issues and potential solutions. The presentation of three novel social enterprise options to provide food assistance enabled participants to think beyond the current system; however, as there are few social enterprise options in Australia [16], they did not have an experience of using these types of services. Only three social enterprise models were presented, with very little description (one image and three to four descriptive sentences), further research is needed to identify and pilot the effectiveness of social enterprise models for food assistance in Australia.

A limitation of the current research is that it was not designed to explore options to address food insecurity other than food assistance. There are numerous social and economic policy actions that should be explored as to their effectiveness in addressing food insecurity, for example, increasing the minimum welfare payments, employment schemes or other economic options that are under the auspice of government. There was a noticeable absence of government policy and/or accountability in the food assistance system in South Australia, and indeed in Australia. Further research is needed to describe options for an integrated food assistance system that includes government, commercial sector and voluntary organisations.

The findings suggest that the retail sector may have an important role to play in addressing food insecurity, outside the current food waste redistribution paradigm. Recipient dissatisfaction with the food currently available suggests that food acquisition and distribution models need to be critically analysed for their ability to address food insecurity. Exploration of effective Corporate Social Responsibility commitments to address food insecurity that are not reliant on redistributing waste food is warranted.

5. Conclusions

Food systems, including charitable food systems, need to work for everyone, especially those who are vulnerable. This study has revealed aspects of the existing South Australian food assistance system that can be disempowering to recipients. Disempowering forms of food assistance can trap recipients in a cycle of food charity. Participants desired empowering forms of assistance that humanise the charitable food system, shift the locus of control and place power back into the hands of users. Improvement in the quality of existing food relief models, should focus on recipient-informed models (co-production) which re-dress existing power differentials. Services which are more strongly recipient-centred, strive to empower clients and provide opportunities for active involvement, social connection and broader support are needed.

Author Contributions: Conceptualisation, S.B., J.C., C.P. and I.G.-S.; Methodology, S.B., J.C., C.P. and I.G.-S.; Focus group facilitation, S.B., I.G.-S., and J.C.; Focus Group Themed Analysis, C.P.; Secondary analysis S.B., Resources, S.B., C.P.; Writing-Original Draft Preparation, S.B. and C.P.; Writing-Review & Editing, S.B., J.C., C.P. and I.G.-S.; Project Administration, I.G.-S.; Funding Acquisition, I.G.-S.

Acknowledgments: The authors would like to acknowledge the service managers, volunteers and recipients of food assistance who participated in the study.

References

1. United Nations. Committee on the Rights of the Child Sixtieth Session 29 May–15 June 2012. Available online: http://docstore.ohchr.org/SelfServices/FilesHandler.ashx?enc= 6QkG1d%2fPPRiCAqhKb7yhsk5X2w65LgiRF%2fS3dwPS4NXPtJlvMuCI3J9Hn06KCDkN8AgEcc% 2bNlwRMULqb84PSl9FicZROAZolAudnAZ3CxmRZ%2fzxW2Yn8qOrVcMCd9xFL (accessed on 21 September 2018).

2. Claeys, P. The right to food: Many developments, more challenges. *Can. Food Stud.* **2015**, *2*, 60–67. [CrossRef]

3. Esping-Andersen, C. *The Three Worlds of Welfare Capitalism*; Polity Press: Cambridge, UK, 1990.

4. Pollard, C.; Begley, A.; Landrigan, T. The rise of food inequality in Australia. In *Food Poverty and Insecurity: International Food Inequalities*; Springer International: Cham, Switzerland, 2016; pp. 89–103.

5. McKee, M.; Reeves, A.; Clair, A.; Stuckler, D. Living on the edge: Precariousness and why it matters for health. *Arch. Public Health* **2017**, *75*, 13. [CrossRef] [PubMed]

6. Pollard, C.M.; Mackintosh, B.; Campbell, C.; Kerr, D.; Begley, A.; Jancey, J.; Caraher, M.; Berg, J.; Booth, S. Charitable food systems' capacity to address food insecurity: An Australian capital city audit. *Int. J. Environ. Res. Public Health* **2018**, *15*, 1249. [CrossRef] [PubMed]

7. Jericho, G. Why South Australians Are Older, Poorer and on Their Way Interstate. *The Guardian Newspaper*. 14 March 2018. Available online: https://www.theguardian.com/business/grogonomics/2018/mar/15/ south-australia-dragged-down-by-demographics (accessed on 18 March 2018).

8. BankSA, Manufacturing South Australia's Future. Trends—November 2017—A Bulletin on Economic Development in South Australia. 2017. Available online: https://www.banksa.com.au/content/dam/bsa/ downloads/bsa-media-trends-nov-2017.pdf (accessed on 18 September 2018).

9. Anglicare. *Improving Individual and Household Outcomes in South Australia—Discussion Paper*; Anglicare SA: Adelaide, Australia, 2017. Available online: https://dhs.sa.gov.au/__data/assets/pdf_file/0007/59812/ Anglicare-SA-Response-to-Food-Security-Discussion-Paper.pdf (accessed on 18 September 2018).

10. Wingrove, K.; Barbour, L.; Palermo, C. Exploring nutrition capacity in Australia's charitable food sector. *Nutr. Diet.* **2017**, *74*, 495–501. [CrossRef] [PubMed]

11. McKay, F.; McKenzie, H. Food aid provision in metropolitan Melbourne: A mixed methods study. *J. Hunger. Environ. Nutr.* **2017**, *12*, 11–25. [CrossRef]

12. Kleve, S.; Davidson, Z.; Gearon, E.; Booth, S.; Palermo, C. Are low to middle income households experiencing food insecurity in Victoria, Australia? An examination of the Victorian Population Health Survey 2006–2009. *Aust. J. Prim. Health* **2017**, *23*, 249–256. [CrossRef] [PubMed]

13. Ramsay, R.; Giskes, K.; Turrell, G.; Gallegos, D. Food insecurity amongst adults residing in disadvantaged urban areas: Potential health and dietary consequences. *Public Health Nutr.* **2012**, *15*, 227–237. [CrossRef] [PubMed]

14. Lindberg, R. Still serving hot soup? Two hundred years of a charitable food sector in Australia: A narrative review. *Aust. N. Z. J. Public Health* **2015**, *39*, 358–365. [CrossRef] [PubMed]

15. Foodbank, W.A. Foodbank WA Annual Report 2015. Available online: https://www.foodbankwa. org.au/wp-content/blogs.dir/5/files/2015/10/Annual-Report-Final-2015_web.pdf (accessed on 14 September 2018).

16. Wills, B. Eating at the limits: Barriers to the emergence of social enterprise initiatives in the Australian emergency food relief sector. *Food Policy* **2017**, *20*, 62–70. [CrossRef]

17. Richards, C.; Kjaernes, U.; Vik, J. Food security in welfare capitalism: Comparing social entitlements to food in Australia and Norway. *J. Rural Stud.* **2016**, *43*, 61–70. [CrossRef]

18. Seligman, H.; Lyles, C.; Marshall, M.; Prendergast, K.; Smith, M.; Headings, A.; Bradshaw, G.; Rosenmoss, S.; Waxman, E. A pilot food bank intervention featuring diabetes appropriate food improved glycemic control among clients in three states. *Health Aff.* **2015** *34*, 1956–1963. [CrossRef] [PubMed]

19. Miewald, C.; Ibanez-Carrasco, F.; Turner, S. Negotiating the local food environment: The lived experience of food access for low-income people living with HIV/AIDS. *J. Hunger. Environ. Nutr.* **2010**, *5*, 510–525. [CrossRef]

20. Hamelin, A.; Beaudry, M.; Habicht, J. Characterization of household food insecurity in Quebec: Food and feelings. *Soc. Sci. Med.* **2002**, *54*, 119–132. [CrossRef]

21. McNeill, K. Talking with Their Mouths Half Full: Food Insecurity in the Hamilton Community. Ph.D. Thesis, The University of Waikato, Hamilton, New Zealand, 2011.

22. Loopstra, R.; Tarasuk, V. The relationship between food banks and household food insecurity among low-income Toronto families. *Can. J. Public Health* **2012**, *38*, 497–514. [CrossRef]

23. Garthwaite, K. Stigma, shame and 'people like us': An ethnographic study of foodbank use in the UK. *J. Poverty Soc. Justice* **2016**, *24*, 277–289. [CrossRef]

24. Purdam, K.; Garrett, E.A.; Esmail, A. Hungry? Food insecurity, social stigma and embarrassment in the UK. *Sociology* **2016**, *50*, 1072–1088. [CrossRef]

25. Middleton, G.; Mehta, K.; McNaughton, D.; Booth, S. The experiences and perceptions of foodbank amongst users in high income countries: An international scoping review. *Appetite* **2018**, *120*, 698–708. [CrossRef] [PubMed]

26. Booth, S. Eating Rough—Food Insecurity Amongst Homeless Young People in Adelaide. Ph.D. Thesis, Flinders University, Adelaide, Australia, 2003.

27. Booth, S.; Begley, A.; Mackintosh, B.; Kerr, D.A.; Jancey, J.; Caraher, M.; Whelan, J.; Pollard, C.M. Gratitude, resignation and the desire for dignity: Lived experience of food charity recipients and their recommendations for improvement, Perth, Western Australia. *Public Health Nutr.* **2018**, *21*, 2831–2841. [CrossRef] [PubMed]

28. Middleton, G. Evaluation of a Community Food Banking Model in South Australia. Honours Thesis, Flinders University, Adelaide, Australia, 2015.

29. Teasdale, S. What's in a name? Making sense of social enterprise discourse. *Public Policy Adm.* **2011**, *27*, 99–119. [CrossRef]

30. Teasdale, S. How can social enterprise address disadvantage? Evidence from an inner city community. *J. Non-Profit Public Sect. Mark.* **2010**, *22*, 89–107. [CrossRef]

31. Shaw, E.; Carter, S. Social entrepreneurship: Theoretical antecedents and empiricle analysis of entrepreneurial processes and outcomes. *J. Small Bus. Enterp. Dev.* **2007**, *14*, 418–434. [CrossRef]

32. Sharir, M.; Lerner, M.; Yitshaki, R. Long term survivability of social ventures: Qualitative analysis of external and internal explainations. In *International Perspectives of Social Entrepreneurship*; Robinson, J., Mair, J., Hockerts, K., Eds.; Palgrave Macmillan: Basingstoke, UK, 2009.

33. Henninck, M.; Hutter, I.; Bailey, A. *Qualitative Reseach Methods*; Sage Publications: Thousand Oaks, CA, USA, 2011.

34. Holweg, C.; Lienbacher, E.; Zinn, W. Social supermarkets-a new challenge in supply chain management and sustainability. *Supply Chain Forum* **2010**, *11*, 50–58. [CrossRef]

35. Hebinck, A.; Galli, F.; Arcuri, S.; Carroll, B.; O'connor, D.; Oostindie, H. Capturing change in european food assistance practices: A transformative social innovation perspective. *Local Environ.* **2018**, *23*, 398–413. [CrossRef]

36. van der Horst, H.; Pascucci, S.; Bol, W. The "dark side" of food banks? Exploring emotional responses of food bank receivers in the netherlands. *Br. Food J.* **2014**, *116*, 1506–1520. [CrossRef]

37. Riches, G. *Food Bank Nations. Poverty, Corporate Charity and the Right to Food*; Routledge: New York, NY, USA, 2018.

38. Mauss, M.T. *The Gift: The Form and Reason for Exchange in Archaic Societies*; Routledge Classics: London, UK, 1990.

39. All-Party Parliamentary Group on Hunger and Food Poverty. *Feeding Britain: A Strategy for Zero Hunger in England, Wales, Scotland and Northern Ireland, the Report of the All-Party Parliamentary Inquiry into Hunger in the United Kingdom*; Children's Society: London, UK, 2014.

40. Paget, A. *Community Supermarkets Could Offer a Sustainable Solution to Food Poverty*; Demos: London, UK, 2015.

41. Caraher, M.; Furey, S. *The Economics of Emergency Food Aid Provision: A Financial, Social and Cultural Perspective*; Springer International: Cham, Switzerland, 2018.

42. Schneider, F. The evolution of food donation with respect to waste prevention. *Waste Manag.* **2013**, *33*, 755–763. [CrossRef] [PubMed]

43.   Cocozza, P. 'If I Shop Here I've Got Money for Gas': Inside the UK's First Social Supermarket. Available online: http://www.theguardian.com/society/2013/dec/09/inside-britains-first-social-supermarket-goldthorpe-yorkshire (accessed on 5 August 2018).

44.   Council of the Ageing. The Voice of Consumers in Home Care: A Practical Guide. 2014. Available online: https://www.cota.org.au/publication/the-voice-consumers-in-home-care-guide/ (accessed on 14 September 2018).

45.   Pantell, M.; Rehkopf, D.; Jutte, D.; Syme, S.L.; Balmes, J.; Adler, N. Social isolation: A predictor of mortality comparable to traditional clinical risk factors. *Am. J. Public Health* **2013**, *103*, 2056–2062. [CrossRef] [PubMed]

46.   Richards, A.; Rohrmann, S.; Vandeleur, C.L.; Schmid, M.; Barth, J.; Eichholzer, M. Loneliness is adversely associated with physical and mental health and lifestyle factors: Results from a Swiss national survey. *PLoS ONE* **2017**, *12*, e0181442. [CrossRef] [PubMed]

47.   Eisenberger, N. The pain of social disconnection: Examing the shared neural underpinnings of physical and social pain. *Nat. Rev. Neurosci.* **2012**, *13*, 421–434. [CrossRef] [PubMed]

48.   Matthews, T.; Danese, A.; Caspi, A.; Fisher, H.L.; Goldman-Mellor, S.; Kepa, A.; Moffitt, T.E.; Odgers, C.L.; Arseneault, L. Lonely young adults in modern Britain: Findings from an epidemiological cohort study. *Psychol. Med.* **2018**, *1*. [CrossRef] [PubMed]

49.   Lambie-Mumford, H.; Dowler, E. Hunger, food charity and social policy–challenges faced by the emerging evidence base. *Soc. Policy Soc.* **2015**, *14*, 497–506. [CrossRef]

50.   Linares, E. Food services for the homeless in Spain: Caritas programme for the homeless. *Public Health Nutr.* **2001**, *4*, 1367–1369. [PubMed]

4

Food Security Experiences of Aboriginal and Torres Strait Islander Families with Young Children in an Urban Setting: Influencing Factors and Coping Strategies

Leisa McCarthy [1,*], Anne B. Chang [1,2,3] and Julie Brimblecombe [1,4]

1   Menzies School of Health Research, 0870 Darwin, Australia; anne.chang@menzies.edu.au (A.B.C.); julie.brimblecombe@monash.edu.au (J.B.)
2   Department of Respiratory Medicine, Queensland Children's Hospital, 4101 Brisbane, Australia
3   Children's Centre for Health Research, Queensland University of Technology; 4101 Brisbane, Australia
4   Department of Nutrition, Dietetics and Food, School of Clinical Sciences, Monash University, 3168 Melbourne, Australia
*   Correspondence: leisa.mccarthy@menzies.edu.au

Abstract: Evidence on Aboriginal and Torres Strait Islander peoples' food security experiences and coping strategies used when food insecurity occurs is limited. Such evidence is important to inform policies that can reduce the consequences of food insecurity. This study investigated factors perceived by Aboriginal and Torres Strait Islander families with young children to influence household food security, and coping strategies used, in an urban setting. A qualitative research inductive approach was used. Data were collected through an iterative process of inquiry through initial interviews with 30 primary care-givers, followed by in-depth interviews with six participants to further explore emerging themes. Major topics explored were: influencing factors, food insecurity experiences, impact on food selection, and coping strategies. Food affordability relating to income and living expenses was a major barrier to a healthy diet with large household bills impacting food choice and meal quality. Access to family support was the main reported coping strategy. Food insecurity is experienced by Aboriginal and Torres Strait Islander families, it is largely intermittent occurring especially when large household bills are due for payment. Family support provides an essential safety net and the implications of this are important to consider in public policy to address food insecurity.

Keywords: food security; food insecurity; Aboriginal and Torres Strait Islander population; children; urban; experiences; coping strategies

1. Introduction

Food security is "access by all people, at all times to sufficient food for an active and healthy life. Food security includes at a minimum: the ready availability of nutritionally adequate and safe foods, and an assured ability to acquire acceptable foods in socially acceptable ways" [1] (p. 337). Irrespective of a country's affluence status, some population groups within high income countries experience food insecurity and varying degrees of hunger. For these groups, strategies to overcome or alleviate food insecurity have been employed, but most measures are thought to be short-lived and a 'stop gap' to temporarily relieve problems [2–11]. Evidence that can inform longer-term solutions are required. Availability of such evidence is important to inform possible practice and policy interventions.

However, literature about people's experiences with household food insecurity is limited, particularly within Indigenous populations of affluent countries, the group most at risk of household food insecurity and poor health [2,7,12–14]. Among families with young children in the United States and Canada, studies reported that although families access food assistance programs, food shortages and hunger are still experienced [2–11]. A study in six Inuit communities of Nunavut, Canada, focused on the availability and accessibility of traditional and market foods (i.e., foods purchased from a shop), found inconsistencies between perceived food security status and experiences in obtaining enough food to eat [7]. In contrast, another study undertaken with a Nunavut Inuit population, found participants who reported food insecurity also reported regular use of community food programs to assist with alleviating hunger [2]. The variance in results likely reflects the different sampling frame of these studies, as one [7] recruited from the broader community and the other [2] through food assistance programs [2,7].

To mitigate household food insecurity, coping strategies (i.e., the mechanisms families have in place to cope with food and money problems) are used [4,5,10,11,15]. A Canadian Quebec-based study described several coping strategies used by participants to overcome household food insecurity: adults reduced size of meals or forwent food so children could eat; modified lifestyle (e.g., forgoing purchases of less essential items and payment of bills to free up money for food); purchased sale item foods and foods close to use by date; and visited a food bank when desperate [10]. An Australian study undertaken in South Western Sydney investigated coping strategies [15]. The most frequent responses of nine coping strategies to select from were, cutting down on the variety of household foods (59.1%); a parent or guardian skipping meals or eating less (58.8%); and putting off paying bills (57.4%) [15]. Other coping strategies reported (among a multicultural group of 90 food pantry users in Washington, USA) include using leftover food, cooking food in bulk and freezing food for later use [11]; and among Latino immigrant families in North Carolina, USA, limiting food purchases considered expensive, e.g., meats and fruits and; shopping for specials and bulk-buying [5].

To alleviate household food insecurity, social support systems are important and include assistance from food programs, food charity organisations, faith communities, neighbours and friends [2–11,13]. Extended family as a social support system is also important [2–4,8,9,11] One study reported support from friends and neighbours as a main coping mechanism in response to food insecurity [5]. Within an Inuit population, living with family as a temporary coping strategy until housing was obtained was identified [2]. Another study, highlighted reciprocity where young mothers would rely on family members for food assistance and then 'return the favour' when other family members experienced difficulties [4].

Among Aboriginal and Torres Strait Islander peoples, the concept of reciprocity is an important component of the social connectedness [16]. This cultural sharing practice is important in maintaining and reinforcing individual and group social bonds and imparting knowledge about good food as related to balance—life, resources, food, knowledge [16,17]. Studies undertaken in Inuit populations have also noted reciprocity has a place in maintaining and reinforcing family and broader community relationship obligations as well as cultural identity and practice [2,7]. 'Cultural sharing' and 'sharing networks' ensure that excess traditional food is provided to the more vulnerable members of the community who cannot obtain these foods [2,7]. Identified in these studies, was that money or other services were exchanged for traditional foods to keep with continuing cultural practices for those who could not hunt [2,7]. Similarly, in a study undertaken with Latino Immigrant Families in North Carolina, USA, money was sent home to families to support food security. This action was justifiable from the belief family back home were in a worse situation to their own and a cultural obligation to look after ones' parents [8].

Despite the importance of knowing coping mechanisms used when household food insecurity occurs within families, there is little to no such data among Aboriginal and Torres Strait Islander people. Obtaining such data provides knowledge on enablers that can inform policies to enhance existing coping strategies and support families. Therefore, this qualitative study explores the experiences of household food insecurity and coping strategies used among Aboriginal and Torres Strait Islander families residing in Darwin and Palmerston, two cities of remote Northern Australia.

2. Materials and Methods

A qualitative research inductive approach was used, where data collection involved an iterative process of inquiry through initial interviews and subsequent in-depth interviews. All interviews were undertaken by the primary author, an Aboriginal woman and nutritionist. An iterative process of data collection and analysis was undertaken. Thematic analysis was applied. The inductive method used was not confined to existing theoretical frameworks [18] or pre-determined categories and allowed for the creation of categories or codes during data collection to arise. These codes were then combined into themes which were mapped to reveal relationships between them. This process of qualitative data collection and analysis makes it particularly suitable to exploring an under-investigated study area.

This qualitative study was part of a larger study that aimed to investigate food security among families with use of a modified study version of the United States Department of Agriculture 18-item Household Food Security Module (mUS 18-item Module). It was during the administration of the mUS 18-item Module, that the initial interviews occurred and were initiated by the participants.

Human Research Ethics approval was obtained from the Human Research Ethics Committee of the Northern Territory Department of Health and Menzies School of Health Research and the Aboriginal Sub Ethics Committee. HREC File Reference Number 09/06.

2.1. Setting

The 2016 Australian Bureau of Statistics Census data estimated Aboriginal and Torres Strait Islander people comprised 3.3% of the Australian population (http://www.abs.gov.au/ausstats/abs@.nsf/mf/3238.0.55.001. 3238.0.55.001—Estimates of Aboriginal and Torres Strait Islander Australians, June 2016. LATEST ISSUE Released at 11:30AM (CANBERRA TIME) 31/08/2018). Darwin is the Northern Territory capital and Palmerston a nearby satellite city. Study data were collected for a period of 7 months between April 2009 and February 2010. At the time of the study population separations for Darwin and Palmerston were unavailable. Therefore, the combined total population of Darwin and Palmerston was 98,152 residents [19], with Aboriginal and Torres Strait Islander peoples comprising 7.5% of the total Palmerston population and 9.4% of the Darwin population [19]. The aim of this study was to investigate the food insecurity experiences of Aboriginal and Torres Strait Islander families in these two main centres of the Northern Territory.

2.2. Sampling

The primary author recruited potential participants through child health clinics in local health services', comprising two Aboriginal health services and two Government health services. A local Aboriginal woman was employed to assist with recruitment at one of the health service sites. Participants were also recruited from the broader community through the assistance of an Aboriginal Research Officer who had extensive networks with Aboriginal families in both Darwin and Palmerston. Convenience sampling through the local health services and known networks was used.

2.3. Participant Recruitment

The inclusion criteria were: care giver of a young Aboriginal and/or Torres Strait Islander child (aged 6 months-4 years); resided in Darwin or Palmerston for ≥12 months; and the child did not have a medical condition requiring food or nutrition supplements. A set of predetermined participant inclusion criteria were developed prior to study commencement with input from the health services during the consultation phase. During recruitment, informed consent was obtained from the eligible child's care-giver to participate in the whole study including qualitative interviews. Recruitment continued until 30 participants had completed the mUS 18-item Module, used to define the presence/absence of food insecurity. As the aim of the larger study was to test the reliability and face validity of the mUS 18-item Module among urban residing Aboriginal and Torres Strait Islander families with children 0.5 to 4 years, 30 participants were deemed a suitable number for this purpose.

2.4. Initial Discussions

Initial discussions, prompted through completion of the mUS 18-item Module, lasted from 30 min to three hours. Notes were taken (audio-recordings were not used) and read back to the participant to confirm the information and typed as a word document. Following each interview, the primary author coded text relating to food security experiences and coping strategies. These codes were explored in subsequent interviews. This iterative process continued until all initial interviews were complete. These codes informed the interview guide for the in-depth interviews (Appendix A).

2.5. In-Depth Interviews

In-depth interviews were audio recorded and notes taken. We purposively invited participants based on gender and identified age groups to reflect the overall study sample. The recordings were transcribed and the transcription read back to the participant either in person or over the telephone to verify the interview content and clarify any queries. Any adjustments or further data collected were agreed to, verified and included. The interview, transcription and analysis process continued iteratively until data saturation was reached i.e., when no new information or new themes emerged [20,21]. To achieve this, six participants were interviewed. Coding of all transcripts was undertaken firstly, by the primary author and then separately by the senior author. A set of themes identified initially by the primary author, was agreed on.

3. Results

Thirty care givers were recruited and engaged in initial discussions. Table 1 shows, the majority were female, Aboriginal and their age ranged between 17 and 58 years. Over half of the participants had partners (married or de facto relationship). The six participants were representative of the main sample in gender and age (Table 1).

Table 1. Demographic characteristics of households.

Characteristic		Initial Discussions (N = 30)	In-Depth Interviews (N = 6)
Parent gender	Female	27	4
Marital Status	Partnered	17	5
Indigenous status	Aboriginal	19	5
	Torres Strait Islander	1	0
	Aboriginal and Torres Strait Islander	6	1
	Non-Indigenous Australian	4	0
Care giver	Parent (mother/father)	27	6
	Other (grandmother/foster carer)	3	0
Parent age (yrs)	Median (range)	44.5 (17–58)	35 (25–39)
Residents in house	Median (range)	6 (3–15)	5.5 (3–10)
Number of children by age group (N = 57)	6 to 24 months	19	3
	25 to 48 months	30	5

3.1. Findings

As shown in Figure 1, themes identified from the initial interviews were grouped according to (i) factors influencing food security and (ii) coping strategies. These were explored further in the in-depth interviews with the following themes identified: *(i) Experiences of Food Insecurity; (ii) Influencing Factors; (iii) Impact on food selection; and (iv) Coping Strategies.* Themes relating to influencing factors are presented as major or minor influencing factors and determined both by the number of participants referring to these themes and whether featured prominently in their responses. (Figure 1).

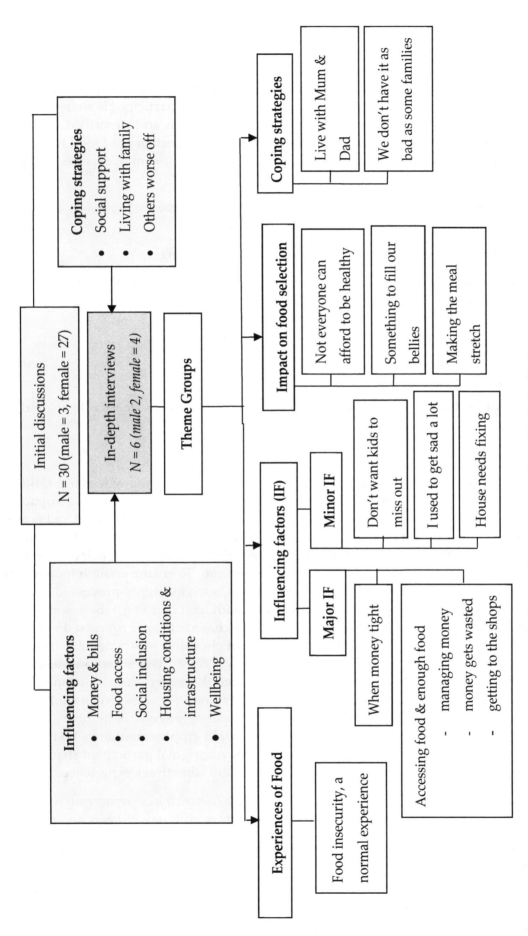

Figure 1. Overview of significant Qualitative Findings.

3.2. Experiences of Food Insecurity

Food Insecurity, a Normal Experience

Participants did not initially identify with being food insecure, although many of their experiences indicated otherwise. Whilst completing the mUS 18-item Module participants shared their own and others' experiences with not having enough food, money or both and described this situation as common among themselves and/or people close to them. The experiences of food insecurity as told by participants implied that food insecurity was seen by most as a 'normal' experience and was also considered 'the norm' within their close social interactions:

There's not enough money, full stop, to pay for food, to last from payday to payday. (Aboriginal mother with four children, aged 34 years and partnered)

Another participant shared his observations when out shopping:

. . . I've seen people put food back. Put things back because they can't get [afford] that. Or take a milk bottle back to get a smaller bottle of milk. Yes, you do see it around. (Aboriginal and Torres Strait Islander father of two children, aged 36 years and partnered).

3.3. Influencing Factors

3.3.1. Major Influencing Factors

These influencing factors were comprised of the sub-themes *"when money is tight"* and *"accessing food and enough food"*.

When Money is Tight

Many participants shared that they prioritised essentials when money was tight. Bills, such as quarterly electricity bills, were a main reason for making "money tight" and this impacted on the amount and type of food purchased. For some ($n = 9$), this situation was intermittent and occurred only when larger bills had to be paid or if there was a temporary change in household income. Whereas others ($n = 11$) described this as an everyday phenomenon. Four of these 11 participants mentioned not having enough money at all times due to an inadequate income. To ensure enough food for the family when 'money was tight' less expensive foods were chosen, such as highly processed foods of lower nutrient quality or cheaper brand options. For example, with fruit and vegetables, some participants purchased these in lesser quantity, did not buy at all, or purchased cheaper processed versions instead of fresh. Approximately half of the participants' spoke of choosing less expensive foods to ensure children had something to eat at each meal when 'money was tight'. This situation was not limited to participants who were recipients of Centrelink (The Centrelink Master Program is one of the Master Programs of the Australian Government Department of Human Services (Australia). The majority of Centrelink's services are the disbursement of social security payments (Source: Wikipedia site *en.wikipedia.org/wiki/Centrelink.*)), as some participants in paid employment, or who had partners in paid employment, also experienced this phenomenon. One Aboriginal participant shared that despite both her and her husband having paid employment, they still sometimes experienced difficulties:

Sometimes we have to be tight [with money] when the big bills (electricity, car repayments) come in and choose less expensive foods to buy. (Aboriginal mother of three children, 25 years and partnered).

This experience was echoed by an Aboriginal man, who as the sole income earner cut back on what he termed 'luxury items' such as snack foods, sweet drinks or desserts, when 'money was tight'.

Don't have real problems with food [having enough to eat] or with money. Only time may have to get tight with the budget is when the big bills come in. This just means cutting back on luxury items. (Aboriginal father of one child, 38 years and partnered).

This participant also revealed other measures used to immediately relieve a "money tight" situation and ensure adequate food, although this measure had greater cost implications:

Often the bill would come in and we would go and do a shop and then make that shop stretch to the next pay to pay the bill. I would consider putting food in people's guts (stomachs) more important than paying bills. If you don't pay the bill on time, there's a late fee $30, $40 dollars. Might as well pay it late, that's how I would look at it. (Aboriginal father of one child, 38 years, partnered).

Of the 30 participants, the sole income for nine were Centrelink payments and four of these individuals were being income managed (Income Management is an Australian Government initiative to assist individuals receiving Centrelink social security payments in managing money to meet essential household needs and expenses, and learn to better manage finances in the long term. (Source: http://www.humanservices.gov.au/customer/services/centrelink/income-management)). Three of the four participants considered these payments as inadequate in meeting their households' basic living costs. A participant told of her experience in being income managed. She viewed income management as good for families who needed help with budgeting. In her case however it was not helpful as she 'looked after her children properly' and the payment was not enough to feed her family:

I have three boys and you know, they eat a lot. One loaf of bread eaten for breakfast! I don't think we get enough money and I can't pay for all the food from my basic card Basic card (similar to a bank key card. A portion of income managed individuals' payments are deposited into a basic card to purchase food and other essential household items only. (Source: http://www.humanservices.gov.au/customer/services/centrelink/income-management). (Aboriginal mother of four children, 34 years and partnered).

Another participant, who stated that she had money problems all the time, worked full-time and had a regular income, but her partner had been having problems with securing permanent full-time employment:

I work full-time, but don't get paid much. My partner works when he gets work and we also rely on government money [Centrelink payments]. The money that we do get seems to just cover the rent, food and basic necessities. Rent and food are expensive in Darwin. We also have a car to run and that's also expensive. (non-Indigenous mother of four children, 30 years and partnered).

Some participants shared that they experienced money problems temporarily due to a sudden change in their income, such as irregular timing in child maintenance payments:

Sometimes they [ex-partners] don't pay [child maintenance] regularly and that throws us out with budgeting for the fortnight. I don't think they [ex-partners] understand how hard it makes things sometimes. (Aboriginal and Torres Strait Islander mother of three children, 38 years, single)

Other participants spoke of full-time employment and being paid well as an enabler of food security. An Aboriginal woman who was a full-time student expressed that her husband was in secure full-time employment, earned a "good wage" that was able to meet the family's needs:

If my husband wasn't on a good wage and he didn't earn enough to cover the bills and other expenses, we would definitely be struggling. (Aboriginal mother of one child, 27 years and partnered).

Nineteen of the 30 participants identified as food secure (63.3%), raised concerns about the rising cost of living and how this would impact on their families in the future. In particular, a man of both Aboriginal and Torres Strait Islander heritage spoke of not having money issues but mentioned the rising cost of living and the impact this could have on his household:

... it's becoming very expensive. Everything has just gone up ... and not just food prices. It's electricity, phone, fuel [for car], the cost of living in general has gone up a lot. You know,

we [participant and his wife] are aware of how difficult it could be if one of us lost our job. And we don't have much in savings. And if there is an economic downturn that affects us, that's why we're trying to pay off as much of our mortgage now just to make sure that we have a buffer. (Aboriginal and Torres Strait Islander father of two children, 36 years, partnered).

Accessing Food and Enough Food

This sub-theme encompassed findings relevant to budgeting and managing money; misuse of money; and food access.

Managing Money

At least five participants spoke of how important it is to budget or "manage money" to ensure enough money for food and bills. An Aboriginal woman shared her experience:

. . . I've always planned a budget to include extras to make sure money for additional expenses such as car maintenance, power bills, etc. Though, power bills have gone up. Not because we're using more power, just the cost of power. Other things (essential items) are going up as well. You know, price of food, petrol, rent. So much pressure on families just to live. In our budget we always make sure the rent and bills are paid and there's money for food. You know, the kids come first. Make sure they're clothed, fed, school fees paid. Sometimes I may need new clothing, shoes, or whatever, but will go without to make sure the kids have what they need. Just make sure I have what I need budgeted for and save for it. (Aboriginal mother with three children, 25 years and partnered).

For some though, budgeting did not always prevent "money being tight":

. . . Sometimes things [budget] blows out and I think I mentioned it before. One month you might get your electricity bill and that. Plus, we have child care fees and that's a big chunk out of that as well. (Aboriginal and Torres Strait Islander father of two children, 36 years and partnered).

Four participants were income managed by Centrelink and had a portion of their income automatically quarantined for food and other household essentials accessed through use of a Basics card. There were mixed experiences with this system and two mentioned post-introduction of income management that money problems still occurred, whilst another two experienced improvements:

It's ok. I don't get much humbug (Humbug is a term predominantly used by Indigenous Australians in a way that means 'to pester', as in being pestered (humbugged) by someone for money) now [since introduction of basics card] for money and have enough money for food. (Aboriginal grandmother, carer of 10 grandchildren, 44 years, widowed).

Money Gets Wasted

Although participants referred to their own struggles with managing money to meet family needs, many participants expressed that there were families in worse situations than themselves, particularly when anti-social behaviour such as gambling, excessive alcohol and illicit drug use were involved. Participants defined anti-social behaviour as that of 'social problems' and associated these with food and money problems:

. . . there are also problems with drinking [alcohol] and gambling. It makes me wonder sometimes, when people say they have no money to pay bills or buy food. They smoke [cigarettes], drink [alcohol] and gamble and don't seem to understand this causes problems. When you have limited money, need to be smart about how to use it. (Aboriginal and Torres Strait Islander mother of three, 38 years and single).

"Other families find it hard too [money problems]. That's why some people sell drugs. Need more money. . . . have problems with gambling and drinking [alcohol]. Maybe drugs. A lot of money gets

wasted. Make me sorry for the kids". (Aboriginal and Torres Strait Islander mother of five, 29 years, partnered).

Food security for some participants' households were directly affected by others' social problems:

My brother is bad. All he wants to do is drink grog [alcohol]. Then he gets hungry and comes here. Eats all my kids' tucker [food]. He takes money from me and Nanna. Other people after him cos' he steal grog [alcohol] from them. (Aboriginal mother of two, 25 years and partnered).

Getting to the Shops

This sub-theme covered the ability to access food (shops) and reliable transport. Eleven participants mentioned their experience with accessing shops and how this impacted on food purchasing as well as seeking out food specials and bargains. Having access to supermarkets was considered by most participants as important to obtain affordable food items. Supermarkets were considered as cheaper and offering a wider variety of goods when compared to the smaller convenience type stores. During the study period a major supermarket chain outlet accessed by a quarter of the participants closed. The only other food outlet option locally available to these participants and within walking distance was the service station (a service station is a motor vehicle fuel outlet and often provides a small range of grocery items, including bread, milk, juice and a few dry goods lines.) which had only a small range of goods and was expensive. The impact of the supermarket closure on food security was expressed by an Aboriginal and Torres Strait Islander woman:

[I] find it hard with shopping since local supermarket closed. Shopping Centre not within walking distance but was a short drive from my house and [I] relied on a lift or taxi that didn't cost very much. Now [I] have to pay more for taxis, as [I] travel further to go shopping. (Aboriginal and Torres Strait Islander mother of four children, 33 years and single)

Different modes of transport were used for food shopping by participants. Access to a reliable car, particularly a privately-owned car, was said to help the most and enabled access to larger supermarkets for food specials and buying food in bulk:

We didn't have a car before but have one now. Made it easier to get around and do the shopping. (Aboriginal and Torres Strait Islander mother of five children, 29 years and partnered).

I don't have transport problems and can go to the places I want to shop. Usually follow the bargains and try to buy in bulk. (Aboriginal and Torres Strait Islander mother of three, 38 years and single).

Participants who accessed public transport, particularly buses, found it difficult when travelling with small children. Using taxis was another option, though this was expensive particularly when funds were limited:

Hard to take the bus with a baby and a two year old to go shop or clinic. (Aboriginal mother of two children, 25 years and partnered).

3.3.2. Minor Influencing Factors

Social pressures, emotional wellbeing and housing featured in discussions of food security with at least one-third of the participants.

Don't Want the Kids to Miss out

Four participants spoke in detail about their school-aged children needing money for entertainment and social occasions, of which put a strain on family income. They did not want their children "to go without" or miss out on social experiences that their children's peers were perceived to have:

We have problems sometimes with having enough money . . . only when we have visitors or things the kids want to go to, like the [Darwin] Show. All the other kids going to the Show and our kids don't want to miss out. It's only fair for them, they only kids and should enjoy themselves. (Aboriginal Grandmother of 10 grandchildren, 44 years and widowed).

Kid's like to buy from the school shop [tuckshop] like the other kids. Sometimes I really don't have enough money but, give them anyway. I don't want other kids at school to think my kids are poor. (Aboriginal mother of seven children, 26 years and single).

I Used to Get Sad a Lot

At least two thirds of participants openly discussed their feelings of how they felt emotionally in relation to food insecurity. Eleven participants expressed feelings of being stressed, down, sad, lonely and of frustration or feeling inadequate in being a good provider for their children. Two of the four participants receiving Centrelink payments referred to the stigma of shopping with a Basics Card and the feeling of frustration and 'shame' (shame is a term used by Aboriginal and Torres Strait Islander peoples as feeling embarrassed either about themselves or others. I.e. feeling shame because no money on the card to purchase groceries and others looking on. Or, feeling shame for someone else in a similar situation.) in having little control over managing their finances. These two participants also believed they did not need to be income managed and described feelings of public humiliation when not having enough money on the Basic card for groceries:

Real shame job [embarrassed] for me to go shop and find out don't have enough money on the card [Basic card] to pay for groceries. Have to leave everything—trolley and all—with everyone watching. Make me real shame. (Aboriginal mother of two children, 25 years and partnered).

Other participants raised and spoke about wellbeing related issues with relevance to food and money. In particular these were emotions of feeling down or sad due to relationship breakdowns and family stresses:

I used to get sad a lot and not able to look after the kids properly. (Aboriginal mother of three children, 34 years and single).

The House Needs Fixing

Of the 30 participants, four were owner-occupiers with seven renting privately and nineteen renting through public housing. One-third of the participants in rental properties discussed problems with general home maintenance, specifically with kitchen maintenance including problems with window fly screens, kitchen benches, kitchen cupboards and stoves:

. . . There are no flyscreens on some of the windows and in others there are holes. The rats get in at night and sometimes [we] can see and hear them running in the house. Sometimes they run over us in our sleep! (Aboriginal mother of four children, 34 years and partnered).

A number of participants expressed frustration in home maintenance:

. . . We've told him [owner] about the kitchen cupboards falling apart and other problems in the house. Just doesn't seem to want to do anything about it . . . . (Aboriginal mother of two children, 29 years and partnered).

We can't use the benches properly 'cause the tiles are broken and dirty (bench top is tiled). The stove doesn't work either". We told housing [public housing authority] we have problems months ago, but they still haven't come to fix them. All we do is wait and see what happens. (Aboriginal mother of four children, 34 years and partnered).

One participant who owned their home, indicated that having adequate food storage space helped with always having food on hand:

. . . we buy frozen vegies as well, because they last longer and we have them on hand to put in our food [cooking]. Well that helps with us. So, having a freezer helps as well [with food storage]. (Aboriginal and Torres Strait Islander father of two children, 36 years and partnered).

Whereas a participant who did not have adequate cold food storage had to shop more frequently:

I have what I need in the house. [I] Need a freezer. That way can buy more meat and put away, instead of going to the shop every day to buy meat for dinner. (Aboriginal mother of seven children, 26 years and single).

3.4. Impact on Food Selection

Within this theme are sub themes that encompass participants' views regarding food affordability; relationship between food and health; and food behaviour in association with food insecurity.

3.4.1. Not Everyone Can Afford to be Healthy

Many references to food and health were made by participants. In particular, the benefits of consuming home prepared meals rather than take-away meals perceived as high in fat and sugar. Four of the 30 participants spoke in-depth about fresh fruit and vegetables being 'healthy' foods and important in the prevention of illnesses such as type 2 diabetes. These foods though were considered by these participants as expensive and not always affordable when compared with other less healthy food options. At least half of the participants referred to the high cost of food influencing food choice.

An Aboriginal woman for example understood the relationship with food and good health, yet felt she was unable to put this knowledge into practice due to limited money and high food costs:

[I] Find it hard sometimes to eat healthy like have fruit and vegetables every day. Sometimes [it's a] bit tight with money and [I] buy food that fills you up. Fruit doesn't [fill you up] and it's expensive. . . . . Always hear about why important to eat healthy to stop diseases like diabetes, but when you try to, it's very expensive. (Aboriginal mother of three children, 29 years and partnered).

We're told to eat right, exercise and be healthy, but it's hard when everything costs so much to be healthy. Not everyone can afford to be healthy. (Torres Strait Islander mother of four children, 30 years and partnered).

One participant, where money for food was not considered an issue, spoke of not wanting her children to eat too much processed foods and have more natural foods in their diets:

I like my children to eat fresh food and foods that are not over processed. Also, processed foods tend to have a lot of sugar and that's no good. (Aboriginal mother of two children, 29 years and partnered).

3.4.2. Something to Fill Our Bellies

Participants referred to compromising food quality for quantity to ensure that there was enough to eat at each meal. Most participants spoke of the importance of eating healthy food at meal times. However, for some this was not always feasible and most important to these participants was ensuring enough food to eat "to fill bellies":

I make sure my kids are fed and don't go without. Some of our meals are not that healthy, but at least we have something to fill our bellies. (Aboriginal and Torres Strait Islander mother of three, 38 years and single).

We can afford food, but not always healthy food. Sometimes, have hamper [tinned corned beef] and rice with bread for dinner. It's filling and the kids are not hungry. (non-Indigenous mother of four children, 30 years and partnered).

Some participants referred to strategies used to ensure the family did not go without a meal:

. . . Usually try to buy in bulk and cook meals in bulk to freeze and use later. Therefore, make sure my daughter never goes without food. (non-Indigenous mother of one, 28 years and single).

3.4.3. Making the Meal Stretch

Most participants mentioned the use of low cost starchy foods, such as rice, pasta and bread to 'fill children up between meals' or add quantity to 'bulk up' meals when unexpected visitors joined in a meal or to use up leftover foods:

. . . If not enough food for each meal, cook more rice or have bread. This fills you up. Only time this happens is when we have unexpected visitors at dinnertime [evening meal] and we have to stretch the food so everyone has something". (Aboriginal mother of three children, 34 years and single).

I make sure kids always eat weet-bix [wheat biscuits breakfast cereal] in the morning before go to school. Have something at school from the shop [school tuckshop] and when they get home usually have bread with something on it. Boys eat a lot and bread is cheap and fills them up. (Aboriginal mother of seven children, 26 years and single).

A male participant spoke of his family's experience with using up left over food and filler foods to bulk up meals:

It's sort of a standard way (having rice) of making the meal stretch. Not that having enough food is an issue. But when we have leftovers, it's a, way of making sure we have enough. (Aboriginal and Torres Strait Islander father of two, 36 years and partnered).

3.5. Coping Strategies

As a coping strategy, social support in the form of accessing extended family was the most prominent form of assistance sought by participants to prevent or help alleviate food insecurity.

3.5.1. Live with Mum and Dad, They Help Out a Lot

Extended family provided the most common form of support and the types of support sought were mainly for money and food, but for some families it was assistance with looking after children. For four participants, assistance was sought regularly where others sought assistance only when there were additional demands placed on the household income. Running out of money and/or food were the most common reasons for accessing social support which usually occurred during 'money tight' times when the 'big bills' were due for payment. An Aboriginal woman with a family who lived with her parents, spoke of how this living arrangement assisted with expenses and provided support with looking after her children:

Sometimes have problems with money. Especially when the bills come in at once and don't always have enough to buy food. My three kids and me live at home with my mum and dad. This makes it easier for when I run out of money. Mum and dad have money for food. (Aboriginal mother of three children, 34 years and single).

Other participants shared their experiences with accessing family for assistance when experiencing difficulties and this support being reciprocated:

My partner has family here and if we don't have food, or money for food, we go over to family's place for dinner [evening meal]. Or if someone has money, we'll lend money. Our home is open to family if we have food and someone wants something to eat or money. But I always make sure we have enough for ourselves first. (non-Indigenous mother of four, 30 years and partnered).

We do have problems with food sometimes. Especially when we get big bills and there's not enough money for food. Usually, go to my mum and dad to ask for money or food. Glad I have them. Don't know where I would go otherwise for help. (Aboriginal and Torres Strait Islander mother of five children, 29 years and partnered).

There were instances where participants who had limited or no social support found it difficult:

I am not from Darwin and don't really have family here. My mother is visiting and I know some people from the community where I come from. Bit lonely sometimes. (Aboriginal mother of seven children, 26 years and single).

For one participant however, a falling out with a family member led to this young mother of two to seek support elsewhere which was limited and resulted in food and money problems.
Four participants received support from family with household chores and looking after children:

We haven't relied on family to help us out with feeding us, only with looking after the baby and other household chores when my wife was sick. (Aboriginal father of one child, 38 years and partnered).

Most participants mentioned that living with immediate family members (parents or siblings) reduced the financial burden of expenses and assisted with raising of children. Almost one third of the participants lived with extended family and seemed to be in this arrangement for similar reasons. A participant shared her situation where she and her family had recently moved in with her parents:

We used to be in government housing, but now me and my partner earn too much and had to give up our house and find a private house to rent. But we can't afford to pay private rent. Too much and won't have much money left for food and other things we need. Me, my partner and the kids moved in with my mum and dad. That way we can save money to buy our own house. (Aboriginal mother of three children, 29 years and partnered).

A mother of one, recently separated from her partner spoke of having to move in with her family to cope with expenses:

My ex [partner] moved out about 2 months ago and it was hard paying the rent and bills, so [I] decided to move out to Palmerston and be with my family. Too expensive living in Darwin. [I] Don't know how other people like me can live there. (non-Indigenous mother of one child, 28 years and single).

3.5.2. We Don't Have It as Bad as other Families

Most participants experiencing food insecurity expressed that others were in a worse situation than their own:

We don't have it bad as some families. At least we always have something to eat, bills are paid and [have] petrol for the car". (Non-Indigenous mother of four children, 30 years and partnered).

"We are doing better than some other families. I know some have to ask for food vouchers [from Centrelink] to buy groceries. (Aboriginal and Torres Strait Islander mother of three children, 38 years and single).

It makes you feel a bit easier to know that your situation is bad, but that someone else is worse off to make yourself feel better or make light of your current situation. I don't know, but I think that it's across the board [whole population]. (Aboriginal father of one child, 38 years and partnered).

4. Discussion

This study examined issues relating to food insecurity within a cohort of urban-based care-givers of Aboriginal and Torres Strait Islander children and found common features that contributed to household food security issues and mechanisms of coping. The most striking finding was that participants did not initially identify with being food insecure, although many participants' experiences indicated otherwise. In general, participants accepted the situation of running out of money, food or both, and having to seek assistance from relatives as a normal experience. This finding has also been described in a study involving six Inuit communities of Nunavut, Canada which described an incongruence between perceived food security status and experiences in obtaining enough food to eat [7]. In contrast, another study undertaken within an Inuit population from Nunavut, found participants who reported food insecurity also reported regular use of community food programs to assist with alleviating hunger [2]. Unlike Chan et al.'s (2006) study, Ford et.al. (2012) recruited participants who were registered with food assistance programs and these participants may have shared characteristics with those considered by this study's participants as "worse off" [2,7].

A second finding was that for most, food insecurity was experienced occasionally and usually when larger bills were due for payment. Food insecurity for some however was a chronic problem and seemed to be often due to an inadequate or irregular income. Two Australian studies have found that the Commonwealth Government New Start Allowance does not provide an adequate income for families, or anyone, to meet healthy living standards [22,23]. The authors did raise whether introducing an independent mechanism, similar to that of the Minimum Wage Panel that assesses its adequacy, to review and set the New Start Allowance level [23]. Participants that reported to have enough money to meet their needs, tended to be in paid employment. Secure employment and stable housing have been shown in other studies to be strongly associated with food security [2,4,5]. In contrast seasonal employment [5,8], unemployment and underemployment (the underemployment classification includes those workers that are highly skilled but work in low paid jobs; workers that are highly skilled but work in low skill jobs and part-time workers that would prefer to be full-time. This is different from unemployment in that the individual is working but isn't working at their full capability. (Source: http://www.investopedia.com/terms/u/underemployment.asp)) [2–4,7,10,11] have been reported as problematic in ensuring a regular income to afford food and other expenses among those experiencing food insecurity. Noted in the findings, a small proportion of participants were income managed and shared mixed views of their experiences. These were, not having enough money to meet the family's groceries requirements; feeling anxious wondering if there was enough money on the card for food; and finally, that it stopped the 'humbugging' from others wanting a loan. A study undertaken by Brimblecombe et al. (2010) in ten remote communities of the Northern Territory where income management had been introduced, investigated the impact of income management on store sales [24]. Stores sale data were reviewed over a 35-month period and included 18-months of data prior to the introduction of income management. Focusing on fruit and vegetable sales and turnover, Brimblecombe et al. (2010) found income management did not have an effect on store sales over the study period [24]. However, the Government stimulus payment between November 2008 to January 2009 did have a positive effect on fruit and vegetable sales [24].

In our study, participants with and without employment, referred to the cost of living as contributing to their food insecurity experiences. In some instances, participants purposely lived with extended family to mitigate potential food insecurity with the rising cost of living, even though they reported to earn an adequate income. Chan et al. also found the cost of living and cash flow among the 'working poor' to negatively impact food security in Nunavut communities [7]. A study undertaken in a United States urban centre found the cost of home rental was the single biggest factor identified among a group of young mothers as contributing to food insecurity [4]. In the current study, not only were high rent and large bills contributing factors to the high cost of living and food insecurity experiences, but issues with housing maintenance and inadequate kitchen facilities were also associated with experiences of food insecurity.

The experience amongst this study population of "money tight" due to the payment of large bills and general cost of living has also been reported by other researchers investigating food security experiences and influencing factors [4,5,8]. Participants in these studies were either low income earners or recipients of welfare (government payments) and received support through government and non-government food and nutrition assistance programs. Food insecurity occurred when money 'ran out' before the next pay period and food and nutrition assistance was accessed at these times to alleviate food insecurity over the short term. This contrasts to the findings of this study, where participants did not report to access food assistance programs.

Whilst participants dealt with intermittent food insecurity through various coping strategies, they did not appear to seek assistance from relevant agencies to alleviate food insecurity. Instead, strategies participants put in place during the "money tight" times were to delay payment of bills or undertake part payment of larger bills through staggered payments, or to cut back "luxury foods", such as sweets, soft drinks and desserts. Similar coping strategies were reported by a study among a group of 90 food pantry users in Washington, USA, where coping strategies included putting off paying bills and using up leftover food, preparing food in bulk and freezing food for later use [11]. A study among Latino immigrant families in North Carolina, USA, also reported participants coped with times of food insecurity by reducing purchase of foods considered expensive, such as meats and fruits and unnecessary foods, such as 'soft drinks, snacks and eating out' [8].

The strategies employed to cope with "money tight" times in this study were seen to be both positive (such as limiting purchase of sweets and soft drinks) and negative (compromising quality for quantity) in respect to food behaviour and health. In other studies, shopping for specials, bulk-buying, cooking in bulk and freezing food portions are examples of other pragmatic responses [4,5,8,11] to food insecurity which were also employed by participants within this study. Negative responses to food insecurity, similar to that reported by this study, have also been reported by others including forgoing healthier food options and choosing cheaper less healthier foods, reducing meal size or going without to ensure children eat [4–6,8,11].

There is debate to whether the behavioural purchase of unhealthy foods in preference to healthy foods is driven by need, due to healthy food not being affordable [2,6,7,25] or by poor dietary habits, established food preferences and poor food purchasing knowledge [7,9]. Poor eating habits among high and low-income earners have been considered as being due to laziness [25] and time constraints [11,26]. In the current study, as similar to other studies, participants perceived healthier food to be more expensive to less healthy food and expressed frustrations at not always being able to afford healthier food options and bewilderment as to why unhealthier foods appeared cheaper. Other studies have reported the cost of healthy food options as a barrier to healthy eating and have commented that low income gave participants little option but to buy highly refined, energy dense foods that provide calories at less cost than low-calorie nutrient rich foods [4,7,15]. Similarly, a study undertaken within a low income urban Australian Aboriginal population, found participants understood what were healthy foods, but were not always able to afford these foods [13]. The same was reported for a study undertaken in an Aboriginal population in remote Australia where participants perceived healthy food to be unaffordable [17].

A fourth finding is participants' concerns for their children's needs often characterised their food behaviour responses to food insecurity. Hamelin and others (2002) also noted experiences of anxiety by some participants in ensuring enough food for the children and the accompanying feelings of despair [10]. Upon similar lines, within this study several participants expressed concerns for the acceptance and social inclusion of their children by peers and how this exacerbated the risk of food insecurity due to allocation of limited food money to non-food items or entertainment. Participants also spoke of the experiences of others' they knew, specifically with drug and alcohol use and how this impacted on families' food security situation. Temple's (2018) study looking at the association between stressful events and food insecurity in Australia, found between the food secure and food insecure respondents there was a prevalence greater than 10% that included among other stressors, drug or alcohol related problems [27].

Use of a private vehicle, as reported within the current study to access food outlets, enabled people to seek out food bargains and specials. Specifically, access to a private vehicle was advantageous in accessing larger supermarkets where food was often cheaper and of more variety. This was also noted by other studies where public transport (buses and taxis) were considered by participants as unreliable, inconvenient or expensive and therefore, found to negatively impact on food security [4,5,9,28,29].

Finally, unlike the variety of social support systems accessed by other populations experiencing food insecurity, including food assistance programs, food charity organisations, faith communities, neighbours and friends [2–11,26], this study is unique in that family support was the only resource reported to be accessed for assistance. Other studies have also identified the extended family as a social support system [2–4,8,9,11] and identified support from friends and neighbours as a main coping strategy in response to food insecurity [5]. Only one study however, mentioned living with family as a temporary measure [2]. Residing with family members, particularly parents, was mentioned within the current study as a way for families to cope with living expenses. For some, this arrangement also provided support with child care. However, we did not the food security of all family members and it is possible that other members have influence perceptions of food security e.g., food insecure members moving in with food secure persons may heighten the odds of the later experiencing food insecurity.

Central to the study participants' social support system, was the action of reciprocity where families coped through inter-reliance on each other for food, money and other necessities. For instance, participants reported that when they had food, they would provide for other extended family members. Then when they would 'run out', extended family assisted in return. Reciprocity was also mentioned in a study, where young mothers would rely on family members for assistance with food and then 'return the favour' when family members experienced difficulties [4].

Within this study, as with other literature, reciprocity forms a cultural practice of sharing among Aboriginal and Torres Strait Islander peoples that is important in maintaining and reinforcing cultural social bonds with individual and group relationships [14]. As noted by Chan et al. and Ford et al., reciprocity has a place in maintaining and reinforcing family and broader community relationship obligations as well as cultural identity and practice among Inuit [2,7]. Among the Inuit these sharing networks extended to hunted traditional foods where excess was provided to the more vulnerable members of the community who cannot obtain these foods [2,7]. For those who could not hunt, money or other services were exchanged for traditional foods to keep with continuing cultural practices [2,7]. This concept of sharing traditional foods in a reciprocated environment to help each other out is also evident in this study where food and monetary assistance was sought and provided within families.

Discussions with participants within our cohort identified reciprocation as an expectation, and a given cultural practice to maintain family relationships. Such sharing support structures however are also fragile and relationship upsets can result in limited or no support as experienced by one participant in this study. In contrast, a food insecurity study undertaken in an Aboriginal and Torres Strait Islander population living in Victoria, indicated that accessing family and friends for assistance was not reported by this population [13]. External programs providing assistance in the forms of food vouchers, as well as charity organisations providing meals and food parcels, are available within the study location. However, these services were not mentioned by participants as being accessed for assistance. This finding however should be interpreted with caution as participants may have chosen not to share this information and seeking knowledge about access to such services was not the purpose of our study.

Finally, unlike studies [4,5] indicating the importance of furthering education to gain employment or improve opportunities for higher paid work as a long-term solution to overcoming food insecurity, this was not found within our cohort. A possible reason is, as identified in this cohort being food insecure is normal i.e., 'normalisation of a pathology'. When problems with food security are encountered, reciprocated arrangements with family as a coping strategy provide an immediate solution and reinforce traditional Aboriginal and Torres Strait Islander relationships. Therefore, furthering education or skill development for employment as an option to alleviate food insecurity may not be considered by participants in our cohort. This is an important issue and further understanding of what constitute food security will be useful in the future.

5. Conclusions

We found that Aboriginal and Torres Strait Islander families in our cohort had varying direct experiences with household food insecurity. A major contributor to this is their limited financial resources in conjunction with rising living costs. For the majority, this was intermittent and occurred when the larger bills were due for payment. For some, however, food insecurity is a chronic problem where expenses outweighed income. Not having enough money to buy food and take care of living expenses is a universal experience for those on limited incomes. Similarly, for the participants in this study having a limited income impacted on their circumstances and other factors also impacted on food security, including transport and concern for social image.

We also found that the extended family was the major form of support for assistance and played possibly a broader cultural role in sharing as also identified among Inuit populations [2,7]. This was also a reciprocated arrangement where families would help each other out. However, it could also be considered fragile as support was very reliant on harmonious relationships between family members and may be considered only functional when relationships are.

5.1. Strengths and Limitations

Unlike other similar published research, a strength of this study is participant sampling in that recruitment was not undertaken through food assistance programs. This study therefore, provides a broader view of food security experiences from a perspective where people are either experiencing food insecurity or not. As previously referred to, this qualitative study is one part of a larger study. Although the sample size is small, initial discussions followed by in-depth interviews consolidated themes, as a point was reached during data collection where no new information was forthcoming and data saturation was reached. The majority of participants were however, from well-established families within the two study locations. Therefore, the findings are more applicable to families who are long term residents of Darwin and Palmerston with extended family networks. Caution is required in generalising findings to all families in the Darwin and Palmerston regions and other similar populations. There are also possibilities of bias with findings reflecting the views of one gender more so than the other. Future studies may need to consider recruitment and sampling strategies that address gender balance.

The interviews were undertaken by an Aboriginal Public Health Nutritionist which was positive in communicating and establishing a trusting relationship with participants of which was captured within the interviews. The study design and methodology could be considered for future qualitative research investigating unexplored topics to generate new knowledge in learning more about Aboriginal and Torres Strait Islander peoples' understandings and experiences of food security. Finally, this qualitative research has unveiled 'new' understandings of food insecurity experiences and coping strategies from an urban Aboriginal and Torres Strait Islander population perspective that otherwise, may have remained unknown to the broader community.

5.2. Implications

A possible solution to assist with meeting payment of expenses is support to families to set up direct debit options of smaller regular payments to offset larger bills and undue financial pressure.

Transport, preferably access to a private car, was also deemed essential by some to undertake food shopping. There could be possible scope for services and other assistance programs to consider these needs. For instance, food shopping assistance for older Australians and the disabled is provided through government and non-government services [28]. Major supermarket chains in Australia such as Coles and Woolworths provide an online shopping and delivery service for a fee. This may not be available by all stores and may not appeal to all consumers. However, it could be considered by government and non-government services to provide food shopping assistance, including a subsidised or free food shopping delivery service, for low income families with young children.

There is a widely held perception that the cost of healthy foods makes a healthy diet unaffordable for families. Participants of this study referred specifically to the cost of fresh fruit and vegetables and the importance of these in prevention of chronic disease, such as type 2 diabetes. Consideration of economic access to healthy foods in public policy seems critical for improved health outcomes. A potential solution may involve food subsidies or similar. There are also opportunities for local councils to consider availability of public allotments to encourage community or family group food gardening to supplement diets though, this was not an option identified by study participants. The perception of fresh fruit and vegetables being costly is worth further research investigation, particularly in assessing the affordability of healthy foods within the study location.

In ensuring appropriate and sustainable safety nets that provide assistance to families, it is important to acknowledge the existence of support services accessed by families that are not recognised within the mainstream and are specific to Indigenous Australians. These include positive family associations. Potential scope for current services is to consider an approach in connecting with family networks for provision of support services, such as financial counselling. Such services have potential to provide peer support family counselling where members experiencing difficulties are supported by family member(s) to engage with services and work through issues.

This study has clearly identified food insecurity experiences among the study population to be related to monetary expenditure outweighing income, particularly with the payment of larger bills. Being in a situation where money is limited and expenses out way available funds, fulfilling a family's social, cultural and physical needs requires a fragile balance of continually adjusting food access and purchasing behavior at time when 'money is tight', maintaining family support structures, and upholding social status.

Author Contributions: L.M., J.B. and A.B.C. jointly conceptualized the study, prepared, reviewed, edited and authored the manuscript. L.M. conducted data collection and analysis under the supervision of J.B. and A.B.C., J.B. finalised data analysis and consolidated findings. For research articles with several authors, a short paragraph specifying their individual contributions must be provided.

Acknowledgments: The authors acknowledge the participants, Aboriginal and Torres Strait Islander families of Darwin and Palmerston, NT; Bagot Community Health Clinic, Darwin NT; Danila Dilba Health Service child health clinic, Palmerston NT; Northern Territory Department of Health child health clinics Darwin and Palmerston; Sian Graham, Aboriginal Research Officer, Menzies School of Health Research, Darwin NT; Helen Fejo-Frith, Aboriginal Research Assistant, Bagot Community; Bagot Community Council; and Associate Jan Ritchie, School of Public Health and Community Medicine, University of New South Wales for reviewing the qualitative chapter of LM's Ph.D. thesis.

Appendix A

Table A1. Inductive development processes towards key guiding questions for the in-depth qualitative interview.

Theme	Notes	Guiding Questions
Influencing factors		
Income quarantining (Basic Card)	Limited control over own money. Anxious when going shopping, as don't know how much money available on basic card for spending. Feelings of shame/embarrassment/anger when: - can't pay for it (not enough money on card) and don't have extra cash. - On the scheme and have no say in being on it or not.	Tell me more about your experiences with the Basic Card. Why do you like/dislike being Income managed? How does this make you feel?
Housing problems (more around maintenance)	House needs fixing, takes a long time before something is done, participant has little control over the situation. Limited availability of public housing, hard to find a place to live. Sense of feeling powerless, beyond people's control	Tell me about your house. Is everything good? i.e., windows, benches, etc.? Does anything need to be fixed?
Food preparation and cooking facilities	Food storage, preparation and cooking facilities: - Need for working stove - Need for a freezer	Do you like to cook? Can you tell me about your experiences with cooking (good/ok). What stops you from cooking?
Money problems	About not having enough money to fulfil own and families' needs/wants/requirements. Impact of the cost of living in Darwin and Palmerston—everything is expensive. Limited money, prioritise what spending on Always make sure the children are fed, don't go without.	Do you have enough money for what you need? If no money problems/worries, what do you do to make sure everything is good? Can you tell me about your money problems/worries? How often do you have money problems/worries? Are money problems ongoing (all the time)? When you have money problems, how do you prioritise spending? Are there things that do you do to cope with the problem?
Social Inclusion	Not wanting money problems to impact on children's lives to point where excluded from social events, outings, what their peers have, etc.	Is it important to you and your kids that you don't miss out on what other families have? What are some of the things you do to make sure you and your kids don't miss out on having what others have?
Budgeting	Always make sure money for food, even if not healthy. An already tight budget for food and regular expenses. Additional expenses puts a strain on the budget therefore, spend less on food and tend to eat less healthy.	How do you make sure there is enough money for things you/your family need between paydays? Does this always work, or do you sometimes find it hard? What else do you do to try and make it work?

Table A1. *Cont.*

Theme	Notes	Guiding Questions
Influencing factors		
Filler Foods	Low cost, high calorie foods to stretch meals and 'fill you up'—bread and rice. E.g of filler foods for a meal—cheap tinned meats (hamper) and rice with bread.	Do you have enough food at each meal for everybody? What do you do to make sure everyone has enough food? Tell me about these foods (filler foods) and the reasons you choose them? - Cheaper, feed more people (stretch meals) and fill you up. - Comfort, familiar food
Wellbeing	2 participants talked about feeling sad. As mentioned previously, feelings of shame, embarrassment, anger, anxiety, powerless.	*If possible, find out more if these feelings are related to money worries/problems.* How do you feel when you don't have enough money? Do you think about having enough money a lot?
Other's worse off	Acknowledge other families experiences similar problems and probably more worse off. However, also put this down to possible use of drug and alcohol and this is where money is diverted to.	From what you know, do you think your family 'has it hard' compared to other families?
Transport	Few transport issues to go places to shop, particularly when relying on public transport and travelling with small children	What are your experiences with having regular transport to go shopping?
Social problems	Identify money (income) diverted to social problems such as drug, alcohol and gambling impact on having enough food.	What are your thoughts on why some families may experience problems with having enough food?
Food Shopping	Transport and the amount of shopping undertaken impacts on where people shop. Others that 'plan' where they shop according to where bargains are—buy bulk.	Do you worry about going food shopping (regularly)? Do you plan where you will shop and what you will buy before you go? Are you able to go to the shops when you want to?
Coping Strategy		
Support Networks	Families rely on extended family and friends' networks for support and 'fill the gaps'	Tell me more about the support you have when you are having difficulties? Do you think you rely on this support network? Where would you go if you didn't have this support network?

References

1. American Dietetic Association. Position of The American Dietetic Association: Domestic food and nutrition security. *J. Am. Diet. Assoc.* **1998**, 337–342. [CrossRef]
2. Ford, J.; Lardeau, M.P.; Vanderbilt, W. The characteristics and experience of community food program users in arctic Canada: A case study from Iqaluit, Nunavut. *BMC Public Health* **2012**, *12*, 464. [CrossRef] [PubMed]
3. Sim, M.S.; Glanville, T.N.; McIntyre, L. Food management behaviours in food insecure, lone mother-led families. *Can. J. Diet. Pract. Res.* **2011**, *72*, 123–129. [CrossRef] [PubMed]
4. Stevens, C.A. Exploring food insecurity among young mothers (15–24 Years). *J. Spec. Pediatr. Nurs.* **2010**, *15*, 163. [CrossRef] [PubMed]
5. De Marco, M.; Thorburn, S.; Kue, J. "In a country as affluent as America, people should be eating": Experiences with and perceptions of food insecurity among rural and urban oregonians. *Qual. Health Res.* **2009**, *19*, 1010–1024. [CrossRef] [PubMed]
6. Hamelin, A.M.; Mercier, C.; Bedard, A. Perception of needs and responses in food security: Divergence between households and stakeholders. *Public Health Nutr.* **2008**, *11*, 1389–1396. [CrossRef] [PubMed]
7. Chan, H.M.; Fediuk, K.; Hamilton, S.; Rostas, L.; Caughey, A.; Kuhnlein, H.; Egeland, G.; Loring, E. Food security in Nunavut, Canada: Barriers and recommendations. *Int. J. Circumpolar Health* **2006**, *65*, 416–431. [CrossRef] [PubMed]
8. Quandt, S.A.; Shoaf, J.I.; Tapia, J.; Hernandez-Pelletier, M.; Clark, H.M.; Arcury, T.A. Experiences of Latino immigrant families in North Carolina help explain elevated levels of food insecurity and hunger. *J. Nutr.* **2006**, *136*, 2638–2644. [CrossRef] [PubMed]
9. Kempson, K.; Palmer Keenan, D.; Sadani, P.S.; Adler, A. Maintaining food sufficiency: Coping strategies identified by limited-resource individuals versus nutrition educators. *J. Nutr. Educ. Behav.* **2003**, *35*, 179–188. [CrossRef]
10. Hamelin, A.M.; Beaudy, M.; Habicht, J.P. Characterisation of household food insecurity in Quebec: Food and feelings. *Soc. Sci. Med.* **2002**, *54*, 119–132. [CrossRef]
11. Hoisington, A.; Armstong Shultz, J.; Butkus, S. Coping strategies and nutrition education needs among food pantry users. *J. Nutr. Educ. Behav.* **2002**, *34*, 326–333. [CrossRef]
12. Temple, J.B.; Russell, J. Food insecurity among older Aboriginal and Torres Strait islanders. *Int. J. Environ. Res. Public Health.* **2018**, *15*, 1766. [CrossRef] [PubMed]
13. Adams, K.; Burns, C.; Liebzeit, A.; Ryschka, J.; Thorpe, S.; Browne, J. Use of participatory research and photo-voice to support urban Aboriginal healthy eating. *Health Soc. Care Community* **2012**, *20*, 497–505. [CrossRef] [PubMed]
14. Markwick, A.; Ansari, Z.; Sullivan, M.; McNeil, J. Social determinants and lifestyle risk factors only partially explain the higher prevalence of food insecurity among Aboriginal and Torres Strait islanders in the Australian state of Victoria: A cross-sectional study. *BMC Pubic Health* **2014**, *14*, 598. [CrossRef] [PubMed]
15. Nolan, M.; Rikard-Bell, G.; Mohsin, M.; Williams, M. Food insecurity in three socially disadvantaged localities in Sydney, Australia. *Health Promot. J. Austr.* **2006**, *17*, 247–254. [CrossRef] [PubMed]
16. Broome, R. *Aboriginal Australians: Black Responses to White Dominance 1788–1994*, 2nd ed.; Allen and Unwin: Sydney, Australia, 1994; pp. 9–21. ISBN 186373760X.
17. Brimblecombe, J. Enough for Rations and a Little Bit Extra: Challenges of Nutrition Improvements in an Aboriginal Community in North–East Arnhem Land. Ph.D. Thesis, Charles Darwin University, Darwin, Australia, 2007.
18. Braun, V.; Clarke, V. Using thematic analysis in psychology. *Qual. Res. Psychol.* **2006**, *3*, 77–101. [CrossRef]
19. Australian Bureau of Statistics. *2006 Census of Population and Housing Quickstats: Australia*; Australian Bureau of Statistics: Canberra, Australia, 2007.
20. Tuckett, A.G. Applying thematic analysis theory to practice: A researcher's experience. *Contemp. Nurse* **2005**, *19*, 75–87. [CrossRef] [PubMed]
21. Attride-Stirling, J. Thematic networks: An analytic tool for qualitative research. *Qual. Res.* **2001**, *1*, 385–401. [CrossRef]
22. Saunders, P.; Bedford, M. New minimum healthy living budget standards for low-paid and unemployed Australians. *Econ. Labour. Relat. Rev.* **2018**, *29*, 273–288. [CrossRef]

23. Saunders, P. Using a budget standards approach to assess the adequacy of newstart allowance. *Aust. J. Soc. Issues* **2018**, *53*, 4–17. [CrossRef]

24. Brimblecombe, J.K.; McDonnel, J.; Barnes, A.; Dhurrkay, J.G.; Thomas, D.P.; Bailie, R.S. Impact of income management on store sales in the Northern Territory. *MJA* **2010**, *192*, 549–554. [CrossRef] [PubMed]

25. Eikenberry, N.; Smith, C. Healthful eating: Perceptions, motivations, barriers, and promoters in low-income Minnesota communities. *J. Am. Diet. Assoc.* **2004**, *104*, 1158–1161. [CrossRef] [PubMed]

26. Inglis, V.; Ball, B.; Crawford, D. Why do women of low socioeconomic status have poorer dietary behaviours than women of higher socioeconomic status? A qualitative exploration. *Appetite* **2005**, *45*, 334–343. [CrossRef] [PubMed]

27. Temple, J.B. The association between stressful events and food insecurity: Cross-sectional evidence from Australia. *Int. J. Environ. Res. Public Health* **2018**, *15*, 2333. [CrossRef] [PubMed]

28. Coveney, J.; O'Dwyer, L.A. Effects of mobility and location on food access. *Health Place* **2009**, *15*, 45–55. [CrossRef] [PubMed]

29. Martin, K.S.; Rogers, B.L.; Cook, J.T.; Joseph, H.M. Social Capital is associated with decreased risk of hunger. *Soc. Sci. Med.* **2004**, *58*, 2645–2654. [CrossRef] [PubMed]

5

Food Insecurity among Older Aboriginal and Torres Strait Islanders

Jeromey B. Temple [1],* [ID] and Joanna Russell [2]

[1] Demography and Ageing Unit, Melbourne School of Population and Global Health, University of Melbourne, Melbourne 3010, Australia

[2] School of Health and Society, University of Wollongong, Wollongong 2522, Australia; jrussell@uow.edu.au

* Correspondence: Jeromey.Temple@unimelb.edu.au

Abstract: It is well established that Indigenous populations are at a heightened risk of food insecurity. Yet, although populations (both Indigenous and non-Indigenous) are ageing, little is understood about the levels of food insecurity experienced by older Indigenous peoples. Using Australian data, this study examined the prevalence and correlates of food insecurity among older Aboriginal and Torres Strait Islanders. Using nationally representative data, we employed ordinal logistic regression models to investigate the association between socio-demographic characteristics and food insecurity. We found that 21% of the older Aboriginal and Torres Strait Islander population were food insecure, with 40% of this group exposed to food insecurity with food depletion and inadequate intake. This places this population at a 5 to 7-fold risk of experiencing food insecurity relative to their older non-Indigenous peers. Measures of geography, language and low socio-economic status were highly associated with exposure to food insecurity. Addressing food insecurity offers one pathway to reduce the disparity in health outcomes between Aboriginal and Torres Strait Islanders and non-Indigenous Australians. Policies that consider both remote and non-remote Australia, as well as those that involve Aboriginal people in their design and implementation are needed to reduce food insecurity.

Keywords: food insecurity; food security; Indigenous population; ageing; Indigenous

1. Introduction

Like many Indigenous populations, the Aboriginal and Torres Strait Islander population in Australia has considerably poorer health outcomes when compared to their non-Indigenous peers, experiencing a range of health conditions at an earlier age of onset and considerably lower life expectancy [1–4]. The health issues facing many older people is an issue of increasing importance given persisting inequalities in socio-economic outcomes, as well as the ageing of this population [5]. In the 10 years to 2026, the population of Aboriginal and Torres Strait Islanders aged 45 and over is projected to increase by 35%, accounting for 22% of this population [6].

Importantly, many of the health conditions prevalent among older Aboriginal and Torres Strait Islanders are preventable, notwithstanding the levels of socio-economic disadvantage faced by this population. The Australian Institute of Health and Welfare (2016) estimates that the burden of disease in the Aboriginal population is 2.3 times of that experienced by non-Indigenous Australians [2]. Through reducing exposure to modifiable risk factors, such as tobacco and alcohol use and poor dietary behaviors, they estimate that about half of the difference in disease burden between Aboriginal and non-Indigenous Australians could be removed. In total, poor dietary behaviors were estimated to account for 10% of the total burden of disease faced by Aboriginal and Torres Strait Islanders.

An important proximate determinant and risk factor of poor nutrition outcomes is food insecurity. Food insecurity refers to the "limited or uncertain availability of nutritionally adequate and safe foods or limited or uncertain ability to acquire acceptable foods in socially acceptable ways" [7]. A growing number of studies have shown that Indigenous populations around the world are at a heightened risk of food insecurity [8–12]. For example, Canadian research has shown that Aboriginal people living on reservations were at 2.6 times the risk of being food insecure when compared to their non-Indigenous peers [8]. Research from the USA shows that levels of food insecurity experienced by American Indians are double that reported by non-Indigenous people [9]. Within the American population, food insecurity rates among the Navajo Nation were the highest reported within the USA to date, with just under 80% of this population experiencing some form of food insecurity [10]. Evidence from Australia shows that about 22% of Aboriginal and Torres Strait Islanders were exposed to food insecurity compared with 4% of non-Indigenous Australians [13].

Despite evidence of heightened risk of food insecurity within Indigenous populations, little is known about the prevalence and correlates of food insecurity in the older Aboriginal and Torres Strait Islander population. However, studies have examined food insecurity among the older non-Indigenous population, concluding the strength of socio-economic factors in explaining food insecurity in later life [14–16]. The aim of this study is to address this research gap through an examination of food insecurity among older Aboriginal and Torres Strait Islanders. Firstly, we assess the prevalence of food insecurity in Aboriginal and Torres Strait Islander older adults and secondly, we examine the risk factors for food insecurity in this population. We conclude with a discussion of the implications of our findings.

2. Materials and Methods

2.1. Survey Data

Data for this study are from the 2012–2013 Australian Aboriginal and Torres Strait Islander Nutrition and Physical Activity Survey (NATSINPAS) conducted by the Australian Bureau of Statistics (ABS) from August 2012 to July 2013 [17]. The survey is based on a sample of 2900 private dwellings across Australia, with a response rate of 79% (3661 households were approached). Within each dwelling, one adult (aged 18 and over) and one child (where applicable) were randomly selected for interview. The survey excluded those living in non-private dwellings such as hospitals, nursing homes and hotels. The survey also excluded all non-Indigenous persons including non-Indigenous born Australians, non-Australian diplomats, and overseas visitors.

An important advantage of the NATSINPAS is the geographic coverage of the survey, including remote and non-remote areas as well as discrete Aboriginal and Torres Strait Islander communities. Remote areas include very remote Australia and remote Australia under the Australian Statistical Geography Standard [18]. Non-remote areas include those residing in major cities, inner or outer regional Australia. The final sample included data on 1792 individuals living in non-remote areas and 2317 individuals in remote areas in Australia. ABS interviewers conducted face to face interviews, collecting information on health, nutrition and characteristics of the household and dwelling.

NATSINPAS was part of the larger Australian Aboriginal and Torres Strait Islander Health Survey (AATSIHS). The sampling design of NATSINPAS sought to provide reliable estimates at the national level, as well as for remote and non-remote Australia. The in-scope population was divided into two broad populations. The first group included those living in discrete Aboriginal and Torres Strait Islander communities in remote Australia, defined as the 'community frame'. The second group included the remainder of the in-scope population, referred to as the 'non-community frame'. The Indigenous Community Frame (ICF) was used to target respondents for the community frame, and was built from a combination of Census data as well as data from the Discrete Indigenous Communities Database. The non-community frame was formed using Census data at a low geographic level (SA1). For some States and Territories, the non-community sample was disaggregated into non-remote and remote non-community areas. Survey weights at the person level were calculated by the ABS to calibrate the probability of selection into the survey relative to estimated resident population counts (less those in non-private dwellings).

Data from NATSINPAS were collected under the Census and Statistics Act 1905. As NATSINPAS included a biomedical component, ethics approvals were sought at both the national level (by the Australian Government Department of Health and Ageing) and at the state and Territory level (by a range of medical and Aboriginal ethics committees). Data for this study were made available by the ABS through the Universities of Australia agreement. NATSINPAS survey data are available to registered users of ABS microdata.

2.2. Measurement

In this study, we consider the prevalence and risk factors for food insecurity among older Aboriginal and Torres Strait Islanders aged 45 years and over ($n = 1062$). Defining the sample aged 45 years and over as 'older' is common in studies of ageing among Aboriginal and Torres Strait Islander people for several reasons [4,19,20]. Firstly, there is a considerable gap in life expectancy of about one decade between Aboriginal and non-Indigenous Australians, reducing the proportion of the population living into advanced old age [3,21]. Second, many conditions and comorbidities as well as frailties commonly associated with aging are early onset in this population [2,3,22]. Third, in recognition of the above two points, government programs such as those governing access to specific aged care services are available to Aboriginal and Torres Strait Islanders from earlier ages when compared to non-Indigenous Australians.

The measurement of food insecurity in NATSINPAS consists of two questions. The household spokesperson (adult aged 18 or over) was asked, "In the last 12 months was there any time when you (or members of this household) ran out of food and couldn't afford to buy more?" A follow up question was asked, "When this happened, did you (or members of this household) go without food?" Following other Australian studies, we use these two questions to create a variable which views food insecurity on a continuum [23]. Those answering 'no' to the first question are coded as 'food secure'. Those who answer 'yes' to the first question, but 'no' to the second are coded as 'food insecure—food depletion'. That is, they ran out of money for food, but did not go without food. The final group, 'food insecure—food depletion and inadequate intake' are those who ran out of money for food and went without food consequently. Although there are a number of limitations to this measure (as discussed in Section 4.4), this is the most detailed measure of financially attributable food insecurity that is collected by the ABS on an irregular basis.

2.3. Statistical Model

To model the association between socio-economic characteristics and food insecurity, we utilized Stata 14.0. As the dependent variable is ordinal, standard logistic regression is inappropriate. We utilized ordered logistic regression fitted by maximum likelihood [24]. Initial variable selection was informed by the growing literature on food insecurity among older Australians [14–16]. Variables entered the regression model and improvement to model fit assessed using the Bayesian Information Criteria following Raftery's (1995) procedure [25]. With the full model specified, we check the conditioning of the matrix of independent variables to investigate any collinearity influence [26]. The condition numbers were very small providing support for the model specification. An important assumption underlying ordinal logistic regression is the parallel lines or proportional odds assumption. This assumption states that the coefficients of variables associated with the probability of food security versus food insecurity with depletion and food security versus depletion and inadequate intake are constant. We follow Brant's (1990) procedure and the non-significant test result provides strong support for modeling the severity of food insecurity within an ordinal framework [27].

Independent Variables

Informed by the literature on food insecurity in Australia and using model selection techniques outlined above, variations in food insecurity were identified by a range of socio-economic characteristics. The final variables included in the model were:

- Age: Measured in aggregate categories (45–54, 55–64, 65–74, 75+)
- Marital Status: Married or not married. Unfortunately, more detailed items such as widowed, never married or separated were unavailable on the data set.
- Gender: Male or Female.
- Household Size: Categorized as 1, 2, 3 or 4, 5 or more.
- Household Composition: Whether the household includes Aboriginal and Torres Strait Islander members only, or with non-Indigenous members also present.
- Indigenous Language Speaking: Whether the persons speaks an Australian Indigenous language.
- Remoteness: Whether the household resides in remote or non-remote parts of Australia, as defined by the Australian Statistical Geography Standard (ASGS).
- Household Income: The measure of household income provided by the ABS was equivalized household income (adjusted or equivalized using an equivalence scale) and collapsed into deciles. This adjusted form of household income allows for welfare and financial wellbeing comparisons between households of different sizes and compositions.
- Self-Reported Health: A dichotomous variable indicating whether the person self-reported their health as being excellent or good versus fair or poor.

3. Results

3.1. Prevalence of Food Insecurity

Table 1 displays the weighted estimates of the severity of food insecurity among Aboriginal and Torres Strait Islanders aged 45 and over. In 2012–2013, approximately 21% of this population reported being food insecure. Of this group of food insecure persons, about 41% reported both food depletion and inadequate intake, that is, they ran out of money and went without food consequently. This group accounted for about 8% of the Aboriginal and Torres Strait Islander population aged 45 years and over.

There is considerable socio-economic and demographic variation in exposure to food insecurity among older people (Table 1). Important to this analysis of food insecurity among older Aboriginal and Torres Strait Islanders is Indigenous language speaking, living in a remote area, and Indigenous household composition. Interestingly, we observe differences in exposure to food insecurity by discrete categories of English language speaking and geography. In this sample, almost all respondents in non-remote areas speak English in the household. Approximately 19% of this group were food insecure, as were those who spoke English in remote areas of Australia. However, for those who speak Indigenous languages residing in remote areas, the prevalence of food insecurity was almost double (about 37%). Indeed, 12% of Indigenous language speakers in remote areas were severely food insecure (or one third of all food insecure people).

Similarly, strong differences in food insecurity by Aboriginal household composition are observed. Those living in a household with both Aboriginal and non-Indigenous members have a food insecurity prevalence of about 7%, compared with 28% of those in Aboriginal only households. Overall, we identify several population sub-groups with a food insecurity prevalence rate of around 30%: Indigenous speakers in remote communities (37%), Aboriginal and Torres Strait Islander only households (28%), smokers (31%), persons in households with a large number of occupants (32%), non-married females (35%), and income earners in the lowest centile (31%).

Although these descriptive results indicate significant differences in exposure to food insecurity by socio-economic characteristics, it is important to control for confounding effects to measure the association between each covariate and the probability of food insecurity.

Table 1. Food Insecurity (%) by Socio-Economic Characteristics, 2012–2013.

	Food Secure	Insecure: Depletion	Insecure: Depletion & Intake	Food Insecure[1]	Unweighted n=
Age					
45–54	76.3 -	14.2 -	9.5 -	23.7	435
55–64	82.6	9.8	7.6	17.4	356
65–74	80.6	11.0	8.4	19.4	200
75+	89.7	8.7	1.6	10.3	71
Self-Reported Health					
Excellent or Good	81.4 -	9.9 -	8.7 -	18.6	667
Fair or Poor	76.1 *	16 *	7.9 *	23.9	395
Language & Remoteness					
Non-remote	81.3 -	10.6 -	8.1 -	18.7	451
Remote-English	80.9	11.6	7.4	19.0	374
Remote-Indigenous[2]	62.7 ***	25.1 ***	12.2 ***	37.3	236
Household Income[3]					
Lowest 20%	69.1 -	16.7 -	14.3 -	31.0	472
20–40%	86.9 **	7.9 **	5.2 *	13.1	215
40–60%	90.5 ***	5.0 ***	4.5 *	9.5	109
60–80%	84.1 ***	7.1 ***	8.8 ***	15.9	77
80–100%	94.7 ***	5.3 ***	0.0 ***	5.3	57
Unknown	77.1	18.9	3.9	22.8	132
Household Composition					
Aboriginal only	72.1 -	15.6 -	11.9 -	27.5	779
Aboriginal and Non[4]	92.6 ***	5.4 ***	2.0 ***	7.4	283
Smoker Status					
Yes	68.8 -	16.1 -	15.1 -	31.2	420
No	86.9 ***	9.4 *	3.7 **	13.1	642
Household Size					
1	75.1 -	14.6 -	10.3 -	24.9	422
2	88.3 **	7.5 *	4.2 *	11.7	413
3–4	72.8	14.1	13.2	27.3	176
5+	68.1 *	24.0 *	7.9	31.9	51
Marital Status					
Female, Unmarried	65.4 -	17.7 -	16.9 -	34.6	393
Female, Married	90.5 ***	5.7 ***	3.7 **	9.4	225
Male, Unmarried	79.3 *	13.6 *	7.0 *	20.6	247
Male, Married	87.3 ***	9.7 ***	9.7 ***	19.4	197

Table 1. *Cont.*

	Food Secure		Insecure: Depletion	Insecure: Depletion & Intake		Food Insecure [1]	Unweighted n =
Non-school Qual [5]							
Yes	79.2	-	11.4	9.4	-	20.8	370
No	79.6	*	12.7	7.7		20.4	692
Weighted 45+ (%)	79.5		12.2	8.4		20.6	
Unweighted 45+ (%)	78.2		13.5	8.3		21.8	
Unweighted (n)	831		143	88		231	1062

[1] Includes respondents indicating food insecurity with food depletion and those indicating food insecurity with food depletion and inadequate intake; [2] Indigenous language; [3] Equivalized household income (to allow for welfare comparisons across households of different sizes) placed into quintiles; [4] Non-Indigenous household members present; [5] Has received post-school education or training; *** $p < 0.001$, ** $p < 0.01$, * $p < 0.05$; - omitted category for tests of proportions. Weighted estimates.

3.2. Regression Results

With a range of demographic and economic controls, English speaking and remoteness remain strong predictors of food insecurity (Table 2). Those speaking Indigenous languages were about 57% more likely to experience food insecurity compared with those in non-remote areas (OR 1.57 95% CI: 1.01–2.44). Again, there was no difference in food insecurity between English speakers in remote and non-remote areas (OR = 0.99 $p < 0.10$). In a similarly sized effect, households with both Aboriginal and non-Indigenous residents were about 60% less likely to experience food insecurity compared with Aboriginal only households, even with controls for geography (OR 0.4 95% CI: 0.22, 0.69).

Table 2. Ordered Logistic Regression Model of Food Insecurity, 2012–2013.

Covariate	Odds Ratio (OR)	95% CI [1]	
Age			
45–54	1.00		
55–64	0.81	0.56, 1.16	
65–74	0.61	0.39, 0.96	*
75+	0.46	0.23, 0.91	*
Marital Status			
Female, Unmarried	1.00		
Female, Married	0.52	0.30, 0.89	*
Male, Unmarried	0.73	0.49, 1.08	
Male, Married	0.62	0.36, 1.05	+
Labor Force Status			
Employed	1.00		
Unemployed	1.58	1.05, 2.36	*
Smoker Status			
Yes	1.00		
No	0.61	0.44, 0.84	***
Self-Reported Health			
Excellent or Good	1.00		
Fair or Poor	1.53	1.10, 2.11	*
Household Income [2]			
Lowest 20%	1.00		
20–40%	0.69	0.45, 1.06	+
40–60%	0.62	0.32, 1.19	
60–80%	0.24	0.08, 0.71	**
80–100%	0.12	0.02, 0.95	*
Unknown	0.89	0.56, 1.42	
Language & Remoteness			
Non-Remote	1.00		
Remote-English	0.99	0.68, 1.47	
Remote-Indigenous [3]	1.57	1.01, 2.44	*
Household Composition			
Aboriginal only	1.00		
Aboriginal and Non [4]	0.40	0.22, 0.69	***
Household Size			
1	1.00		
2	1.27	0.80, 2.01	
3–4	1.95	1.17, 3.25	**
5+	2.64	1.28, 5.46	**

[1] 95% Confidence Interval for the Odds Ratio; [2] Equivalized household income (to allow for welfare comparisons across households of different sizes) placed into quintiles; [3] Indigenous language; [4] Non-Indigenous household members present; *** $p < 0.001$, ** $p < 0.01$, * $p < 0.05$, + $p < 0.1$.

Non-smokers remained 39% less likely to experience food insecurity (OR 0.61 95% CI: 0.44, 0.84) and persons in large households were at a high risk, particularly those in household with 5 or more occupants (OR 2.64 95% CI: 1.28, 5.46). Those in the top 20% of the income distribution were about

88% less likely (OR 0.12 95% CI: 0.02, 0.95) to suffer food insecurity and those in the 60–80 percentile were about 76% less likely (OR 0.24 95% CI: 0.08, 0.71) when compared to lowest income earners.

Gender and social marital status also remains significant in the regression models. Compared to unmarried females, married females were about 48% less likely to experience food insecurity (OR 0.52 95% CI: 0.30, 0.89). Married males were 38% less likely to experience food insecurity relative to non-married females, but the estimate is only significant at the 90% level.

4. Discussion

Although several Australian studies have examined food insecurity in the older population, little is known about the prevalence and risk factors of food insecurity among older Aboriginal and Torres Strait Islanders specifically. In this paper, we have used nationally representative survey data to measure the prevalence and correlates of food insecurity among Aboriginal and Torres Strait Islanders aged 45 and over.

4.1. High Prevalence of Food Insecurity among Older Aboriginal and Torres Strait Islanders

Firstly, we find the prevalence of food insecurity among older Aboriginal and Torres Strait Islanders is high with about 21% reporting exposure, and 41% of this group reporting food depletion and inadequate intake. These estimates are in line with published results from the ABS showing that about 22% of Aboriginal and Torres Strait Islanders experience food insecurity compared to 4% of non-Indigenous Australians (ABS, 2015). The prevalence of food insecurity among older non-Indigenous Australians using a similar measure has previously been reported at 3% [14,28]. That is, older Aboriginal and Torres Strait Islanders are at about a 5–7 fold risk of food insecurity relative to their non-Indigenous peers.

This finding is important for several reasons. There is now a significant body of evidence on the implications of food insecurity for individual health and wellbeing. International studies show exposure to food insecurity is associated with symptoms of depression and anxiety, multimorbidity, lower levels of self-reported health status, lower nutrient diets, a greater likelihood of reporting social isolation, long standing health problems and activity limitations, and a greater likelihood of reporting heart disease, diabetes, and high blood pressure [29–37]. Among non-Indigenous Australians, food insecurity has also been shown to be associated with self-reported depression, reduced quality of life and poor diet quality [14,23,38]. More broadly, food insecurity may be related to decreased productivity and social interaction and contribute to increased economic inequality [39].

The high prevalence of food insecurity among older Aboriginal and Torres Strait Islanders is also important in the context of the gap in health outcomes that persists between Aboriginal and non-Indigenous Australians. 'Closing the Gap' is an Australian Government strategy whereby a key goal is to improve the health outcomes of Aboriginal and Torres Strait Islander populations. Specifically, the strategy seeks to reduce mortality by 2030 to levels experienced by the non-Indigenous population [40]. Addressing food insecurity among Aboriginal and Torres Strait Islanders by providing appropriate access to safe and nutritious foods has the potential to improve dietary behaviors that ultimately would contribute to increased life expectancy.

The 'Closing the Gap' strategy recognizes that the likelihood of co-morbidities is higher in the Aboriginal population when compared to the non-Indigenous population [41]. For example, about 38% of Aboriginal adults with either cardiovascular disease (CVD), diabetes or chronic kidney disease (CKD) had two or more health conditions compared to 26% of non-Indigenous people [2,41]. Coronary heart disease and diabetes are major contributors to the disease burden in Indigenous populations aged 45 years and over [2]. Poor dietary habits are known risk factors for poor health outcomes, with poor dietary habits contributing 50.1% towards the burden of CVD in Aboriginal populations [2,41]. Improving access to food is one factor that could affect the ability to choose a nutritious diet and improve dietary behaviors thereby improving health outcomes in Aboriginal and Torres Strait Islander population.

4.2. Socio-Economic Characteristics Are Strongly Associated with Food Insecurity

The prevalence of food insecurity is not evenly spread throughout the population and we find socio-economic factors are strongly associated with food insecurity and that specific demographic groups report higher rates of food insecurity. In the model of food insecurity formulated here, socio-economic factors are viewed as moderating food insecurity through the degree of resource-constrained access to the food supply.

Specifically, we identify a number of population sub-groups with a food insecurity prevalence rate of around 1 in 3: Indigenous speakers in remote communities (37%), Aboriginal and Torres Strait Islander only households (28%), smokers (31%), persons in households with a large number of occupants (32%), non-married females (35%) and income earners in the lowest centile (31%).

Differences in food insecurity status by socio-economic factors is consistent with studies in community dwelling non-Indigenous older Australians showing food insecurity differs by a range of socio-demographic risk factors, such as income, marital status, and smoker status [14–16]. The strength of socio-economic factors in explaining heightened food insecurity among Indigenous populations has also been noted elsewhere. For example, Pardilla et al. (2013), in their study of the Navajo Nation, note "Low socio-economic status, which is highly prevalent on the Navajo Nation and which we found to be significantly associated with food insecurity, must be considered in future endeavors to improve food security and decrease the risk of chronic disease" ([10] p. 64).

The strength of socio-economic factors as risk factors in experiencing food insecurity is concerning given the continued economic deprivation experienced by many Aboriginal and Torres Strait Islanders. For example, considerable disparities in socio-economic outcomes persist between non-Indigenous and Aboriginal persons across all age groups through lower levels of education, employment and living in areas with greater socio-economic disadvantage, while also being at considerable risk of experiencing interpersonal racism [5,42]. Not only do socio-economic factors provide greater access to the food supply (e.g., due to greater resources with which to purchase food), but these resources may also enable families to better cope with unexpected shocks (e.g., unexpected unemployment or disability) that could be a precursor to food insecurity.

4.3. Food Insecurity is High in Both Urban and Remote Settings

Results presented here also underscore differences in food insecurity risks between remote and non-remote areas of Australia. Interestingly, we find that non-English speaking persons in remote areas (37.3%) are at double the risk of exposure to food insecurity than English speakers in either remote (19%) or non-remote (18.7%) Australia.

Part of this disparity may reflect the lack of detailed geographical measures on NATSINPAS due to confidentialization. That is, non-English speakers are more likely to be resident in particularly isolated areas of remote Australia—with limited access to affordable food sources and health facilities. Notwithstanding, a considerable literature has emerged on the disparity in food prices between urban, regional, and remote regions in Australia. In one study, a 47% difference in prices was reported between remote and urban supermarkets for healthier foods [43]. Solutions to this complex problem include improvements to freight and transport costs, as well as improving low levels of demand for nutritious foods [44]. Indeed, one of the key drivers of food choice in remote Aboriginal communities is poverty [45]. These transport and demand issues are exacerbated by the lack of availability and variety of healthier food choices and lack of locally grown food in remote areas of Australia [45,46]. Combining the high cost of food and high poverty levels in remote regions likely explains the increased likelihood of being food insecure for non-English speaking Aboriginal and Torres Strait Islanders.

However, it was interesting to note that the likelihood of being food insecure did not differ between non- remote and remote English-speaking Aboriginal and Torres Strait Islanders with about 1 in 5 at risk of exposure to food insecurity. This is important as 75% of the Aboriginal and Torres Strait Islander population live in urban and regional areas [47]. Furthermore, projections of the Aboriginal and Torres Strait Islander population indicate future growth of the older population to be more prevalent in cities and regional areas. Between 2016 and 2026, the population aged 45 years and over is projected to grow by 36% in major cities, 39% in Inner and Outer regional areas and by 24% in remote and very remote areas of Australia [6]. These findings suggest that solutions to addressing food insecurity in older Aboriginal and Torres Strait Islander populations need to focus on all geographical locations. Indeed, recent efforts have tended to focus on food insecurity in remote areas, with less focus given to people living in urban areas [48,49].

Despite the focus of recent programs, a greater awareness of the linguistic and cultural needs in remote areas is required for effective solutions to food insecurity. In a systematic review of Aboriginal food and nutrition programs, Browne and colleagues (2018) conclude that "the most important factor determining success of Aboriginal and Torres Strait Islander food and nutrition programs is community involvement in (and ideally, control of) program development and implementation" [50]. As further argued by Bramwell et al. (2017), "given the sensitivity and shame often associated with food insecurity, more needs to be known about how health professionals can broach the issue to ensure dignity and cultural safety" ([48] p. 7). Herein lies a major problem for the implementation of food insecurity programs, as there is a considerable underrepresentation of Aboriginal and Torres Strait Islander people in the health sector—including at the programmatic design level [51].

4.4. Study Limitations

In interpreting our results, it is important to consider the study's limitations. Our findings potentially underestimate the degree of food insecurity in this population for several reasons. Firstly, the NATSINPAS population is limited to Aboriginal and Torres Strait Islanders residing in private dwellings and excludes a range of other vulnerable populations such as the homeless, those in poor health living in care facilities or hospitals. Indeed, there is a considerable need for further research on food insecurity risk in non-community based settings, among both Indigenous and non-Indigenous populations [52]. Secondly, the measure of food insecurity we employ is primarily an indicator of food insecurity as it only addresses access to food by economic means and does not include physical or mobility access. For example, research has shown that along with financial barriers, storage, transportation, health, and functional barriers are associated with experiencing food insecurity [53,54]. Using a more comprehensive tool that addressed issues of anxiety, quality and quantity of food suggested the prevalence of food insecurity in non-Indigenous older adults was 13% compared to 2% resulting from responses to the single item tool [16]. Furthermore, qualitative research suggests that many older people engage in "precarious nutritional self-management strategies" that are important indicators of food insecurity, and are not captured in the measures used herein [55]. Specific to this population, access to and availability of skills to use traditional foods or 'bush tucker' is also likely to be an important component of overall food security [12]. The food insecurity of older Aboriginal and Torres Strait Islanders would undoubtedly be higher according to these broader definitions. Finally, the prevalence and severity of food insecurity may be cyclical and cannot be captured in cross sectional data [56,57]. Longitudinal data are necessary to measure complex movements in and out of food insecurity and unfortunately this data is not collected. Moreover, as these data are cross sectional, we cannot and do not draw a causal relationship between the independent variables and food insecurity.

5. Conclusions

Noting these limitations, this paper was the first to examine food insecurity among older Aboriginal and Torres Strait Islanders. We found that food insecurity is experienced by a sizeable minority of older persons (1 in 5), that 41% of this group go without food consequently and that specific demographic groups are at a considerably heightened risk. In total, older Aboriginal and Torres Strait Islanders are at about a 5–7 fold risk of experiencing food insecurity relative to their non-Indigenous peers.

These findings offer information with which to identify food insecure persons and to inform nutrition programs in place to improve health and wellbeing. Existing studies note the importance of involving Aboriginal and Torres Strait Islander people in the management, design, and implementation of such programs and considerably more needs to be done in this area. However, nutrition programs alone are likely to be ineffective. The strength of socio-economic factors in explaining the prevalence of food insecurity, suggest that policies must improve economic and social wellbeing (through the 'Closing the Gap' strategy) in tandem with targeted nutrition programs and policies aimed at providing an affordable, healthy food supply. Recent evaluation studies, unfortunately, show slow progress with the 'Closing the Gap' strategy, with improvements in some but not all health and economic outcomes for Aboriginal and Torres Strait Islanders over the past decade [58,59].

Our findings further suggest solutions to addressing food insecurity in older Aboriginal and Torres Strait Islander populations need to focus on all geographical locations—not just on remote Australia, which has been the focus to date. In both remote and non-remote Australia, greater awareness of linguistic and cultural needs as well as the involvement and management of programs for and by Aboriginal and Torres Strait Islanders is required to improve levels of food security. Addressing food insecurity through these means offers one pathway for reducing nutrition related disease and co-morbidities, thereby assisting the 'Closing the Gap' strategy to achieve its aim of improving health outcomes for Aboriginal and Torres Strait Islanders.

Author Contributions: J.B.T. and J.R. jointly conceived the study and authored the manuscript. J.B.T. completed the data analysis. Both authors read and approved the final manuscript.

Acknowledgments: Data for this study were provided to the authors by the Australian Bureau of Statistics (ABS) through the ABS Universities Australia agreement.

References

1. Valeggia, C.R.; Snodgrass, J.J. Health of Indigenous People. *Annu. Rev. Anthropol.* **2015**, *44*, 117–135. [CrossRef]
2. Australian Institute of Health and Welfare. *Australian Burden of Disease Study: Impact and Causes of Illness and Death in Aboriginal and Torres Strait Islander People 2011*; Australian Burden of Disease Study Series No. 6. (Cat. no. BOD 7); Australian Institute of Health and Welfare: Canberra, Australia, 2016.
3. Australian Institute of Health and Welfare. *Trends in Indigenous Mortality and Life Expectancy, 2001–2015: Evidence from the Enhanced Mortality Database*; Cat. No. AIHW 174; Australian Institute of Health and Welfare: Canberra, Australia, 2017.
4. Gubhaju, L.; McNamara, J.; Banks, E.; Joshy, G.; Raphael, B.; Williamson, A.; Eades, S. The overall health and risk factor profile of Australian Aboriginal and Torres Strait Islander participants from the 45 and up study. *BMC Public Health* **2013**, *13*, 661. [CrossRef] [PubMed]
5. Cunningham, J.; Paradies, Y. Socio-demographic factors and psychological distress in Indigenous and non-Indigenous Australian adults aged 18–64 years: Analysis of national survey data. *BMC Public Health* **2012**, *12*, 95. [CrossRef] [PubMed]
6. Australian Bureau of Statistics. *Estimates and Projections, Aboriginal and Torres Strait Islander Australians, 2001 to 2026*; Catalogue Number 3238.0; Australian Bureau of Statistics: Canberra, Australia, 2014.
7. American Dietetic Association. Domestic food and nutrition security: Position of the American Dietetic Association. *J. Am. Diet. Assoc.* **1998**, *98*, 337–342. [CrossRef]
8. Willows, N.D.; Veugelers, P.; Raine, K.; Kuhle, S. Prevalence and sociodemographic risk factors related to household food security in Aboriginal peoples in Canada. *Public Health Nutr.* **2009**, *12*, 1150–1156. [CrossRef] [PubMed]
9. Gundersen, C. Measuring the extent, depth and severity of food insecurity: An application to American Indians in the USA. *J. Popul. Econ.* **2007**, *21*, 191–215. [CrossRef]
10. Pardilla, M.; Prasad, D.; Suratkar, S.; Gittelsohn, J. High levels of food insecurity on the Navajo Nation. *Public Health Nutr.* **2013**, *17*, 58–65. [CrossRef] [PubMed]

11. Skinner, K.; Hanning, R.; Tsuji, L.J.S. Prevalence and severity of household food insecurity of First Nations people living in an on-reserve, sub-Arctic community within the Mushkegowuk Territory. *Public Health Nutr.* **2014**, *17*, 31–39. [CrossRef] [PubMed]

12. Skinner, K.; Pratley, E.; Burnett, K. Eating in the city: A review of the literature on food insecurity and Indigenous people living in urban spaces. *Societies* **2016**, *6*, 7. [CrossRef]

13. Australian Bureau of Statistics. *Australian Aboriginal and Torres Strait Islander Health Survey: Nutrition Results—Food and Nutrients (Catalogue Number 4727.0.55.005)*; Australian Bureau of Statistics: Canberra, Australia, 2015.

14. Temple, J. Food insecurity among older Australians: Prevalence, correlates and well-being. *Aust. J. Ageing* **2006**, *25*, 158–163. [CrossRef]

15. Quine, S.; Morrell, S. Food insecurity in community-dwelling older Australians. *Public Health Nutr.* **2006**, *9*, 219–224. [CrossRef] [PubMed]

16. Russell, J.; Flood, V.; Yeatman, H.; Mitchell, P. Prevalence and risk factors of food insecurity among a cohort of older Australians. *J. Nutr. Health Aging* **2014**, *18*, 3–8. [CrossRef] [PubMed]

17. Australian Bureau of Statistics. Microdata. In *National Aboriginal and Torres Strait Islander Nutrition and Physical Activity Survey (Catalogue Number 4715.0.30.002)*; Australian Bureau of Statistics: Canberra, Australia, 2015.

18. Australian Bureau of Statistics. *Australian Standard Geographical Classification (ASGC) 2011 (Catalogue Number 1216.0)*; Australian Bureau of Statistics: Canberra, Australia, 2011.

19. Cotter, P.; Anderson, I.; Smith, L.R. Indigenous Australians: Ageing without longevity. In *Longevity and Social Change in Australia*; Borowski, A., Encel, S., Ozanne, E., Eds.; University of New South Wales Press Ltd.: Sydney, Australia, 2007; pp. 65–98.

20. Waugh, E.; Mackenzie, L. Ageing well from an urban Indigenous Australian perspective. *Aust. Occup. Ther. J.* **2011**, *58*, 25–33. [CrossRef] [PubMed]

21. Australian Bureau of Statistics. *Life Tables for Aboriginal and Torres Strait Islander Australians, 2010–2012 (Catalogue Number 3302.0.55.003)*; Australian Bureau of Statistics: Canberra, Australia, 2013.

22. Hyde, Z.; Flicker, L.; Smith, K.; Atkinson, D.; Fenner, S.; Skeat, L.; Lo Giudice, D. Prevalence and incidence of frailty in Aboriginal Australians, and association with mortality and disability. *Maturitas* **2016**, *87*, 89–94. [CrossRef] [PubMed]

23. Temple, J. Severe and moderate forms of food insecurity in Australia: Are they distinguishable? *Aust. J. Soc. Issues* **2008**, *43*, 649–668. [CrossRef]

24. McCullagh, P. Regression models for ordinal data. *J. R. Stat. Soc. Ser. B (Methodological)* **1980**, *42*, 109–142.

25. Raftery, A. Bayesian model selection in social research. *Sociol. Methodol.* **1995**, *25*, 111–163. [CrossRef]

26. Belsley, D.; Kuh, E.; Welsch, R. *Regression Diagnostics: Identifying Influential Data and Sources of Collinearity*; John Wiley & Sons, Inc.: New York, NY, USA, 1980.

27. Brant, R. Assessing proportionality in the proportional odds model for ordinal logistic regression. *Biometrics* **1990**, *46*, 1171–1178. [CrossRef] [PubMed]

28. Radimer, L.; Allsopp, R.; Harvey, P.; Friman, D.; Watson, E. Food insufficiency in Queensland. *Aust. N. Zeal. J. Public Health* **1997**, *21*, 303–310. [CrossRef]

29. Kendall, A.; Olson, C.; Frongillo, E. Relationship of hunger and food insecurity to food availability and consumption. *J. Am. Diet. Assoc.* **1996**, *96*, 1019–1024. [CrossRef]

30. Rose, D.; Oliveria, D. Nutrient intakes of individuals from food insufficient households in the United States. *Am. J. Public Health* **1997**, *87*, 1956–1961. [CrossRef] [PubMed]

31. Heflin, C.; Siefert, K.; Williams, D. Food insufficiency and women's mental health: Findings from a 3 year panel of welfare recipients. *Soc. Sci. Med.* **2005**, *61*, 1971–1982. [CrossRef] [PubMed]

32. Sharkey, J. Risk and presence of food insufficiency are associated with low nutrient intakes and multimorbidity among housebound older women who receive home-delivered meals. *J. Nutr.* **2003**, *133*, 3485–3491. [CrossRef] [PubMed]

33. Stuff, J.; Casey, P.; Szeto, K.; Gossett, G.; Robbins, J.; Simpson, P.; Connell, C.; Bogle, M. Household food insecurity is associated with adult health status. *J. Nutr.* **2004**, *134*, 2330–2335. [CrossRef] [PubMed]

34. Tarasuk, V. Household food insecurity with hunger is associated with women's food intakes, health and household circumstances. *J. Nutr.* **2001**, *131*, 2670–2676. [CrossRef] [PubMed]

35. Vozoris, N.; Tarasuk, V. Household food insufficiency is associated with poorer health. *J. Nutr.* **2003**, *133*, 120–126. [CrossRef] [PubMed]

36.   Laraia, B.; Siega-Riz, A.; Gundersen, C.; Dole, N. Psychosocial factors and socioeconomic indicators are associated with household food insecurity among pregnant women. *J. Nutr.* **2006**, *136*, 177–182. [CrossRef] [PubMed]

37.   German, L.; Kahana, C.; Rosenfeld, V.; Zabrowsky, I.; Wiezer, Z.; Fraser, D.; Shahar, D. Depressive symptoms are associated with food insufficiency and nutritional deficiencies in poor community-dwelling elderly people. *J. Nutr. Health Aging* **2011**, *15*, 3–8. [CrossRef] [PubMed]

38.   Russell, J.C.; Flood, V.M.; Yeatman, H.; Wang, J.J.; Mitchell, P. Food insecurity and poor diet quality are associated with reduced quality of life in older adults. *Nutr. Diet.* **2016**, *73*, 50–58. [CrossRef]

39.   Hamelin, A.; Habicht, J.; Beaudry, M. Food insecurity: Consequences for the household and broader social implications. *J. Nutr.* **1999**, *129*, 525s–528s. [CrossRef] [PubMed]

40.   Council of Australian Governments. *Closing the Gap in Indigenous Health Outcomes*; Council of Australian Governments: Canberra, Australia, 2009.

41.   Australian Institute of Health and Welfare. *Cardiovascular Disease, Diabetes and Chronic Kidney Disease—Australian Facts: Aboriginal and Torres Strait Islander People*; Cardiovascular, Diabetes and Chronic Kidney Disease Series No. 5. (Cat. No. CDK 5); Australian Institute of Health and Welfare: Canberra, Australia, 2015.

42.   Cunningham, J.; Paradies, Y. Patterns and correlates of self-reported racial discrimination among Australian Aboriginal and Torres Strait Islander adults, 2008–09: Analysis of national survey data. *Int. J. Equity Health* **2013**, *12*, 47. [CrossRef] [PubMed]

43.   Ferguson, M.; King, A.; Brimblecombe, J.K. Time for a shift in focus to improve food afford ability for remote customers. *Med. J. Aust.* **2016**, *204*, 409. [CrossRef] [PubMed]

44.   Pollard, C.; Nyaradi, A.; Lester, M.; Sauer, K. Understanding food security issues in remote Western Australian Indigenous communities. *Health Prom. J. Aust.* **2014**, *25*, 83–89. [CrossRef] [PubMed]

45.   Brimblecombe, J.K.; Ferguson, M.M.; Libert, S.C.; O'Dea, K. Characteristics of the community-level diet of Aboriginal people in remote northern Australia. *Med. J. Aust.* **2013**, *198*, 380–384. [CrossRef] [PubMed]

46.   Pollard, C. Selecting interventions for food security in remote indigenous communities. In *Food Security in Australia: Challenges and Prospects for the Future*; Farmar-Bowers, Q., Higgins, V., Millar, J., Eds.; Springer: New York, NY, USA, 2013; ISBN 978-1-4614-4484-8.

47.   Browne, J.; Laurence, S.; Thorpe, S. Acting on Food Insecurity in Urban Aboriginal and Torres Strait Islander Communities: Policy and Practice Interventions to Improve Local Access and Supply of Nutritious Food. 2009. Available online: http://www.healthinfonet.ecu.edu.au/health-risks/nutrition/other-reviews (accessed on 1 October 2017).

48.   Bramwell, L.; Foley, W.; Shaw, T. Putting urban Aboriginal and Torres Strait Islander food insecurity on the agenda. *Aust. J. Primary Health* **2017**, *23*, 415–419. [CrossRef] [PubMed]

49.   Browne, J.; Hayes, R.; Gleeson, D. Aboriginal health policy: Is nutrition the 'gap' in 'Closing the Gap'? *Aust. N. Zeal. J. Public Health* **2014**, *38*, 362–369. [CrossRef] [PubMed]

50.   Browne, J.; Adams, K.; Atkinson, P.; Gleeson, D.; Hayes, R. Food and nutrition programs for Aboriginal and Torres Strait Islander Australians: An overview of systematic reviews. *Aust. Health Rev.* **2018**. [CrossRef] [PubMed]

51.   LoGiudice, D. The health of older Aboriginal and Torres Strait Islander peoples. *Aust. J. Ageing* **2016**, *35*, 82–85. [CrossRef] [PubMed]

52.   Vahabi, M.; Martin, L. Food insecurity: Who is being excluded? A case of older people with dementia in long-term care homes. *J. Nutr. Health Aging* **2014**, *18*, 685–691. [CrossRef] [PubMed]

53.   Radermacher, H.; Feldman, S.; Bird, S. Food security in older Australians from different cultural backgrounds. *J. Nutr. Educ. Behav.* **2010**, *42*, 328. [CrossRef] [PubMed]

54.   Wolfe, W.; Frongillo, E.; Valois, P. Understanding the experience of food insecurity by elders suggests ways to improve its measurement. *J. Nutr.* **2003**, *133*, 2762. [CrossRef] [PubMed]

55.   Quandt, S.; Arcury, T.; McDonald, J.; Bell, R.; Vitolins, M. Meaning and management of food security among rural elders. *J. Appl. Gerontol.* **2001**, *10*, 356–376. [CrossRef]

56.   Bhargava, V.; Lee, J. Food insecurity and health care utilization among older adults. *J. Appl. Gerontol.* **2017**, *36*, 1415–1432. [CrossRef] [PubMed]

57.   Wolfe, W.; Olson, C.; Kendall, M.; Frongillo, E. Understanding food insecurity in the elderly: A conceptual framework. *J. Nutr. Educ.* **1996**, *28*, 92–100. [CrossRef]

58. Department of Prime Minister and Cabinet. *Closing the Gap: Prime Ministers Report 2018*; Department of Prime Minister and Cabinet: Canberra, Australia, 2018.

59. Biddle, N.; Gray, M.; Schwab, J. *Measuring and analyzing success for Aboriginal and Torres Strait Islander Australians (CAEPR Working Paper 122/2017)*; Centre for Aboriginal Economic Policy Research ANU: Canberra, Australia, 2017.

6

Food Insecurity and Mental Health among Females in High-Income Countries

Merryn Maynard [1,*], Lesley Andrade [2], Sara Packull-McCormick [2], Christopher M. Perlman [2], Cesar Leos-Toro [2] and Sharon I. Kirkpatrick [2,*]

[1] Meal Exchange Canada, Toronto, ON M5V 3A8, Canada
[2] School of Public Health and Health Systems, University of Waterloo, Waterloo, ON N2L 3G1, Canada; landrade@uwaterloo.ca (L.A.); srpackul@uwaterloo.ca (S.P.M.); chris.perlman@uwaterloo.ca (C.M.P.); cesar.leos-toro@uwaterloo.ca (C.L.-T.)
[*] Correspondence: merryn@mealexchange.com (M.M.); sharon.kirkpatrick@uwaterloo.ca (S.I.K.)

Abstract: Food insecurity is a persistent concern in high-income countries, and has been associated with poor mental health, particularly among females. We conducted a scoping review to characterize the state of the evidence on food insecurity and mental health among women in high-income countries. The research databases PubMed, EMBASE, and psycINFO were searched using keywords capturing food insecurity, mental health, and women. Thirty-nine articles (representing 31 unique studies/surveys) were identified. Three-quarters of the articles drew upon data from a version of the United States Department of Agriculture Household Food Security Survey Module. A range of mental health measures were used, most commonly to measure depression and depressive symptoms, but also anxiety and stress. Most research was cross-sectional and showed associations between depression and food insecurity; longitudinal analyses suggested bidirectional relationships (with food insecurity increasing the risk of depressive symptoms or diagnosis, or depression predicting food insecurity). Several articles focused on vulnerable subgroups, such as pregnant women and mothers, women at risk of homelessness, refugees, and those who had been exposed to violence or substance abuse. Overall, this review supports a link between food insecurity and mental health (and other factors, such as housing circumstances and exposure to violence) among women in high-income countries and underscores the need for comprehensive policies and programs that recognize complex links among public health challenges.

Keywords: food insecurity; mental health; depression; women; scoping review

1. Introduction

Food insecurity is a growing and persistent concern in high-income countries [1,2]. In North America, rates of household food insecurity have remained stable or risen in the last several years [3,4]. High rates have also been documented in the UK and Australia [5,6]. According to the Food and Agriculture Organization, "food security exists when all people, at all times, have physical, social, and economic access to sufficient safe and nutritious food that meets their dietary needs and food preferences for an active and healthy life" [7].Conceptualizations of food insecurity in high-income countries primarily focus on the economic aspect; for example, the Household Food Security Survey Module (HFSSM) [8], which is commonly used in the United States and Canada, measures uncertain or inadequate access to food due to financial constraints. This conceptualization aligns with literature linking vulnerability to food insecurity to high rates of poverty, particularly among population subgroups, such as single-parent households, racial/ethnic minorities, and those relying on social assistance [2–4,9–13].

Among population subgroups in high-income countries, food insecurity has been shown to be associated with compromised nutrition [14], poor general health, and a myriad of chronic health conditions [15,16]. Food insecurity has also been shown to be a marker of poor mental health, with studies identifying associations with mood and anxiety disorders and suicidal ideation, particularly among women [16–18]. Indeed, severity of household food insecurity appears to be linked with poor mental health in a dose–response manner, with experiences of severe food insecurity representing extreme chronic stress [19] and possibly acting as an independent determinant of suicidal ideation [20].

The relationship between food insecurity and poor mental health among women is of particular concern given that they are disproportionately impacted by food insecurity [2–4,21]. Women are overrepresented among low-income groups compared to men, with visible minority women and single mothers experiencing high rates of poverty in Canada and the United States [9–11]. Further, the existing literature suggests that women may be particularly vulnerable to poor mental health in conjunction with poverty and food insecurity [12] and for women with children, that the stress associated with these experiences has possible ripple effects, negatively impacting their children's physical and mental health as well [13].

To identify future research needs and inform policy and program responses, we conducted a scoping review to examine the state of the literature on food insecurity and mental health among women living in high-income countries.

2. Materials and Methods

The scoping review was conducted according to steps outlined by Arksey and O'Malley [22]. Scoping reviews, which use systematic search techniques, are appropriate when the aim is to address a broad question, such as querying the state of the evidence on a topic (especially when study designs may vary) and identifying gaps in that evidence [22] to inform future research and practice. As per Arksey and O'Malley [22], steps in the process include identifying the research question, identifying relevant studies, study selection, charting the data, and collating, summarizing, and reporting the results. Reporting follows the PRISMA guidelines [23].

2.1. Identifying Relevant Studies

The systematic search, developed in consultation with a librarian who is an expert in systematic searching, was conducted using the research databases PubMed, EMBASE, and psycINFO to capture records published up to May 2016. Given the range of possible mental health conditions, the search strategy was quite broad. Key words and Medical Subject Headings (MeSH) included "food" OR "nutrition" OR "diet" AND "security" OR "insecurity" OR "insufficiency" OR "scarcity" OR "*adequacy" OR "hunger" OR "poverty" OR "food supply" OR "nutritional requirements/status" AND "anxiety" OR "depression" OR "mental health" OR "mental health disorder" OR "mental health illness" OR "psychosis" OR "emotional disorder" OR "mania" OR "mental disease" OR "phobia" OR "mental disturbance/health/psychology". The key words and MESH headings to capture women included "women" OR "woman" OR "female" OR "pregnancy" OR "sex factors" OR "women's rights" OR "mothers" OR "girl" (note: * indicates a wildcard, which allows searching a range of terms related to a root word). The initial search elicited a total of 13,645 citations (excluding duplicates) (Figure 1).

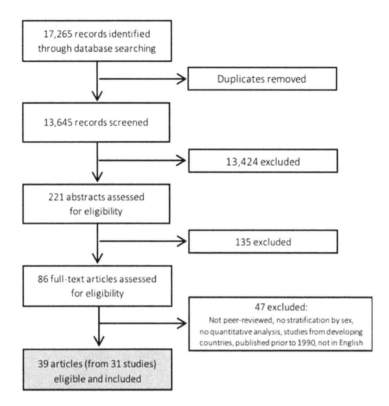

Figure 1. Overview of identification and screening of records for scoping review of literature on food insecurity and mental health among women in high-income countries.

2.2. Study Selection

Articles deemed eligible quantitatively examined associations between food insecurity and indicators of mental health, with a focus on females in high-income countries; studies that included both males and females but reported analyses stratified by sex were also considered. Specific criteria related to age were not applied, allowing consideration of studies reporting on adolescent girls as well as women. Studies published since 1990 (to provide insights into relatively recent research on the topic of food insecurity) were considered.

An initial screening of titles and abstracts was conducted by one author (S.P.-M.) to identify potentially relevant peer-reviewed articles that addressed food insecurity and health, leaving 221 citations for further review (Figure 1). Abstracts for these 221 citations were screened independently by a second author (M.M. or S.I.K.) and discrepancies resolved, leaving 86 citations for full-text review. After full-text screening (conducted independently by two authors), 39 articles remained, representing 31 unique studies/surveys. Separate articles making use of data from the same study or survey were examined and charted to identify salient characteristics related to measurement of food security and mental health and the examination of associations between the two.

2.3. Charting the Data

A data abstraction form guided extraction of the characteristics of interest, including study setting and population, study design, main study objectives, measures used to assess food security and mental health and specific mental health states considered, and analytic approach and findings.

2.4. Collating, Summarizing, and Reporting the Results

The abstracted data were assessed in terms of patterns in measures and tools used and associations between food insecurity and depression (the most frequently examined mental health measure) and other mental health markers. Given that we conducted a scoping rather than a systematic review, formal quality appraisal of studies was not conducted [22]. However, in addition to synthesizing the evidence emerging from this literature, we comment on the characteristics of the available research, in terms of study design for example, to inform future research.

3. Results

3.1. Overview of Included Articles

The characteristics of the 39 articles are outlined in Appendix A. Over half (n = 23) were published from 2010 on [15–17,24–43]. The majority (n = 34) analyzed data from studies conducted in the United States, three focused on studies conducted in Canada [16,17,32], one was focused on a sample in New Zealand [43], and one was conducted in England [44]. Twenty-eight articles reported on cross-sectional analyses (one also included qualitative data collection [28]) and eleven reported longitudinal analyses (one included qualitative data collection [45]) (Appendix A). Although all studies assessed the association between food insecurity and a mental health condition or state in some manner, the particular research questions and analytic approaches varied. Some studies examined food insecurity and mental health among general samples of the population, whereas others focused on particularly vulnerable population subgroups or sought to assess the feasibility or other properties of tools. Half (n = 20) focused on mothers or caregivers, another five studied pregnant women, and several focused on other specific subpopulations, including rural women, those living with disabilities, older women, refugees, women experiencing insecure housing or homelessness, and women at risk for HIV (Appendix A).

3.2. Food Insecurity Measures

Three-quarters (n = 30) of the reviewed articles drew upon data collected using a version of the Household Food Security Survey Module (HFSSM), developed by the United States Department of Agriculture [8] (Table 1). The full HFSSM contains 18 items and yields a single score indicating the severity of household food insecurity over the past 12 months or 30 days; ten items refer to adults and eight refer to children in the household [8]. Scores are typically used to categorize households as food secure or food insecure with different levels of severity (since a review of the measure conducted in the early 2000s [46], the categories of food insecurity have been referred to as low and very low food security, replacing earlier labels of food insecure with/without hunger). The HFSSM was compared to household food expenditures and income [8] and associated with compromised dietary intakes [14], supporting its validity in capturing constrained food access due to inadequate finances. Fourteen articles drew upon abbreviated versions of HFSSM, including the six-item subset developed by USDA and the ten adult-referenced items, as well as other adaptations (Table 1).

One article reported on data using a single item drawn from the 12-item Radimer–Cornell scale [47], and another used data collected using the Community Childhood Hunger Identification Project (CCHIP) instrument [48]. Both the Radimer–Cornell and CCHIP tools are used to categorize food security status and were shown to have good specificity and sensitivity compared to evaluations of food security status based on household food inventories, dietary recall data, and other measures among a sample of women living with children in rural New York [49]. These tools were drawn upon in the development of the HFSSM [8].

Three articles drew upon data collected using a single item from the National Health and Nutrition Examination Survey-III (NHANES-III) to assess food insufficiency (defined as "an inadequate amount of food intake due to a lack of money or resources") [50]. As opposed to more comprehensive instruments, measures of food insufficiency are less detailed and may misclassify some households [49,51]. Finally, four articles drew upon data from other single- or multi-measures adapted from prior literature (Table 1).

Table 1. Overview of measures of food security drawn upon in articles ($n = 39$) examining associations between food insecurity and mental health among women in high-income countries.

Measure	Description	Abbreviated and Modified Versions	Articles Using Full Version	Articles Using Modified Versions
Community Childhood Hunger Identification Project	An 8-item scale developed by Wehler et al. [48]. Part of a survey instrument to examine the prevalence of hunger among low-income families. The items address qualitative and quantitative compromises among adults and children. Shown to have good specificity and sensitivity compared to evaluations of food security status based on household food inventories, dietary recall data, and other measures among a sample of women living with children in rural New York [49].	None	None	Wehler et al. 2004 [52]
Household Food Security Survey Module	An 18-item measure developed by the United States Department of Agriculture [8] and used to monitor household food security in the US and Canada. Measures the food security status of a household in the last 12 months. Items ask an adult respondent about anxiety related to the household food supply, running out of food, providing inadequately nutritious food, and substitutions or restrictions in food consumption by adults and/or children in the household due to lack of financial resources. Items are compiled to form a continuous, linear scale that categorizes households into one of four groups; food secure, marginal food secure, low food secure, and very low food secure [8]. Data from the HFSSM have been compared to household food expenditures and income [8] and dietary intakes [14], supporting its validity in capturing constrained food access due to inadequate financial resources.	Six-item short form: uses a subset of the 18-item survey. Does not characterize severe food insecurity and does not contain child-specific items. 10-item adult scale: includes only items referenced to adults in the household. Health Canada modifications: Refers to low food security as "moderate food insecurity" and very low food security as "severe food insecurity". Less stringent than USDA coding, in that 2+ affirmative responses place an individual into a food insecure category.	Bronte-Tinkew et al. 2007 [53]; Casey et al. 2004 [54]; Chilton et al. 2013 [28]; Corman et al. 2016 [24]; Garg et al. 2015 [25]; Hanson et al. 2012 [15]; Hernandez et al. 2014 [26]; Huddleston-Casas et al. 2009 [55]; Laraia et al. 2006 [56]; Laraia et al. 2015 [27]; Lent et al. 2009 [45]; McCurdy et al. 2015 [29]; Sun et al. 2016 [30]; Trapp et al. 2015 [31] Health Canada coding: Muldoon et al. 2013 [32]; Tarasuk et al. 2013 [16]	Dressler et al. 2015 [37]; Kaiser et al. 2007 [57]; Laraia et al. 2009 [58]; Martin et al. 2016 [17] (Health Canada coding); Mathews et al. 2010 [34]; Peterman et al. 2013 [38]; Sharpe et al. 2016 [39]; Whitaker et al. 2006 [59]; 15-item adaptation for pregnant Latinas: Hromi-Fielder et al. 2011 [36] Other non-standard adaptations (3-, 4-, or 7-items): Ajrouch et al. 2010 [35]; Davey-Rothwell et al. 2014 [40]; Harrison et al. 2008 [60]; Melchior et al. 2009 [44]; Sidebottom et al. 2014 [33]
National Health and Nutrition Examination Survey-III (NHANES-III) food sufficiency indicators	NHANES-III was a health and nutrition survey conducted by the US Center for Disease Control (CDC). A food sufficiency component was included in the in-home adult questionnaire. Respondents were classified as "food insecure" if they "sometimes" or "often" did not have enough food to eat. Other questions included how many days in the prior month the respondent did not have money for food, reasons for not having enough food, and whether the respondent or child in the household had restricted their food intake due to lack of food [61].	None	Heflin et al. 2005 [62]; Siefert et al. 2007 [63]; Siefert et al. 2001 [64]	None

Table 1. *Cont.*

Measure	Description	Abbreviated and Modified Versions	Articles Using Full Version	Articles Using Modified Versions
New Zealand measure of individual deprivation (NZiDep)	An 8-item scale measuring individual socioeconomic deprivation, specific to New Zealand. The scale has been validated among Maori, Pacific, and White New Zealand citizens [65]; criterion validity relied upon associations with tobacco smoking. Includes three-item composite measure of food security: "In the last 12 months have you personally made use of special food grants or food banks because you did not have enough money for food?" (yes/no), "In the last 12 months have you personally been forced to buy cheaper food so that you could pay for other things you needed?" (yes/no), "In the last 12 months have you personally gone without fresh fruit and vegetables often so that you could pay for other things you needed?" (yes/no).		Carter et al. 2011 [43]	None
Radimer–Cornell scale	A 12-item scale developed by Radimer et al. [47] at Cornell University based on qualitative research with low-income women. Twelve items cover aspects of household, adult, and child food insecurity. The content of the items address food anxiety, monotony of diet, financial constraints, food restriction, insufficient intake, and acquiring food in socially acceptable ways [47,66]. Shown to have good specificity and sensitivity compared to evaluations of food security status based on household food inventories, dietary recall data, and other measures among a sample of women living with children in rural New York [49]. Further information about the evolution of the instrument is available [67].	Single item	None	Sharkey et al. 2011 [41]
Other Multi- or Single-Item Measures			Birmingham et al. 2011 [42]; Klesges et al. 2001 [68]; Sharkey et al. 2003 [69]	None

3.3. Mental Health Measures

Depression and depressive symptoms were the most prevalent mental health states assessed. Associations between food insecurity and depression were examined in 36 articles (Appendix A). Ten articles drew upon measures assessing clinical diagnoses, while the remainder relied upon self-reported symptoms.

Measures are described in Table 2, along with information about their validation. In reviewed articles, authors sometimes noted that measures have been tested for psychometric properties such as internal consistency, in some cases, in the context of the particular study (Appendix A). Data from the short form of the World Health Organization World Mental Health Composite International Diagnostic Interview (CIDI) [70] were drawn upon to establish a clinical diagnosis of depression or anxiety in six articles. To assess depressive symptoms, the Centre for Epidemiologic Studies Depression Scale (CES-D) [71] was used most frequently, drawn upon in 14 articles. For anxiety, one article drew upon data from Spielberger's Trait Anxiety Inventory [72] and another the Hopkins Symptom Checklist Subscale (HSCL) [73]. Some measures targeted specific life stages such as pregnancy and older age; for example, maternal depressive symptoms were assessed with the Kemper three-item screen [74] and the Edinburgh Postpartum Depression Scale [75], while depressive symptoms among older women were assessed using the Geriatric Depression Scale [76].

Various other mental health markers were measured, including perceived control over one's life, perceived stress, quality of life, self-esteem, mastery, general mental health, psychosis, substance abuse, post-traumatic stress disorder, and disordered eating (Appendix A).

Table 2. Overview of measures of mental health drawn upon in articles ($n = 39$) examining associations between food insecurity and mental health among women in high-income countries.

Measure	Description	Abbreviated Versions	Articles Using Full Version	Articles Using Abbreviated Versions
Center for Epidemiologic Studies, Depression Scale (CES-D)	A 20-item self-report scale measuring depressive symptoms in the general population. Components assess depressed mood, feelings of guilt and worthlessness, feelings of helplessness and hopelessness, psychomotor retardation, loss of appetite, and sleep disturbance in the prior week. Validity of the CES-D has been established through correlations with self-reported measures, clinical scores for depression, and other construct validity variables. Reliability and validity has been demonstrated across diverse characteristics of general population samples [71].	10-item short form 12-item short form	Ajrouch et al. 2010 [35]; Davey-Rothwell et al. 2014 [40]; Dressler et al. 2015 [37]; Hanson et al. 2012 [15]; Hromi-Fielder et al. 2011 [36]; Huddleston-Casas et al. 2009 [55]; Laraia et al. 2006 [56]; Laraia et al. 2009 [58]; Lent et al. 2009 [45]; McCurdy et al. 2015 [29]; Siefert et al. 2007 [63]	Bronte-Tinkew et al. 2007 [53]; Garg et al. 2015 [25]; Sharpe et al. 2016 [39]
Cohen's Perceived Stress Scale (PSS)	A 14-item self-report Likert scale that measures the degree of unpredictability of the respondents' life and the degree to which the respondent feels stress regarding these situations. Validated in young adult and post-secondary student population, the PSS correlated with physical and mental health related outcomes [77].	PSS-4 (4-item subset) 10-item short form	Laraia et al. 2006 [56]	Trapp et al. 2015 [31]; Laraia et al. 2015 [27]
Diagnostic Interview Schedule (DIS)	A structured interview designed for non-clinicians to assess and diagnose psychiatric disorders in respondents according to criteria in the Diagnostic and Statistical Manual of Mental Disorders, Fourth Edition (DSM-IV). The DIS has 19 diagnostic modules that cover different types of mental disorders. Within each module, respondents answer whether they have particular symptoms at the present, or have experienced them in the past [78].	None	Melchior et al. 2009 [44]	None
Edinburgh Postpartum Depression Scale (EPDS)	A 10-item self-report scale used to measure risk of postpartum depression in mothers within eight weeks of delivery. Items assess feelings of guilt, sleep deprivation, lack of energy, suicidality, and other general depressive symptoms experienced within the last 7 days. Validity has been examined in a sample of postpartum mothers, 6-weeks post-delivery, and compared with clinician diagnosis of depression [75].	3-item short form	None	Birmingham et al. 2011 [42]
Geriatric Depression Scale (GDS)	A 30-item self-report scale that assesses depression in geriatric populations ($\geq$55 years). Items assess motivation, self-esteem, helplessness, mood, and agitation [76].	15-item short form	Klesges et al. 2001 [68]	Sharkey et al. 2003 [69]
Hopkins Symptom Checklist Subscale (HSCL)	A 58-item self-report scale used primarily with psychiatric outpatients, capturing five symptom dimensions including somatization, obsessive-compulsive, interpersonal sensitivity, depression, and anxiety [73]. Authors discuss a variety of studies in which the validity of the HSCL has been evaluated.	None	Klesges et al. 2001 [68]	None

Table 2. *Cont.*

Measure	Description	Abbreviated Versions	Articles Using Full Version	Articles Using Abbreviated Versions
Kemper 3-Item Screen	A 3-item self-report screening tool designed to assess maternal depressive symptoms. Validity examined with English-speaking mothers with children under 6 years of age, demonstrated 100% sensitivity and 88% specificity [74].	None	Casey et al. 2004 [54]; Chilton et al. 2013 [28]; Sun et al. 2016 [30]	None
Kessler-10 Scale	A 10-item screen developed for the US National Health Interview Survey. Designed to assess symptoms of general psychological distress through items on level of nervousness, hopelessness, lack of energy, depressive feelings, and worthlessness. Validity was examined with adults living in Australia, aged 18 years and older [79].	None	Carter et al. 2011 [43]	None
Patient Health Questionnaire (PHQ-9)	A 9-item questionnaire administered in a primary care setting by clinicians, designed to provide a diagnosis of major depressive disorder according to DSM guidelines. Items assess depressive symptoms and anhedonia experienced within the past 2 weeks. Validity was assessed among patients recruited through primary care offices, with 73% sensitivity and 94% specificity [80].	PHQ-2 (2-item subset)	Harrison et al. 2008 [60]; Sidebottom et al. 2014 [33]	Trapp et al. 2015 [31]
Pearlin's Mastery Scale	A 7-item self-report Likert scale that measures the degree of control respondents feel they have over their lives. Authors note validation with individuals aged 18 to 65 years [81].	None	Heflin et al. 2005 [62]; Laraia et al. 2006 [56]	None
Rosenberg's Self-Esteem Scale	A 10-item self-report Likert scale that assesses level of self-esteem in respondents [82].	None	Laraia et al. 2006 [56]; Laraia et al. 2009 [58]	None
SF-36 Health Survey	A 36-item health survey that consists of 5 physical health scales and 5 mental health scales. The mental component summary score is calculated from scores on 4 subscales; social functioning, role emotional, vitality, and mental health scales [83]. When tested on individuals 16–74 years of age, the SF-36 demonstrated good construct validity in patient population. Authors noted promise in use with the general population [83]	SF-12 (12-item short form)	Lent et al. 2009 [45]	Mathews et al. 2010 [34]
Spielberger's Trait Anxiety Inventory	The Spielberger State-Trait Anxiety Inventory is a 20-item tool commonly used to measure anxiety, with higher scores indicating greater levels of anxiety [72]. The American Psychological Association has noted sensitivity of this inventory to predict distress overtime in caregivers [72].	None	Laraia et al. 2006 [56]	None
World Health Organization World Mental Health Composite International Diagnostic Interview (CIDI)	A comprehensive interview designed to diagnose major depressive disorder, other depressive disorders, anxiety disorders, substance abuse, and impulse control disorders according to the World Health Organization International Classification of Disease (ICD) and DSM criteria [70]. Evaluation studies suggested good test-retest and interrater reliability, and its use in different settings and countries was deemed acceptable [84].	CIDI short form (CIDI-SF), also referred to as screening version	None	Corman et al. 2016 [24]; Heflin et al. 2005 [62]; Hernandez et al. 2014 [26]; Martin et al. 2016 [17]; Siefert et al. 2001 [64]; Whitaker et al. 2006 [59]

3.4. Overview of Findings on Food Insecurity and Mental Health

The majority of cross-sectional analyses examining depression and food insecurity (or food insufficiency) reported some form of association deemed to be significant [16,28,29,32,34–36,38–44,54,56–60,63,64,68,69,85]. Several longitudinal analyses likewise observed relationships between depression and food insecurity, with food insecurity increasing the risk of experiencing depressive symptoms or a depression diagnosis [44,53,62], or changes in food insecurity associated with changes in depression [62]. For example, a longitudinal analysis of data from 8693 parent–child dyads by Bronte-Tinkew et al. [53] found that mothers affected by food insecurity were more likely to report depressive symptoms compared to food-secure mothers. Some authors reported that the relationship functioned in the opposite direction, with depression leading to food insecurity [15,24–26,45], or was bidirectional [55]. For example, Garg et al., who analyzed data from the Early Childhood Longitudinal Study Birth Cohort ($n = 2917$), found that mothers who experienced depression were at greater risk of remaining food insecure over time compared to mothers without depression [25]. Food insecurity and depression were also investigated in relation to other markers of material deprivation; for example, Corman et al. [24] found that women who experienced a major depressive episode at baseline had greater odds of experiencing food insecurity and inadequate housing at follow-up.

Several articles focused on pregnant women and revealed associations between prenatal and postpartum depression and food insecurity [33,36,42,56,60]. Food-insecure pregnant women were at increased risk of experiencing prenatal depressive symptoms compared to their food-secure counterparts [33,36]. Although a comprehensive measure of food insecurity was not used, Birmingham et al. [42] tested depression screening methods in a cross-sectional analysis of 195 mothers of newborns and found that those who had concerns about food were 5.5 times more likely to have a positive postpartum depression screen result.

Anxiety and stress were associated with food insecurity in multiple studies [16,17,32,56,59]. Analyses of cross-sectional data from the 2007–2008 Canadian Community Health Survey (CCHS) by Tarasuk et al. ($n = 77,053$) [16] and Muldoon et al. ($n = 5588$) [32] indicated that severe food insecurity and a self-reported diagnosis of mood or anxiety disorders were associated among women. Siefert et al. [64] found an association between food insecurity and generalized anxiety disorder in a cross-sectional study of 724 US women receiving welfare, but the relationship was not significant when covariates were taken into account. In two studies, one cross-sectional ($n = 606$) [56] and one longitudinal ($n = 526$) [27], Laraia et al. found that food-insecure pregnant women had higher perceived stress compared to food-secure women, and those who had experienced any level of food insecurity during pregnancy or at three months postpartum were more likely to have high perceived stress scores at 12 months postpartum. Martin et al. [17] investigated perceived stress among Canadian adults and found that the prevalence of high levels of stress increased with lower food security status. However, Trapp et al. [31] explored food insecurity among a group of 222 low-income mothers and their children in a cross-sectional analysis and found that levels of perceived stress did not differ between food-insecure and food-secure groups.

Three recent articles explored disordered or emotional eating among women experiencing food insecurity [27,37,39]. Laraia et al. [27] and Sharpe et al. [39] found bivariate associations between food insecurity and disordered or emotional eating; however, in models adjusted for sociodemographic characteristics, Laraia et al. [27] did not observe significant associations between food insecurity and disordered eating behaviors. Dressler et al. [37] examined associations between emotional eating and depression and suggested that emotional eating may mediate associations among food insecurity, mental health, and other food-related outcomes, such as dietary intakes and weight status.

Moreover, some studies examined multiple mental and physical health conditions suggesting comorbid physical and mental health problems increased vulnerability to food insecurity [16,34] and that food insecurity increased vulnerability to poor physical and mental health [41,69]. There was also a focus on implications for others, including children, in the household. For example,

Bronte-Tinkew et al. [53] found that mothers living in food-insecure households reported high rates of depression, which was correlated with fair and poor health in children.

Given that the precise focus of the studies varied, a range of covariates was examined. Several studies examined various forms of social support [15,17,35,52,60,63]. Instrumental social support (e.g., ability to borrow money, help with childcare and transportation) was examined in a study conducted by the Detroit Centre for Oral Health Disparities. Cross-sectional analyses by Siefert et al. [63] (n = 824) indicated that the effect of food insufficiency on depression could be reduced with the availability of instrumental social support, while Ajrouch et al. [35] (n = 736) found that this protective effect was dampened when respondents experienced high levels of food insecurity-related stress. Using cross-sectional Canadian data, Martin et al. [17] (n = 100,401) found associations between food insecurity and feelings of community belonging; for example, the prevalences of living in severely food-insecure households were 18% and 25.6% among women reporting high and low community belonging, respectively. In a cross-sectional analysis, Wehler et al. [52] (n = 354) found that financial social support from a sibling reduced the odds of mothers experiencing hunger but did not reduce the odds of children in the same household experiencing hunger. Further, Hanson and Olson [15] (n = 225) found that parenting social support (e.g., having someone to talk to and having help in an emergency) did not reduce the odds of a household experiencing persistent vs. discontinuous food insecurity over a period of three years.

The role of childhood and adulthood adverse experiences, including abuse, was also examined. In multivariable models, Wehler et al. [52] found that sexual abuse in childhood increased the odds of adult hunger, and that this appeared to be mediated by experiences of intimate partner violence in adulthood. Sun et al. [30] examined Adverse Childhood Experiences, including abuse, neglect, and household dysfunction, and found that mothers reporting four or more adverse experiences were more likely to report food insecurity, with adjustment for demographic factors. In bivariate analyses, Harrison et al. [60] found that each of food insecurity, intimate partner violence and depressive symptoms were correlated. In multivariable models accounting for demographic factors, Melchior et al. [44] found that intimate partner violence was higher among women who had reported indications of food insecurity two years prior.

4. Discussion

Overall, the evidence reviewed here supports a link between food insecurity and compromised mental health among women in high-income countries. Although longitudinal data were limited, associations between food insecurity and depression appear to operate in both directions. There are multiple plausible potential pathways by which food insecurity and poor mental health may be linked. The experience of food insecurity itself is characterized by worry and anxiety about the household food supply. Toxic stress, which refers to chronic and unyielding stress without adequate social and environmental supports [13], may be one pathway through which food insecurity and mental health are intertwined. Depending on the availability and regularity of finances, periods of household food insecurity can occur repeatedly or chronically; households in the United States that were food insecure in 2016 experienced food insecurity in seven months on average [3]. Therefore, food insecurity may represent a chronic stressor that could contribute to the development of poor mental health. Conversely, a mental health condition could inhibit an individual from maintaining steady employment, thereby increasing vulnerability to food insecurity. Further, Seligman and Schillinger [86] posit that the relationship between food insecurity and poor health is cyclical; food insecurity increases the likelihood of trade-offs in food choices among those who receive low income and challenges the self-management of health conditions. Poor self-management results in higher health care and medication costs for the individual, which further contribute to financial instability and food insecurity [86]. Once an individual enters this cycle, it may be very difficult to exit, particularly in countries where there are disparities in access to health care and social supports, impacting access. Additionally, studies found an association between instances of abuse and depression and food insecurity [26,44,52,60]. The early life stress hypothesis argues that stressors experienced during key developmental periods can enhance vulnerability to mental health outcomes in adult life [87].

The majority of the available literature is cross-sectional, and further longitudinal research could shed light on the nature of the observed relationships and factors that underlie them. For example, research is needed to examine the interconnections among various markers of mental health and experiences of food insecurity across the lifespan, as well as to further examine the influence of potential mediating factors, such as social support or experiences of abuse. Many existing studies have focused on women with children, and pregnant women have also been investigated. A population of growing interest in regards to food insecurity is postsecondary students [88–91]; given that this is a life stage during which vulnerability to poor mental health is also high [89,92,93], research examining the root causes of both issues and how they interact is of public health importance. At the other end of the spectrum, we also identified little research focused on older women.

Food insecurity is a complex and multidimensional phenomenon [51,94] and its measurement is also complex. Many of the reviewed studies relied upon data from the HFSSM, or an adaptation, to assess food security. The HFSSM is considered the standard in household food insecurity measurement in North America and is used widely in research and surveillance [3,4]. While this tool provides an indicator of quantitative deprivation, it focuses on economic access to food and does not capture aspects that are likely to be relevant to mental health, such as the social acceptability of food acquisition strategies [51]. For example, Hamelin et al. have described alienation that accompanies lack of access to adequate food [67], as well as the social implications [95]. Nonetheless, the HFSSM has been widely-used and, within the North American context, provides data that are comparable to those from national surveys [4,8,21]. The Household Food Insecurity Access Scale (HFIAS) [94] is a standardized tool that uses similar questions as the HFSSM and is designed to differentiate food-secure from food-insecure households across cultural contexts; this tool may be appropriate depending on the setting and populations of interest. Whenever feasible, a comprehensive tool is recommended over single or brief measures that may not accurately classify households and cannot provide insights into severity of food insecurity (thus potentially missing the opportunity to shed insights into those who are most vulnerable). Additionally, studies using mixed methods can generate unique information not yielded by a standardized measure such as the HFSSM.

There was greater variety in measures used to assess mental health compared with those used to determine household food security status, the majority involving screening for depressive symptoms, along with diagnostic measures that use more stringent criteria. Many authors noted that these tools had been tested and are widely used, but the range of tools used makes it difficult to compare across studies. As with food insecurity, abbreviated measures, such as those assessing depression and depressive symptoms, may have been limited in sensitivity and specificity compared to full measures, potentially dampening observed relationships or creating spurious effects. While the use of comprehensive measures and greater standardization of tools used to assess depression and other mental health conditions may allow for greater comparability across this body of literature and more robust inferences, it is critical for any study that the measure be well suited to the research question and the population/setting.

Furthermore, much of the existing research has focused on depression; widening this scope could enable policy and program responses that consider the potential range of mental health conditions related to inadequate food access. An emerging area of research is the link between food insecurity and disordered eating; in addition to the studies reviewed here focused on women, recent findings from a study of US adult men and women accessing a food pantry indicated a positive association between food insecurity and indicators of eating disorder pathology, such as binge eating and engaging in compensatory behaviors [96]. Additionally, few studies examined food security in relation to schizophrenia/psychosis or bipolar disorder among females.

The findings of the reviewed articles should be interpreted in light of several considerations. Most of the available research is based on US populations. While several studies were conducted among subpopulations such as women with children and African-American women, more research is needed to assess how food insecurity and mental health interact with other markers of vulnerability (such as single parenthood, insecure housing, drug use, experiences of violence, and immigrant/refugee status) in diverse subgroups. The majority of studies were cross-sectional, and causal inferences were not possible. Additionally, for longitudinal studies, in some cases, it was challenging to ascertain the timing of baseline and follow-up data collections. Adherence to checklists such as STROBE (Strengthening the Reporting of Observational Studies in Epidemiology) [97] could help promote transparency and accurate interpretation. Many authors noted limitations of self-reported data on mental health outcomes and food insecurity [16,17,26,29–32,34,40,44,55,62]. Some also noted temporal incongruence between measures of food insecurity and indicators of mental health [25,39,41] that may have affected their findings. Due to the varied emphases of the studies (including assessing feasibility and other characteristics of measures), a range of covariates and potential confounders were examined; in some cases, they were used to characterize samples whereas in others, they were included in statistical models such that it is difficult to compare estimates from one study to another. Finally, explicit approaches to account for the potential conceptual overlap between food insecurity and mental health indicators, such as feelings of worry or anxiety that are conceptualized as part of the experience of food insecurity and are also markers of psychological distress, were not common.

Considerations related to the review itself also warrant highlighting. We followed methodology for a scoping study [22] and, thus, did not conduct a formal appraisal of the quality of the included evidence, nor weight the evidence. Rather, our objective was to characterize the existing literature as to identify directions for future research. Further, although we employed a systematic search strategy and careful screening, our search was broad and it is possible that some relevant articles were inadvertently excluded. Additionally, we did not consider studies that presented pooled estimates for males and females. Although our interest was in females, this does not preclude the existence of associations between food insecurity and mental health among males, as observed in some reviewed studies that include stratified analyses. Additionally, given that we relied upon published articles, we did not account for publication bias in that research not supporting relationships between food insecurity and mental health may be less likely to have been identified.

5. Conclusions

Overall, this review supports a link between food insecurity and poor mental health among women in high-income countries. Despite gaps, the existing evidence is sufficient to warrant policy and program interventions to address these major public health challenges in a coordinated manner. An underlying theme of the literature is the complex ways in which food insecurity and mental health are connected both to each other and to an array of other issues, such as experiences of violence, housing circumstances, and life transitions such as pregnancy. These links underscore the need for coordinated approaches that consider how policy and program interventions can best address these complex issues and their interactions. Such approaches may be informed by systems methods [98–100] that consider the interplay among factors and how interventions to address one issue may affect another issue, influencing overall health and well-being.

Strategies to address financial inadequacy, such as a guaranteed basic income, have been called for to reduce vulnerability to food insecurity [19,101,102], and could play a role in ameliorating mental health conditions [103]. Additionally, food security screening has been recommended within clinical settings to enable referral to available community resources [13,104–106] (although it is imperative that practitioners have effective resources to which they can make referrals). While addressing the financial circumstances that underlie food insecurity is critical, screening for food access issues among those seeking treatment for mental health conditions could help build momentum in addressing the whole person instead of tackling issues in isolation, for example, helping health practitioners to understand, and potentially address, reasons for non-adherence to recommendations related to diet or other factors. Health and social service settings with integrated care models, in which women have access to a range of services that provide support during periods of food insecurity and poor mental health, may allow complex challenges to be addressed simultaneously [107]. In addition, health care providers are uniquely positioned to support individuals in accessing services such as government income-related benefits, dietary allowance benefits, or legal supports [16,106,108], and alongside individuals with lived experience of vulnerability, to advocate for increased financial supports and access to mental health care.

Author Contributions: S.P.-M., S.I.K., and M.M. developed and conducted the search and screened articles. S.P.-M. and M.M. extracted data and C.L.-T., L.A., and S.I.K. verified data extraction. M.M., L.A. and S.I.K. led the manuscript development and all authors contributed critical revisions.

Acknowledgments: The authors are grateful to Jackie Stapleton for her guidance on the search strategy and Mona Qutub for her assistance with referencing.

Appendix A

Table A1. Key characteristics of articles ($n = 39$ from 31 studies/surveys) included in scoping review of food insecurity and mental health among women in high-income countries, by measure of food insecurity.

Reference	Sample (Participants (Age), Setting, Race/Ethnicity, Data Source)	Study Design (Sample Size)	Purpose	Food Security Measure	Mental Health Measure	Mental Health States/Conditions	Covariates Considered	Analytic Approach and Key Findings
				Household Food Security Survey Module (HFSSM)				
				Longitudinal analyses				
Bronte-Tinkew et al. 2007 [53]	Mothers (mean age, 27.5 years), US, race/ethnicity not specified Early Childhood Longitudinal Study-Birth Cohort (ECLS-B)	Longitudinal (8693)	Examine association between food insecurity and child health, and examine parental depression and behaviors as mediators	USDA HFSSM	CES-D 12-item subset Authors note strong psychometric properties	Symptoms of maternal depression	Parent education, maternal employment, maternal age (at birth), family structure, receipt of food subsidy, child exposure to cigarette smoke, number of well-baby visits, household poverty index ratio	Structural equation modeling: Mothers in food-insecure households reported higher levels of depressive symptoms ($\beta = 0.243$, $p < 0.001$), which were associated with parent-reported fair or poor health in children at 24 months.
Corman et al. 2016 [24]	Mothers (mean age, 25 years) from 75 birth hospitals in 20 US cities, included White, African American, Hispanic, and other races/ethnicities Fragile Families and Child Wellbeing Study	Longitudinal (2965)	Examine association between maternal depression in the postpartum year, housing conditions, and food insecurity	USDA HFSSM	CIDI short form Authors note that the measure has been validated	Clinical diagnosis of a MDE (defined as 3+ symptoms of dysphoria or anhedonia for most of the day for a period of at least 2 weeks) during the postpartum year (assessed at 1 year)	Maternal, paternal, and prenatal housing characteristics (measured at baseline), maternal grandparents' mental illness and child characteristics	Multivariable analysis: Compared to women who did not report depression, mothers who reported depression were more likely to experience inadequate housing at 2–3 years due to lack of heat (aOR 1.57, 95% CI 1.11–2.22) and energy insecurity (aOR 1.69, 95% CI 1.24–2.30). Depression was associated with combinations of hardships, including inadequate housing, housing instability, and food insecurity (aOR 3.85, 95% CI 1.34–11.11).
Garg et al. 2015 [25]	Low-income **mothers** (mean age, 25 years) and their young children in the US, non-Hispanic White, non-Hispanic Black, Hispanic, Asian-Pacific Islander, other races/ethnicities Early Childhood Longitudinal Study, Birth Cohort (ECLS-B)	Longitudinal (2917)	To determine impact of maternal depression on future household food insecurity in low-income households with young children.	USDA HFSSM	CES-D 12 item Authors note that the short form has been previously validated.	Depressive symptoms	Maternal and household characteristics including race/ethnicity, age, marital status, employment, education, mothers' foreign-born status, household income, and maternal self-reported health status.	Multivariable analyses: Maternal depression at baseline (9 months) was associated with food insecurity at follow-up (24 months) (aOR 1.50, 95% CI 1.06–2.12). Mothers who reported depressive symptoms and received WIC at baseline were more likely (aOR 1.59, 95% CI 1.15–2.21) to experience food insecurity at follow-up.

Table A1. *Cont.*

Reference	Sample (Participants (Age), Setting, Race/Ethnicity, Data Source)	Study Design (Sample Size)	Purpose	Food Security Measure	Mental Health Measure	Mental Health States/Conditions	Covariates Considered	Analytic Approach and Key Findings
Hanson et al. 2012 [15]	Low income, rural mothers (mean age, 30 years) in US, White and non-White races/ethnicities Rural Low-Income Families: Monitoring Their Well-being and Functioning in the Context of Welfare Reform	Longitudinal (225)	Examine food insecurity and various risk factors, including human capital, social support, and financial situation, among rural low-income families with children.	USDA HFSSM	CES-D 20-item	Depressive symptoms	Education, 3 or more chronic health conditions, food and financial skills, high support for parenting, home ownership at baseline, employment, housing assistance, participation in SNAP assistance, health insurance	Multivariable analyses: Compared to women having no years at risk for depression, women classified as at risk for depression for 2 consecutive years had 4.28 times greater odds of experiencing persistent versus no food insecurity ($p < 0.01$), and 3.65 times greater odds to experience persistent versus discontinuous food insecurity ($p < 0.05$).
Hernandez et al. 2014 [26]	Low-income, urban, unmarried mothers (mean age, 28 years) of newborn children recruited from 75 birth hospitals in 20 US cities, White, African American, Hispanic, and other races/ethnicities Fragile Families and Child Well-being Study	Longitudinal (1690)	Examine association between intimate partner violence, depression, and household food insecurity	USDA HFSSM	CIDI short form	Clinical diagnosis of depression; depressive symptoms	Mothers' age, race/ethnicity, education, employment, relationship status, household income, number of children, baseline food security	Multivariable analyses: Mothers reporting depression were twice as likely to be food-insecure two years later compared to mothers who did not report depression (aOR 2.03, 95% CI 1.45–2.84). The relationship between intimate partner violence and food insecurity among women was mediated by depression ($z = 2.89$, $p < 0.01$).
Lent et al. 2009 [45]	Rural, low-income mothers (18+ years), recruited through local educators, WIC and Even Start programs in New York, US, majority White. Rural Families Speak: Tracking the Well-Being and Functioning of Rural Families in the Context of Welfare Policies Study	Longitudinal (mixed methods) (29)	Examine the temporal/causal relationship and potential mechanisms between mental health conditions such as depression and household food insecurity	USDA HFSSM	CES-D 20-item, SF-36 Health Survey (mental health scales: Vitality, Social Functioning, Role Emotional, Mental Health)	Depressive symptoms	Not applicable	Unadjusted analyses: High levels of depressive symptoms (according to the CES-D) at wave 2 were correlated with remaining food-insecure at wave 3 ($p = 0.009$); reverse relationship not significant. Unhealthy scores on the mental health scores at wave 2 were also associated with remaining food-insecure at wave 3 ($p = 0.01$). Qualitative analyses suggest that poor mental health contributes to persistence of food insecurity by limiting employment.

Table A1. *Cont.*

Reference	Sample (Participants (Age), Setting, Race/Ethnicity, Data Source)	Study Design (Sample Size)	Purpose	Food Security Measure	Mental Health Measure	Mental Health States/Conditions	Covariates Considered	Analytic Approach and Key Findings
Huddleston-Casasin et al. 2009 [55]	Rural mothers (mean age, 30 years) recruited from programs serving low-income populations in 17 US states, included White, African American, Latina, and other races/ethnicities NC-223, Rural Families Speak Study	Longitudinal (413)	Examine direction of the relationship between household food insecurity and depression over three annual waves of data	USDA HFSSM	CES-D 20-item Authors note that reliability in this sample matched that documented for the general population	Depressive symptoms	Age, ethnicity, household income, marital status, education	Structural equation modeling (using data for 413 women, with sensitivity analysis with 184 women who had depression data for three waves): A bidirectional relationship between food insecurity and depression was observed. (χ^2/df = 1.835, RMSEA = 0.068, CFI = 0.989) was observed.
Laraia et al. 2015 [27]	Pregnant women (16+ years), US, included White, Black, other races/ethnicities Pregnancy, Infection, and Nutrition (PIN) Postpartum study, recruited from University of North Carolina Hospitals and private clinics	Longitudinal (526)	To examine relationship between food insecurity and perceived stress, disordered eating, dietary intake, and postpartum weight status	USDA HFSSM, 18 items (between 27 and 30 weeks' gestation) and 6-item short form (12 months postpartum)	Cohen's Perceived Stress Scale (PSS) 10-item, Eating Attitude Test (EAT) 26 item Authors note that Cohen's Perceived Stress has been validated in pregnant women	Perceived stress, disordered eating	Maternal race, age, marital status, education, parity, physical activity, smoking during pregnancy and postpartum, breastfeeding postpartum, poverty level	Multivariable analyses: Women living in food-insecure households during pregnancy had higher levels of perceived stress (β = 3.36, 95% CI 0.79–5.92) and higher scores for disordered eating (β = 1.95, 95% CI 0.25–4.16) at 3 months postpartum and higher levels of perceived stress (β = 3.67, 95% CI 0.94–6.41) at 12 months postpartum compared to those living in food-secure households during pregnancy. Women who experienced any level of household food insecurity during the postpartum period had higher perceived stress (β = 6.12, 95% CI 3.86–8.38), and higher scores for disordered eating (β = 1.79, 95% CI 0.03–3.62) compared to women in food-secure households.

Table A1. *Cont.*

Cross-sectional analyses

Reference	Sample (Participants (Age), Setting, Race/Ethnicity, Data Source)	Study Design (Sample Size)	Purpose	Food Security Measure	Mental Health Measure	Mental Health States/Conditions	Covariates Considered	Analytic Approach and Key Findings
Casey et al. 2004 [54]	Female caregivers (age not specified), US, women of African American, White, and Hispanic race/ethnicity Children's Sentinel Nutrition Assessment Program (C-SNAP), recruited from medical centers in several large US cities	Cross-sectional (5306)	Examine nature of the relationship between depression, food insecurity, and loss of social assistance and its impact on child health	USDA HFSSM	Kemper 3-item screen Authors note sensitivity of 100%, specificity of 88%, and positive predictive value of 66% compared to an 8-item screening instrument	Maternal depressive symptoms	Study site location, race, insurance type, education, and low birth weight	Multivariable analysis: Mothers experiencing food insecurity had greater odds of positive depression screen compared to those from food secure households (aOR 2.69, 95% CI 2.33–3.11). Mothers experiencing a decrease or sanction in food stamp status had increased odds of reporting a positive depression screen, compared to those with no decrease in food stamp status (aOR 1.26, 95% CI 0.97–1.65 and aOR 1.56 95% CI 1.06–2.30, respectively).
Chilton et al. 2013 [28]	Mothers (mean age, 26.7 years) in Philadelphia, US, African American, White, Hispanic races/ethnicities Recruited from public assistance programs through the Children's Health Watch study	Cross-sectional (mixed methods) (44)	Explore aspects of exposure to violence related to food insecurity among lone mother households.	USDA HFSSM	Kemper 3-item screen	Maternal depressive symptoms	Not applicable	Descriptive estimates: A higher proportion of mothers living with very low food security reported depressive symptoms (71%) compared to those with low food security (53%) and food-secure (17%) mothers. Women living with very low food security (53%) were more likely to have experienced life-changing violence in childhood compared to those with low food security (33%) and food secure (33%) mothers.
McCurdy et al. 2015 [29]	Low-income mothers (mean age, 30.1 years) and children recruited from 7 preschools in low-income urban neighborhoods in the US, included Hispanic and non-Hispanic races/ethnicities	Cross-sectional (166)	To determine correlates of weight, including food security, among low-income, ethnically diverse mothers and examine role of mental health	USDA HFSSM	CES-D 20-item Authors note high internal consistency for the measure and note acceptable internal reliability in this sample	Depressive symptoms	Not applicable	Bivariate analyses: Mothers living in food-insecure households had more depressive symptoms compared to food-secure mothers (t = 2.26, p < 0.02).

Table A1. *Cont.*

Reference	Sample (Participants (Age), Setting, Race/Ethnicity, Data Source)	Study Design (Sample Size)	Purpose	Food Security Measure	Mental Health Measure	Mental Health States/Conditions	Covariates Considered	Analytic Approach and Key Findings
Sun et al. 2016 [30]	Mothers (mean age, 24 years) of young children (aged < 4 years), US, non-Hispanic White, non-Hispanic Black, Hispanic, other races/ethnicities, recruited from Philadelphia hospitals.	Cross-sectional (1255)	To examine association between adverse childhood experiences among mothers and household and child food insecurity determine associations with depressive symptoms	USDA HFSSM	Kemper 3-Item Screen, ACEs scale for Adverse Childhood Experiences Authors note that the Kemper 3-item is validated as a proxy for a longer screener with 100% sensitivity, 88% specificity, and 66% positive predictive value, and ACEs scale has been validated and shown to have good test-retest reliability.	Depressive symptoms, adverse childhood experiences, such as abuse, neglect, and household dysfunction	Caregiver's age and self-rated health, caregiver's participation in nutrition programs, race/ethnicity, marital status, employment, education, and child's health insurance,	Depressive symptoms were reported among 18.4% of women in food-secure households, 48.6% of those in households with low food security, and 54.4% of those in households with very low food security ($p < 0.01$). Multivariable analyses: Mothers who reported depressive symptoms and 4+ adverse childhood experiences were 2.3 times (95% CI 1.0–5.3) as likely to report low food security, 6.6 times (95% CI 2.1–20.5) as likely to report indications of very low food security compared to those reporting depressive symptoms but no adverse childhood experiences. In addition, mothers who reported depressive symptoms and 4+ adverse childhood experiences were 17.6 times (95% CI 7.3–42.6) as likely to report child food insecurity compared to those who reported no depressive symptoms and no adverse childhood experiences.
Trapp et al. 2015 [31]	Low-income children (2–4 years) and **mothers** (18+ years), US, Hispanic, African-American races/ethnicities Steps to Growing Up Health study, primary care-based intervention	Cross-sectional (222)	Examine relationship between food security, diet, and weight status among urban preschool children, and examine whether maternal depression and stress acts as a mediator	USDA HFSSM	PHQ-2, Cohen's Perceived Stress Scale 4-item subset (PSS-4) Authors note that the PHQ-2 has good validity, and identified the sensitivity and specificity of the cutoff used for risk for major depression	Depressive symptoms and perceived stress	Household size, primary home language, marital status, employment, household income	Bivariate analyses: Mothers living in food-insecure households were more likely to report depressive symptoms compared to food-secure mothers (27% vs. 9%; $p < 0.001$), but perceived stress scores were not different between food-insecure and food-secure mothers ($p = 0.5$).

Table A1. *Cont.*

Reference	Sample (Participants (Age), Setting, Race/Ethnicity, Data Source)	Study Design (Sample Size)	Purpose	Food Security Measure	Mental Health Measure	Mental Health States/Conditions	Covariates Considered	Analytic Approach and Key Findings
Laraia et al. 2006 [56]	Low-income pregnant women (mean age, 29 years), US, included African American, White, and other races/ethnicities Pregnancy, Infection, and Nutrition (PIN) cohort study, recruited from University of North Carolina Hospitals and private clinics	Cross-sectional (606)	Examine prevalence and determinants of food insecurity among pregnant women from medium- and low-income women	USDA HFSSM	Cohen's Perceived Stress Scale 14-item, Spielberger's Trait Anxiety Inventory 20-item, CES-D 20-item, Rosenberg's Self Esteem Scale 10-item, Pearlin's Mastery Scale 7-item, Levenson's IPC Locus of Control 24-item Authors note stability and internal consistency of measures	Perceived stress, anxiety, depressive symptoms, self-esteem, mastery, locus of control	Mother's age, number of children, household income, education, race, marital status	Multivariable analyses: Perceived stress (aOR 2.24, 95% CI 1.63–3.08), trait anxiety (aOR 2.14, 95% CI 1.55–2.96), depressive symptoms (aOR 1.87, 95% CI 1.40–2.51), and feeling that ones' destiny is up to chance (aOR 1.67, 95% CI 1.20–2.32) were positively associated with household food insecurity. Women living in food-insecure households were less likely to report feelings of mastery over their lives (aOR 0.49, 95% CI 0.35–0.68) and high self-esteem (aOR 0.52, 95% CI 0.38–0.69).
Muldoon et al. 2013 [32]	Adults (18–64 years), Canada 2007–2008 Canadian Community Health Survey	Cross-sectional (sample subset of 5588 reporting indications of food insecurity in the past year)	Examine rates of mental illness among Canadian adults who lived in food-insecure households with and without hunger	USDA HFSSM (Health Canada coding)	Self-reported diagnosis of chronic health conditions diagnosed by a health professional	Clinical diagnoses of mood or anxiety disorders	Education, age, single parent household status, immigrant status	Multivariable analyses: Females experiencing food insecurity with hunger had greater odds (aOR 1.89, 95% CI 1.62–2.20) of reporting a depression diagnosis compared to women who did not report food insecurity with hunger.
Tarasuk et al. 2013 [16]	Adults (18–64 years), Canada 2007–2008 Canadian Community Health Survey	Cross-sectional (77,053)	Examine whether chronic physical and mental conditions health conditions are associated with household food insecurity	USDA HFSSM (Health Canada coding)	Self-reported presence of chronic health conditions diagnosed by a health professional	Clinical diagnoses of mood or anxiety disorders	Age, sex, province, education, household type, median household income, main source of household income, and home ownership	Multivariable analysis: Self-reported diagnoses of 3 or more chronic physical and mental health conditions raised the odds of a woman experiencing severe food insecurity (aOR 2.15, 95% CI 1.50–3.10) compared to fewer or no chronic conditions Among women in food-secure households, 11.6% reported mood or anxiety disorders; among those in marginally food-secure, moderately food-insecure, and severely food-insecure households, the prevalences were 20.3%,

Table A1. *Cont.*

Abbreviated/adapted versions of Household Food Security Survey Module (HFSSM)

Longitudinal analyses

Reference	Sample (Participants (Age), Setting, Race/Ethnicity, Data Source)	Study Design (Sample Size)	Purpose	Food Security Measure	Mental Health Measure	Mental Health States/Conditions	Covariates Considered	Analytic Approach and Key Findings
Melchior et al. 2009 [44]	**Mothers of twins** (average 35.5 years) from England and Wales, Britain, included White and non-White races/ethnicities. Environmental Risk Study	Longitudinal (1116)	Examine the association between food insecurity and maternal depression, psychosis spectrum disorder, alcohol or drug abuse, and intimate partner violence	USDA HFSSM, 7-item short form	Diagnostic Interview Schedule (DIS)	Depressive symptoms, psychotic symptoms	Mother's age, income, ethnicity, marital status, household size, mother's employment, mother's reading ability	Multivariable analyses: Food insecurity increased the odds of depression (OR 2.12, 95% CI 1.61–4.93), intimate partner violence (OR 2.36, 95% CI 1.18–4.73), and psychosis (OR 4.01, 95% CI 2.03–7.94) among women two years later. Food insecurity was associated with mental illness comorbidity in mothers—29% of food-insecure mothers had experienced mental health problems or intimate partner violence.
Sidebottom et al. 2014 [33]	**Pregnant women** (mean age, 22 years) recruited from Health Centres in Minneapolis and St. Paul, US, included African American, American Indian, Asian/Pacific Islander, Hispanic (any race), White, and bi/multiracial women Data from the Twin Cities Healthy Start Program	Longitudinal (prenatal and postpartum assessments) (594)	Examine correlates of depression in pregnancy and postpartum period	USDA HFSSM, 4-item subset	PHQ-9 with modification of the item measuring psychomotor issues (split into 2 questions but scored as one) Authors noted sensitivity of 77%, specificity of 94%, and positive predictive value of 59% in primary care populations, with higher values in populations with a high prevalence of depressive disorder	Depressive symptoms	Age, race/ethnicity, foreign-born, lack of social support, abuse of any kind, child protection involvement, living with child's father, drug, alcohol and cigarette use, lack of phone access, and housing instability	Multivariable analyses: Compared to women who had low depressive symptom levels in both the prenatal and postpartum periods, the odds of elevated depressive symptoms prenatally were higher (aOR 2.44, 95% CI 1.43–4.16) among those with low levels of food security. Food security and depressive symptoms in the postpartum period were not related.

Table A1. *Cont.*

Cross-sectional analyses

Reference	Sample (Participants (Age), Setting, Race/Ethnicity, Data Source)	Study Design (Sample Size)	Purpose	Food Security Measure	Mental Health Measure	Mental Health States/Conditions	Covariates Considered	Analytic Approach and Key Findings
Whitaker et al. 2006 [59]	Mothers (18+ years) of 3-year old children, recruited from 75 birth hospitals in 20 US cities. Included White, African American, Hispanic, other races/ethnicities Fragile Families and Child Wellbeing Study	Cross-sectional (2870)	Examine if food security is associated with prevalence of depression and anxiety in mothers and behavior problems in children	USDA HFSSM, 10 adult-referenced items	CIDI short form administered 3 years after child's birth, modified cut-off for a major depressive episode (MDE) based on symptoms of anhedonia	Clinical diagnosis of a MDE or generalized anxiety disorder (GAD) in the prior 12 months	Mother's education, race/ethnicity, relationship status, employment in previous year, binge drinking, illicit drug use, global health, prenatal smoking, prenatal physical domestic violence, household income/poverty ratio, number of children, non-food related material hardship, and whether father was ever in jail	Multivariable analyses: Compared to fully food-secure mothers, experiencing marginal food insecurity increased the odds of experiencing an MDE or GAD (aOR 1.4, 95% CI 1.1–1.8; and aOR 1.7, 95% CI 1.0–2.7, respectively). Compared to fully food-secure mothers, experiencing food insecurity increased the odds of experiencing an MDE or GAD (aOR 2.2, 95% CI 1.6–2.9; and aOR 2.3, 95% CI 1.5–3.6 respectively). Mothers experiencing food insecurity twice as likely to also experience either MDE or GAD compared to food-secure mothers (aOR 2.2, 95% CI 1.6–2.9).
Laraia et al. 2009 [58]	African American, first-time mothers (18–35 years) recruited from Special Supplemental Nutrition Program for Women, Children, and Infants (WIC) clinics in North Carolina, US Infant Care, Feeding, and Risk of Obesity observational study	Cross-sectional analysis of longitudinal study, focused on 3-month postpartum baseline data (206)	Identify maternal and household correlates of food insecurity among African-American mothers	USDA HFSSM, 6-item short form	CES-D, Rosenberg Self-Esteem Scale	Depressive symptoms and self-esteem	Maternal age, education, work status, depression score, and self-esteem, as well as household composition (presence of father, grandmother and household size)	Bivariate analyses: Women living in food-insecure households had significantly higher scores on the depressive scale compared to food-secure women (p < 0.05). Multivariable analyses: Depressive symptoms were associated with marginal food security and food insecurity (aRRR * 1.04, 95% CI 1.00–1.08 and aRRR * 1.10, 95% CI 1.04–1.16, respectively). Self-esteem scores were negatively associated with risk for marginal food security and food insecurity (aRRR * 0.91, 95% CI 0.84–0.98, and aRRR * 0.89, 95% CI 0.79–0.99, respectively) * aRRR = adjusted Relative Risk Ratio.

Table A1. *Cont.*

Reference	Sample (Participants (Age), Setting, Race/Ethnicity, Data Source)	Study Design (Sample Size)	Purpose	Food Security Measure	Mental Health Measure	Mental Health States/Conditions	Covariates Considered	Analytic Approach and Key Findings
Mathews et al. 2010 [34]	Mothers (<25 years) recruited from the Special Supplemental Nutrition Program for Women, Infants, and Children (WIC) clinics in Butte County, California, US, included White, non-White races/ethnicities	Cross-sectional (155)	Evaluate the prevalence of and associations between food insecurity and health status among women participating in WIC	USDA HFSSM, 6-item short form	SF-12 Health Survey Authors noted that the SF-12 has been validated previously	General mental (and physical) health symptoms	Diet choice score, income, ethnicity, age, education	Bivariate analyses: Women experiencing low or very low food insecurity had significantly lower mental health scores, indicating more mental health symptoms compared to food-secure women ($p < 0.001$). The correlation between food insecurity and mental health scores indicates that as women's food security increased, mental health also increases. Multivariable analyses: The likelihood of having a good mental health score was lower (OR 0.41, 95% CI 0.16–0.73) among those in food-insecure versus those in food-secure households.
Ajrouch et al. 2010 [35]	Female African-American caregivers (mean age, 30.8 years) of young children recruited from high-poverty census tracts in Detroit, US Detroit Centre for Research on Oral Health Disparities.	Cross-sectional (multiple waves of data collection, relevant variables were assessed in wave 2) (736)	Explore link between situational stressors, including food insufficiency, and psychological distress, and examine social support as a potential mediator	USDA HFSSM, 3-item subset (referred to as food insufficiency) Cronbach's alpha reported as 0.79	CES-D 20-item Authors noted high internal reliability in this sample	Depressive symptoms	Age, self-rated health, and education level	Multivariable analyses: Higher food insufficiency associated with higher depressive symptoms (referred to as psychological distress) ($\beta = 2.88$, $p < 0.001$). At high levels of stress, social support was not a mediator of this relationship.
Hromi-Fielder et al. 2011 [36]	Low income, pregnant Latina women (mean age, 25 years), recruited from local agencies and programs in Hartford, Connecticut, US.	Cross-sectional (135)	Assess relationship between household food insecurity and prenatal depressive symptoms	USDA HFSSM, 15-item subset adapted version for pregnant Latinas Authors note that the adapted version was validated for this population	CES-D 20-item Authors note that the CES-D has been validated with multi-ethnic samples, including Mexican-Americans	Prenatal depressive symptoms	Parity, heartburn during pregnancy, self-reported health during pregnancy, history of depression, Latina subgroup, acculturation	Multivariable analyses: Women experiencing food insecurity were more likely to report high levels of prenatal depressive symptoms compared to those who were food secure (aOR 2.59, 95% CI 1.03–6.52).

Table A1. *Cont.*

Reference	Sample (Participants (Age), Setting, Race/Ethnicity, Data Source)	Study Design (Sample Size)	Purpose	Food Security Measure	Mental Health Measure	Mental Health States/Conditions	Covariates Considered	Analytic Approach and Key Findings
Harrison et al. 2008 [60]	Pregnant women in Minneapolis and St. Paul, US, included African American, Asian/Pacific Islander, Hispanic, American Indian, White, bi/multiracial races/ethnicities. recruited from Federally Qualified Health Centres Feasibility study associated with Twin Cities Healthy Start Program	Cross-sectional (1386)	Examine the prevalence, co-occurrence, and inter-correlations of self-reported psychosocial risk factors, including food insecurity.	USDA HFSSM, 4-item subset	PHQ-9, intimate partner violence items, 8 items from the Maternal Social Support Index Authors note high levels of internal reliability, test-retest reliability, sensitivity, and specificity for PHQ-9	Depressive symptoms	Not applicable	Bivariate analyses: Depressive symptoms ($r = 0.267$), social support ($r = 0.194$), and intimate partner violence ($r = 0.173$) were significantly correlated ($p \leq 0.0001$) with household food insecurity.
Martin et al. 2016 [17]	Adults (18–75 years), Canada Data from the 2009–2010 Canadian Community Health Survey	Cross-sectional (100,401)	To examine the co-occurrence of food insecurity and mental illness across varying levels of stress and community belonging	USDA HFSSM, 10 adult-referenced items (Health Canada coding)	Self-reported diagnosis of a mood or anxiety disorder, subsample ($n = 47,942$) completed CIDI short form, one item for each of perceived stress and community belonging	Clinical diagnosis of a mood disorder such as depression, bipolar disorder, mania, or dysthymia; or an anxiety disorder such as phobia, obsessive-compulsive disorder, or panic disorder. Past 12 months of major depression from CIDI short form.	Age, marital status, children in house, household income, education, unemployment, and self-perceived physical health, as well as overall stress level and community belonging.	Multivariable analyses: Women living in severely food-insecure households had 18.4% (95% CI 16.7–20.1) greater adjusted prevalence of a mental disorder compared to those living in food-secure households. The prevalence of women reporting high levels of stress increased with worsening food security. Greater proportions of severely food-insecure women reported low community belonging compared to more food-secure women. Interaction between community belonging, food insecurity, and perceived stress not significant.

Table A1. *Cont.*

Reference	Sample (Participants (Age), Setting, Race/Ethnicity, Data Source)	Study Design (Sample Size)	Purpose	Food Security Measure	Mental Health Measure	Mental Health States/Conditions	Covariates Considered	Analytic Approach and Key Findings
Dressler et al. 2015 [37]	Low-income women (18–64 years) recruited from homeless shelters, food pantries, libraries, soup kitchens, and community centers, US, included African American, White, Native American women	Cross-sectional (330)	Examine depression and its relationship with food insecurity, weight status, emotional eating, and dietary intake among low-income women	USDA HFSSM, 6-item short form	CES-D 20-item, emotional eating questions developed using validated questionnaires Authors note that the CES-D is valid and reliable and note the internal consistency in the sample for both the CES-D and the emotional eating questions	Symptoms of depression and emotional eating	Not applicable	Bivariate analyses: Women categorized as depressed had higher food insecurity scores compared to women who were not depressed (3.2 vs. 1.9, $p < 0.05$). Depression and emotional eating were also associated.
Kaiser et al. 2007 [57]	Women (18+ years) living in California, US, included White, African American, Hispanic/Latino, and other races/ethnicities. 2004 California Women's Health Survey	Cross-sectional (4037)	Identify factors associated with food insecurity	USDA HFSSM, 6-item subset, modified to refer to respondent and not to other adults in household	Indicators of mental or emotional problems	Mental, (physical), or emotional problems that interfere with daily life, feeling depressed or sad, and feeling overwhelmed	Income as a proportion of the federal poverty ratio	Multivariable analyses: Higher food insecurity was associated with feeling depressed or sad for 2+ days in the prior month (aOR 1.61, 95% CI 1.28–2.02), feeling overwhelmed in past 30 days (aOR 3.10, 95% CI 2.49–3.85), and reporting that physical or mental health conditions interfered with normal activities in past 30 days (aOR 1.81, 95% CI 1.45–2.27).
Peterman et al. 2013 [38]	Cambodian women (30–65 years) recruited from clients of the Cambodian Mutual Assurance Association of Lowell, Massachusetts, US Cambodian Community Health Program 2010	Cross-sectional (150)	Examine post-immigration experiences with food, food security status, and correlates among refugee women	USDA HFSSM, 6-item short form	Harvard Program in Refugee Trauma's depression scale; 14 items, previously translated and validated for use in Cambodian refugee populations	Clinical diagnosis of depression	Marital status, receipt of food stamps, income to poverty ratio, acculturation, age	Multivariable analyses: Women experiencing marginal/low/very low food security were more likely (aOR 3.73, 95% CI 1.26–11.05) to be classified as depressed compared to those in food-secure households.

Table A1. *Cont.*

Reference	Sample (Participants (Age), Setting, Race/Ethnicity, Data Source)	Study Design (Sample Size)	Purpose	Food Security Measure	Mental Health Measure	Mental Health States/Conditions	Covariates Considered	Analytic Approach and Key Findings
Sharpe et al. 2016 [39]	Low-income women (25–51 years) recruited from 18 census tracts in which 25% or more of residents had below-poverty income in South Carolina, US, mainly African-American Sisters Taking Action for Real Success (STARS) trial	Cross-sectional (202)	Examine whether on diet quality and psychosocial and behavioral factors are associated with household food security	USDA HFSSM, 6-item short form	CES-D 10 item, emotional eating subscale of the Eating Behavior Patterns Questionnaire Authors noted that the CESD-10 has been validated and that the Eating Behavior Patterns Questionnaire has been shown to have acceptable internal consistency and construct validity in African-American women; authors also identified Cronbach's alphas for both measures in the study sample	Symptoms of depression and emotional eating	Not applicable	Bivariate analyses: Women experiencing food insecurity had significantly higher scores for depressive symptoms (indicating more symptoms) compared to women living in food-secure households (mean score 10.9 (SD 6.1) vs. 8.3 (SD 5.0), t = 3.36, $p < 0.001$). Women experiencing food insecurity had significantly lower emotional eating scores (indicating higher levels of emotional eating) compared to women living in food-secure households (mean score 10.2 (SD 3.1) vs. 11.4 (SD 3.8), t = 2.45, $p < 0.02$).
Davey-Rothwell et al. 2014 [40]	Low-income women (18–55 years) at risk for HIV, recruited through street outreach and public advertisements in the US, majority African-American women Data from the CHAT study	Cross-sectional (based on 6-month visit) (443)	Explore food insecurity among drug-using and non-drug-using women and examine the relationship between depression and food insecurity	USDA HFSSM, 4-item subset Authors noted acceptable internal consistency in this sample	CES-D 20-item Authors noted high internal consistency in this sample	Depressive symptoms	Age, race, income, receipt of food stamps	Multivariable analyses: Drug-users were 2.71 times (aOR, 95% CI 1.51–4.88), and non-drug-users were 5.9 times (aOR, 95% CI 2.80–12.45) more likely to experience depression if they were food insecure compared to food secure.

Table A1. *Cont.*

Reference	Sample (Participants (Age), Setting, Race/Ethnicity, Data Source)	Study Design (Sample Size)	Purpose	Food Security Measure	Mental Health Measure	Mental Health States/Conditions	Covariates Considered	Analytic Approach and Key Findings

Radimer–Cornell Scale

Cross-sectional analyses

| Sharkey et al. 2011 [41] | Urban and rural women (18+ years) living in Brazos Valley, Texas, US, included White and non-White races/ethnicities Brazos Valley Health Status Assessment | Cross-sectional (1367) | Examine health status, mental distress, and household food insecurity among urban and rural women | Radimer–Cornell Scale, first item focused on food deprivation (food we bought did not last and we did not have enough money to buy more) was used to determine presence of household food insecurity Authors noted that the Scale has been shown to be valid for non-white participants | Centre for Disease Control (CDC) and the Behavioral Risk Factor Surveillance Systems (BRFSS) questionnaire to assess health-related quality of life (perceived mental—and general and physical—well-being —thinking about your mental health, which includes stress, depression, and problems with emotions, for how many days during the past 30 days was your mental health not good?) Authors noted that the measures have been shown to be valid for non-white populations | Perceived mental health (stress, depression, problems with emotions), referred to as frequent mental distress | Age, race, education, annual household income, employment, rural vs. urban geographic location | Multivariable analyses: Women experiencing food insecurity in the last 30 days were more likely to frequently experience mental distress compared to food-secure women (aOR 2.25, 95% CI 1.59–3.18). |

Table A1. *Cont.*

Reference	Sample (Participants (Age), Setting, Race/Ethnicity, Data Source)	Study Design (Sample Size)	Purpose	Food Security Measure	Mental Health Measure	Mental Health States/Conditions	Covariates Considered	Analytic Approach and Key Findings
				Community Childhood Hunger Identification Project (CCHIP) measure				
				Cross-sectional analyses				
Wehler et al. 2004 [52]	Homeless and housed women (mean age, 28 years) recruited from Worcester's homeless shelters and welfare hostels and the Department of Public Welfare office, US; included White, African American, Hispanic, and other races/ethnicities. Worcester Family Research Project	Cross-sectional (354)	Examine factors associated with adult or child hunger among low-income housed and homeless female-headed families	CCHIP, 7 items querying adult and child hunger Authors noted high level of internal consistency and factor analysis indicated a single-factor solution	Structured Clinical Interview for Diagnostic Statistical Manual (DSM-III-R non-patient edition), Life Experiences Survey	Clinical diagnosis of substance use, depression, posttraumatic stress disorder (PTSD), major life events in adulthood (e.g., violence)	Age, ethnicity, housing status, marital status, acculturation, parenting status, parent substance abuse, foster care status, number and age of children, income, psychological factors (coping and parental hassles), social service utilization, social network size	Exploratory analytic approach identified factors differentiating families with child hunger from those with no hunger, these did not include the mental health factors. Multivariable analyses: The experience of sexual abuse in childhood increased the odds of adult hunger (aOR: 4.23, 95% CI 2.28–7.82); intimate partner violence in adulthood and a PTSD diagnosis appeared to be mediators of the childhood sexual abuse-current hunger association. Financial support from a sibling reduced the odds of experiencing food insecurity.
				NHANES-III food insufficiency indicators				
				Longitudinal analyses				
Heflin et al. 2005 [62]	Mothers (18–54 years) receiving public assistance in urban Michigan, US; included African American, non-Hispanic White races/ethnicities. Women's Employment Study	Longitudinal (753)	Examine effect of food insecurity on the mental health status of welfare recipients over a 3-year period	NHANES-III food insufficiency question Authors noted that this measure is widely accepted as a valid measure of food insufficiency	CIDI short form, Pearlin Mastery Scale 7 item	Clinical diagnosis of depression, mastery (degree to which individuals perceive themselves to be in control of their own lives)	Household size, marital status, household income, poverty-related stressful life circumstances, neighborhood hazards, domestic violence, experiences of discrimination based on race and gender	Multivariable fixed effects models: Changes in food insecurity significantly predict changes in major depression status after adjusting for changes in household composition and socio-environmental stressors ($\beta = 0.75$, SE 0.24, $p < 0.01$). No association observed between changes in food insufficiency status and changes in mastery.

Table A1. *Cont.*

Reference	Sample (Participants (Age), Setting, Race/Ethnicity, Data Source)	Study Design (Sample Size)	Purpose	Food Security Measure	Mental Health Measure	Mental Health States/Conditions	Covariates Considered	Analytic Approach and Key Findings
Cross-sectional analyses								
Siefert et al. 2001 [64]	Single women receiving welfare (mean age, 28 years) living in urban Michigan, US, included African-American, White women Women's Employment Study	Cross-sectional (724)	Examine relationship between food insufficiency and physical and mental health among low-income women	NHANES-III food insufficiency question Authors noted that this measure is widely accepted as a valid measure of food insufficiency	CIDI short form Authors noted that acceptable test-retest reliability and clinical validity have been observed	Clinical diagnosis of major depressive disorder and generalized anxiety disorder	Self-rated health, physical limitations, age, number of children in the household, education level, poverty level, employment, poverty-related stressful life events and conditions	Multivariable analyses: Food insufficiency significantly predicted major depressive disorder (aOR 2.21, 95% CI 1.48–3.29). The association between food insufficiency and generalized anxiety disorder, adjusted for covariates, was not significant.
Siefert et al. 2007 [63]	African-American mothers (mean age, 28 years) recruited from 39 high-poverty census areas in Detroit, US Detroit Center for Research on Oral Health Disparities	Cross-sectional (multiple waves of data collection, relevant variables were assessed in wave 1) (824)	Determine correlates of depressive symptoms among low-income mothers	NHANES-III food insufficiency questionAuthors noted that this measure is widely accepted as a valid measure of food insufficiency	CES-D, 20-item Authors noted that the CES-D is a reliable and well-validated sale, with standard scoring widely used in research, four-factor structure found in the general population has also been found in African-Americans with low socioeconomic status	Depressive symptoms	Living in poorly maintained housing, not being employed, experiences of everyday discrimination, instrumental and emotional social support, age, education, household size, number of children <18 years of age, income	Bivariate analyses: Mothers with depressive symptoms more likely to report household food insufficiency (14.5%) compared to women without depressive symptoms (6%). Multivariable analyses: In models adjusted for income and education, living in a food-insufficient household was associated with 2.5 greater odds (95% CI 1.25–4.98) of maternal depressive symptoms. Instrumental social support was a protective factor.
Other brief measures								
Cross-sectional analyses								
Birmingham et al. 2011 [42]	Mothers of newborns (mean age, 25 years), US, included African American, Hispanic, White, Asian, other races/ethnicities, recruited from urban pediatric emergency departments	Cross-sectional (195)	To examine the performance of the Edinburgh Postpartum Depression Scale (EPDS) for screening patients in emergency departments, and examine correlates of postpartum depression	2 items querying worry about the food supply and inability to eat the way you should due to lack of money	EPDS 3-item short form	Postpartum depressive symptoms	Maternal age, ethnicity, education, marital status, employment, maternal health problems, health insurance, household income, household size, father's presence in the home, social support, infant health and health insurance,	Multivariable analyses: Having concerns about food increased odds (aOR 5.5, 95% CI 2.2–13.5) of postpartum depression.

Table A1. *Cont.*

Reference	Sample (Participants (Age), Setting, Race/Ethnicity, Data Source)	Study Design (Sample Size)	Purpose	Food Security Measure	Mental Health Measure	Mental Health States/Conditions	Covariates Considered	Analytic Approach and Key Findings
Carter et al. 2011 [43]	General population (15+ years) in New Zealand, included NZ/European, Maori, Pacific, Asian, and other groups. New Zealand Survey of Families, Income, and Employment, 2002–2010	Cross-sectional (18,090)	Examine association between food insecurity and psychological distress	Food security items from measure of individual deprivation (NZiDep): 3 items querying use of food banks and food compromises due to lack of money for food in last 12 months	Kessler-10 scale	Symptoms of psychological distress	Age, ethnicity, legal marital status, family composition, household income, employment, highest level of education, individual-level deprivation	Multivariable analyses: Women who experienced food insecurity were more likely to report moderate to high levels of psychological distress (OR 2.1, 95% CI 1.8–2.4).
Klesges et al. 2001 [68]	Disabled women (65+ years) living in the community in Baltimore, US, primarily White women Women's Health and Aging Study	Cross-sectional (1001)	Examine prevalence and correlates of financial difficulty acquiring food	Single item, self-perception of food sufficiency "How often does it happen that you (and your husband) do not have enough money to afford the kind of food you should have?" Authors note that such single-item measures have shown validity in discriminating energy intake differences, but have poor sensitivity and underestimate prevalence	Geriatric Depression Scale (GDS),Hopkins Symptom Checklist subscale for anxiety, 20-item perceived quality of life scale	Symptoms of depression, anxiety, quality of life	Age, marital status, and number of household members	Multivariable analyses: In non-white women, depression was associated with financial difficulty accessing food (aOR 1.13, 95% CI 1.04–1.22). This association not significant among white women after adjusting for covariates.
Sharkey et al. 2003 [69]	Women (60+ years) who are homebound (as a result of disability, illness, or isolation), recruited from meal delivery programs in North Carolina, US, included African-American and White women Nutrition and Function Study (NAFS)	Cross-sectional (279)	Examine food sufficiency and association with dietary intake and burden of multiple diseases	Four items adapted from a national nutrition evaluation survey, 2 situations related to lack of food, 2 related to making trade-offs between food and other necessities Authors noted that the items were previously used in a national evaluation of elderly nutrition programs	Geriatric Depression Scale (GDS) 15-item short form	Depressive symptoms	Not applicable	Bivariate analyses: Women experiencing food insufficiency had higher prevalence of 6 or more depressive symptoms (52% vs. 26%, $p = 0.03$) and disease multi-morbidity (74% vs. 41%, $p < 0.001$) compared to those who were food sufficient.

References

1. Gregory, C.A.; Coleman-Jensen, A. *Food Insecurity, Chronic Disease, and Health among Working-Age Adults*; Economic Research Report, 235; U.S. Department of Agriculture, Economic Research Service: Washington, DC, USA, 2017. Available online: https://www.ers.usda.gov/webdocs/publications/84467/err-235_summary.pdf?v=42942 (accessed on 27 June 2018).
2. Tarasuk, V.; Mitchell, A.; Dachner, N. Household Food Insecurity in Canada, 2014. 2016. Available online: http://proof.utoronto.ca/resources/proof-annual-reports/annual-report-2014/ (accessed on 27 June 2018).
3. Coleman-Jensen, A.; Rabbitt, M.P.; Gregory, C.; Singh, A. *Household Food Security in the United States in 2016*; Economic Research Report; United States Department of Agriculture: Washington, DC, USA, 2017. Available online: https://www.ers.usda.gov/webdocs/publications/84973/err237_summary.pdf?v=42979 (accessed on 27 June 2018).
4. Tarasuk, V.; Mitchell, A.; Dashner, N. Household Food Insecurity in Canada, 2012. 2014. Available online: http://proof.utoronto.ca/resources/proof-annual-reports/annual-report-2012/ (accessed on 27 June 2018).
5. Bates, B.; Roberts, C.; Lepps, H.; Porter, L. The Food & You Survey: Wave 4. 2017. Available online: https://www.food.gov.uk/sites/default/files/media/document/food-and-you-w4-exec-summary.pdf (accessed on 27 June 2018).
6. Lindberg, R.; Lawrence, M.; Gold, L.; Friel, S.; Pegram, O. Food insecurity in Australia: Implications for general practitioners. *Aust. Fam. Physician* **2015**, *44*, 859–863. [PubMed]
7. FAO. Agriculture and Development Economics Division. *Food Security: Policy Brief*. 2006. Available online: http://www.fao.org/fileadmin/templates/faoitaly/documents/pdf/pdf_Food_Security_Cocept_Note.pdf (accessed on 27 June 2018).
8. Bickel, G.; Nord, M.; Price, C.; Hamilton, W.; Cook, J. *Guide to Measuring Household Food Security*; USDA: Alexandria, VA, USA, 2000. Available online: https://fns-prod.azureedge.net/sites/default/files/FSGuide.pdf (accessed on 27 June 2018).
9. Entmacher, J.; Robbins, K.; Vogtman, J.; Morrison, A. *Insecure and Unequal: Poverty and Income among Women and Families, 2000–2013*; National Women's Law Center: Washington, DC, USA, 2014; Available online: https://nwlc.org/resources/insecure-unequal-poverty-and-income-among-women-and-families-2000-2013/ (accessed on 27 June 2018).
10. Maheux, H.; Chui, T. *Women in Canada: A Gender-Based Statistical Report*; Statistics: Ottawa, ON, Canada, 2011; Available online: https://www150.statcan.gc.ca/n1/pub/89-503-x/89-503-x2010001-eng.htm (accessed on 27 June 2018).
11. Semega, J.L.; Fontenot, K.R.; Kollar, M.A. Income and Poverty in the United States: 2016. Current Population Reports; 2017. Available online: https://www.census.gov/library/publications/2017/demo/p60-259.html (accessed on 27 June 2018).
12. Ivers, L.C.; Cullen, K.A. Food insecurity: Special considerations for women. *Am. J. Clin. Nutr.* **2011**, *94*, 1740S–1744S. [CrossRef] [PubMed]
13. Knowles, M.; Rabinowich, J.; Ettinger de Cuba, S.; Cutts, D.B.; Chilton, M. "Do you wanna breathe or eat?": Parent perspectives on child health consequences of food insecurity, trade-offs, and toxic stress. *Matern. Child Health J.* **2015**, *20*, 25–32. [CrossRef] [PubMed]
14. Kirkpatrick, S.I.; Tarasuk, V. Food insecurity is associated with nutrient inadequacies among Canadian adults and adolescents. *J. Nutr.* **2008**, *138*, 604–612. [CrossRef] [PubMed]
15. Hanson, K.L.; Olson, C.M. Chronic health conditions and depressive symptoms strongly predict persistent food insecurity among rural low-income families. *J. Health Care Poor Underserved.* **2012**, *23*, 1174–1188. [CrossRef] [PubMed]
16. Tarasuk, V.; Mitchell, A.; McLaren, L.; McIntyre, L. Chronic physical and mental health conditions among adults may increase vulnerability to household food insecurity. *J. Nutr.* **2013**, *143*, 1785–1793. [CrossRef] [PubMed]
17. Martin, M.S.; Maddocks, E.; Chen, Y.; Gilman, S.E.; Colman, I. Food insecurity and mental illness: Disproportionate impacts in the context of perceived stress and social isolation. *Public Health* **2016**, *132*, 86–91. [CrossRef] [PubMed]

18.   McIntyre, L.; Williams, J.V.A.; Lavorato, D.H.; Patten, S. Depression and suicide ideation in late adolescence and early adulthood are an outcome of child hunger. *J. Affect. Disord.* **2013**, *150*, 123–129. [CrossRef] [PubMed]

19.   Jessiman-Perreault, G.; McIntyre, L. The household food insecurity gradient and potential reductions in adverse population mental health outcomes in Canadian adults. *SSM Popul. Health* **2017**, *3*, 464–472. [CrossRef] [PubMed]

20.   Davison, K.M.; Marshall-Fabien, G.L.; Tecson, A. Association of moderate and severe food insecurity with suicidal ideation in adults: National survey data from three Canadian provinces. *Soc. Psychiatry Psychiatr. Epidemiol.* **2015**, *50*, 963–972. [CrossRef] [PubMed]

21.   Health Canada. *Canadian Community Health Survey, Cycle 2.2, Nutrition (2004): Income-related Household Food Security in Canada*; No. 4696; HC Publisher: Ottawa, ON, Canada, 2007; Available online: https://www.canada.ca/content/dam/hc-sc/migration/hc-sc/fn-an/alt_formats/hpfb-dgpsa/pdf/surveill/income_food_sec-sec_alim-eng.pdf (accessed on 27 June 2018).

22.   Arksey, H.; O'Malley, L. Scoping studies: Towards a methodological framework. *Int. J. Soc. Res. Methodol.* **2005**, *8*, 19–32. [CrossRef]

23.   Moher, D.; Liberati, A.; Tetzlaff, J.; Altman, D.G.; Grp, P. Preferred reporting items for systematic reviews and meta-analyses: The PRISMA statement (reprinted from annals of internal medicine). *Phys. Ther.* **2009**, *89*, 873–880. [PubMed]

24.   Corman, H.; Curtis, M.A.; Noonan, K.; Reichman, N.E. Maternal depression as a risk factor for children's inadequate housing conditions. *Soc. Sci. Med.* **2016**, *149*, 76–83. [CrossRef] [PubMed]

25.   Garg, A.; Toy, S.; Tripodis, Y.; Cook, J.; Cordella, N. Influence of maternal depression on household food insecurity for low-income families. *Acad Pediatr.* **2015**, *15*, 305–310. [CrossRef] [PubMed]

26.   Hernandez, D.C.; Marshall, A.; Mineo, C. Maternal depression mediates the association between intimate partner violence and food insecurity. *J. Womens Health* **2014**, *23*, 29–37. [CrossRef] [PubMed]

27.   Laraia, B.; Vinikoor-Imler, L.C.; Siega-Riz, A.M. Food insecurity during pregnancy leads to stress, disordered eating, and greater postpartum weight among overweight women. *Obesity* **2015**, *23*, 1303–1311. [CrossRef] [PubMed]

28.   Chilton, M.M.; Rabinowich, J.R.; Woolf, N.H. Very low food security in the USA is linked with exposure to violence. *Public Health Nutr.* **2013**, *17*, 1–10. [CrossRef] [PubMed]

29.   McCurdy, K.; Kisler, T.; Gorman, K.S.; Metallinos-Katsaras, E. Food- and health-related correlates of self-reported body mass index among low-income mothers of young children. *J. Nutr. Educ. Behav.* **2015**, *47*, 225–233. [CrossRef] [PubMed]

30.   Sun, J.; Knowles, M.; Patel, F.; Frank, D.A.; Heeren, T.C.; Chilton, M. Childhood adversity and adult reports of food insecurity among households with children. *Am. J. Prev. Med.* **2016**, *50*, 561–572. [CrossRef] [PubMed]

31.   Trapp, C.M.; Burke, G.; Gorin, A.A.; Wiley, J.F.; Hernandez, D.; Crowell, R.E.; Grant, A.; Beaulieu, A.; Cloutier, M.M. The relationship between dietary patterns, body mass index percentile, and household food security in young urban children. *Child. Obes.* **2015**, *11*, 148–155. [CrossRef] [PubMed]

32.   Muldoon, K.A.; Duff, P.K.; Fielden, S.; Anema, A. Food insufficiency is associated with psychiatric morbidity in a nationally representative study of mental illness among food insecure Canadians. *Soc. Psychiatry Psychiatr. Epidemiol.* **2013**, *48*, 795–803. [CrossRef] [PubMed]

33.   Sidebottom, A.C.; Hellerstedt, W.L.; Harrison, P.A.; Hennrikus, D. An examination of prenatal and postpartum depressive symptoms among women served by urban community health centers. *Arch. Womens Ment. Health* **2014**, *17*, 27–40. [CrossRef] [PubMed]

34.   Mathews, L.; Morris, M.N.; Schneider, J.; Goto, K. The relationship between food security and poor health among female WIC participants. *J. Hunger Environ. Nutr.* **2010**, *5*, 85–99. [CrossRef]

35.   Ajrouch, K.J.; Reisine, S.; Lim, S.; Sohn, W.; Ismail, A. Situational stressors among African-American women living in low-income urban areas: The role of social support. *Women Health* **2010**, *50*, 159–175. [CrossRef] [PubMed]

36.   Hromi-Fiedler, A.; Bermúdez-Millán, A.; Segura-Pérez, S.; Pérez-Escamilla, R. Household food insecurity is associated with depressive symptoms among low-income pregnant Latinas. *Matern. Child Nutr.* **2011**, *7*, 421–430. [CrossRef] [PubMed]

37.   Dressler, H.; Smith, C. Depression affects emotional eating and dietary intake and is related to food insecurity in a group of multiethnic, low-income women. *J. Hunger Environ. Nutr.* **2015**, *10*, 496–510. [CrossRef]

38. Peterman, J.N.; Wilde, P.E.; Silka, L.; Bermudez, O.I.; Rogers, B.L. Food insecurity among Cambodian refugee women two decades post resettlement. *J. Immigr. Minor. Health* **2013**, *15*, 372–380. [CrossRef] [PubMed]

39. Sharpe, P.A.; Whitaker, K.; Alia, K.A.; Wilcox, S.; Hutto, B. Dietary intake, behaviors and psychosocial factors among women from food-secure and food-insecure households in the United States. *Ethn Dis.* **2016**, *26*, 139–146. [CrossRef] [PubMed]

40. Davey-Rothwell, M.A.; Flamm, L.J.; Kassa, H.T.; Latkin, C.A. Food insecurity and depressive symptoms: Comparison of drug using and nondrug-using women at risk for HIV. *J. Commun. Psychol.* **2014**, *42*, 469–478. [CrossRef] [PubMed]

41. Sharkey, J.R.; Johnson, C.M.; Dean, W.R. Relationship of household food insecurity to health-related quality of life in a large sample of rural and urban women. *Women Health* **2011**, *51*, 442–460. [CrossRef] [PubMed]

42. Birmingham, M.C.; Chou, K.J.; Crain, E.F. Screening for postpartum depression in pediatric emergency department. *Pediatr. Emerg. Care* **2011**, *27*, 795–800. [CrossRef] [PubMed]

43. Carter, K.N.; Kruse, K.; Blakely, T.; Collings, S. The association of food security with psychological distress in New Zealand and any gender differences. *Soc. Sci. Med.* **2011**, *72*, 1463–1471. [CrossRef] [PubMed]

44. Melchior, M.; Caspi, A.; Howard, L.M.; Ambler, A.P.; Bolton, H.; Mountain, N.; Moffitt, T.E. Mental health context of food insecurity: A representative cohort of families with young children. *Pediatrics* **2009**, *124*, e564–e572. [CrossRef] [PubMed]

45. Lent, M.D.; Petrovic, L.E.; Swanson, J.A.; Olson, C.M. Maternal mental health and the persistence of food insecurity in poor rural families. *J. Health Care Poor Underserved.* **2009**, *20*, 645–661. [CrossRef] [PubMed]

46. Wunderlich, G.S.; Norwood, J. *Food Insecurity and Hunger in the United States: An Assessment of the Measure*; National Academies Press: Washington, DC, USA, 2006; Available online: https://www.nap.edu/catalog/11578/food-insecurity-and-hunger-in-the-united-states-an-assessment (accessed on 27 June 2018).

47. Radimer, K.L.; Olson, C.M.; Greene, J.C.; Campbell, C.C.; Habicht, J.P. Understanding hunger and developing indicators to assess it in women and children. *J. Nutr. Educ.* **1992**, *24*, 36S–44S. [CrossRef]

48. Wehler, C.A.; Scott, R.I.; Anderson, J. The community child hunger identification project: A model of domestic hunger—Demonstration project in Seattle, Washington. *J. Nutr. Educ.* **1992**, *24* (Suppl. 1), 29S–35S.

49. Frongillo, E.A., Jr.; Rauschenbach, B.S.; Olson, C.M.; Kendall, A.; Colmenares, A.G. Questionnaire-based measures are valid for the identification of rural households with hunger and food insecurity. *J. Nutr.* **1997**, *127*, 699–705. [CrossRef] [PubMed]

50. Briefel, R.R.; Woteki, C. Development of food sufficiency questions for the third national health and nutrition examination survey. *J. Nutr. Educ.* **1992**, *24* (Suppl. 1), 24S–28S. [CrossRef]

51. Tarasuk, V. Discussion Paper on Household and Individual Food Insecurity. 2001. Available online: https://www.canada.ca/en/health-canada/services/food-nutrition/healthy-eating/nutrition-policy-reports/discussion-paper-household-individual-food-insecurity-2001.html (accessed on 27 June 2018).

52. Wehler, C.; Weinreb, L.F.; Huntington, N.; Scott, R. Risk and protective factors for adult and child hunger among low-income housed and homeless female-headed families. *Am. J. Public Health* **2004**, *94*, 109–115. [CrossRef] [PubMed]

53. Bronte-Tinkew, J.; Zaslow, M.; Capps, R.; Horowitz, A.; McNamara, M. Food insecurity works through depression, parenting, and infant feeding to influence overweight and health in toddlers. *J. Nutr.* **2007**, *137*, 2160–2165. [CrossRef] [PubMed]

54. Casey, P.; Goolsby, S.; Berkowitz, C.; Frank, D.; Cook, J.; Cutts, D.; Black, M.M.; Zaldivar, N.; Levenson, S.; Heeren, T.; et al. Maternal depression, changing public assistance, food security, and child health status. *Pediatrics* **2004**, *113*, 298–304. [CrossRef] [PubMed]

55. Huddleston-Casas, C.; Charnigo, R.; Simmons, L.A. Food insecurity and maternal depression in rural, low-income families: A longitudinal investigation. *Public Health Nutr.* **2009**, *12*, 1133–1140. [CrossRef] [PubMed]

56. Laraia, B.A.; Siega-Riz, A.M.; Gundersen, C.; Dole, N. Psychosocial factors and socioeconomic indicators are associated with household food insecurity among pregnant women. *J. Nutr.* **2006**, *136*, 177–182. [CrossRef] [PubMed]

57. Kaiser, L.; Baumrind, N.; Dumbauld, S. Who is food-insecure in California? Findings from the California Women's Health Survey, 2004. *Public Health Nutr.* **2007**, *10*, 574–581. [CrossRef] [PubMed]

58. Laraia, B.A.; Borja, J.B.; Bentley, M.E. Grandmothers, fathers, and depressive symptoms are associated with food insecurity among low-income first-time African-American mothers in North Carolina. *J. Am. Diet. Assoc.* **2009**, *109*, 1042–1047. [CrossRef] [PubMed]

59. Whitaker, R.C.; Phillips, S.M.; Orzol, S.M. Food insecurity and the risks of depression and anxiety in mothers and behavior problems in their preschool-aged children. *Pediatrics* **2006**, *118*, e859–e868. [CrossRef] [PubMed]

60. Harrison, P.A.; Sidebottom, A.C. Systematic prenatal screening for psychosocial risks. *J. Health Care Poor Underserved.* **2008**, *19*, 258–276. [CrossRef] [PubMed]

61. United States Centers for Disease Control and Prevention. Third National Health and Nutrition Examination Survey (NHANES III), 1988–94: NHANES-III Household Adult Data File Documentation, Ages 17+. Available online: https://wwwn.cdc.gov/nchs/nhanes/nhanes3/DataFiles.aspx (accessed on 27 June 2018).

62. Heflin, C.M.; Siefert, K.; Williams, D.R. Food insufficiency and women's mental health: Findings from a 3-year panel of welfare recipients. *Soc. Sci. Med.* **2005**, *61*, 1971–1982. [CrossRef] [PubMed]

63. Siefert, K.; Finlayson, T.L.; Williams, D.R.; Delva, J.; Ismail, A.I. Modifiable risk and protective factors for depressive symptoms in low-income African American mothers. *Am. J. Orthopsychiatr.* **2007**, *77*, 113–123. [CrossRef] [PubMed]

64. Siefert, K.; Heflin, C.M.; Corcoran, M.E.; Williams, D.R. Food insufficiency and the physical and mental health of low-income women. *Women Health* **2001**, *32*, 159–177. [CrossRef] [PubMed]

65. Salmond, C.; Crampton, P.; King, P.; Waldegrave, C. NZiDep: A New Zealand index of socioeconomic deprivation for individuals. *Soc. Sci. Med.* **2006**, *62*, 1474–1485. [CrossRef] [PubMed]

66. Kendall, A.; Olson, C.; Frongillo, E.A., Jr. Validation of the Radimer/Cornell measures of hunger and food insecurity. *J. Nutr.* **1995**, *125*, 2793–2801. [PubMed]

67. Hamelin, A.M.; Beaudry, M.; Habicht, J.P. Characterization of household food insecurity in Québec: Food and feelings. *Soc. Sci. Med.* **2002**, *54*, 119–132. [CrossRef]

68. Klesges, L.M.; Pahor, M.; Guralnik, J.M.; Shorr, R.I.; Williamson, J.D. Financial difficulty acquiring food among elderly disabled women: Results from the Women's Health and Aging Study (WHAS). *Am. J. Public Health* **2001**, *91*, 68–75. [PubMed]

69. Sharkey, J.R. Risk and presence of food insufficiency are associated with low nutrient intakes and multimorbidity among homebound older women who receive home-delivered meals. *J. Nutr.* **2003**, *133*, 3485–3491. [CrossRef] [PubMed]

70. World Health Organization. WHO WMH-CIDI Instruments. *World Health Organization.* 2018. Available online: https://www.hcp.med.harvard.edu/wmhcidi/about-the-who-wmh-cidi/ (accessed on 27 June 2018).

71. Radloff, L.S. The CES-D scale: A self-report depression scale for research in the general population. *Appl. Psychol. Meas.* **1977**, *1*, 385–401. [CrossRef]

72. American Psychological Association. The State-Trait Anxiety Inventory (STAI). 2018. Available online: http://www.apa.org/pi/about/publications/caregivers/practice-settings/assessment/tools/trait-state.aspx (accessed on 27 June 2018).

73. Derogatis, L.R.; Lipman, R.S.; Rickels, K.; Uhlenhuth, E.H.; Covi, L. The Hopkins Symptom Checklist (HSCL): A self-report symptom inventory. *Behav. Sci.* **1974**, *19*, 1–15. [CrossRef] [PubMed]

74. Kemper, K.J.; Babonis, T.R. Screening for maternal depression in pediatric clinics. *Am. J. Dis. Child.* **1992**, *146*, 876–878. [CrossRef] [PubMed]

75. Cox, J.L.; Holden, J.M.; Sagovsky, R. Detection of postnatal depression: Development of the 10-item Edinburgh Postnatal Depression Scale. *Br. J. Psychiatry* **1987**, *150*, 782–786. [CrossRef] [PubMed]

76. Yesavage, J.A.; Brink, T.L.; Rose, T.L.; Lum, O.; Huang, V.; Adey, M.; Leirer, V.O. Development and validation of a geriatric depression screening scale: A preliminary report. *J. Psychiatr. Res.* **1982**, *17*, 37–49. [CrossRef]

77. Cohen, S.; Kamarck, T.; Mermelstein, R. A global measure of perceived stress. *J. Health Soc. Behav.* **1983**, *24*, 385–396. [CrossRef] [PubMed]

78. Weiner, I.B.; Craighead, W.E. Diagnostic Interview Schedule for DSM-IV (DIS-IV). In *The Corsini Encyclopedia of Psychology*; John Wiley & Sons Inc.: Hoboken, NJ, USA, 2009.

79. Andrews, G.; Slade, T. Interpreting scores on the Kessler Psychological Distress Scale (K10). *Aust. N. Z. J. Public Health* **2010**, *25*, 494–497. [CrossRef]

80. Kroenke, K.; Spitzer, R.L.; Williams, J.B.W. The PHQ-9: Validity of a brief depression severity measure. *J. Gen. Intern. Med.* **2001**, *16*, 606–613. [CrossRef] [PubMed]

81.	Pearlin, L.I.; Menaghan, E.G.; Lieberman, M.A.; Mullan, J.T. The stress process. *J. Health Soc. Behav.* **1981**, *22*, 337–356. [CrossRef] [PubMed]

82.	Rosenberg, M. *Society and the Adolescent Self-Image*; Princeton University Press: Princeton, NJ, USA, 1965.

83.	Brazier, J.E.; Harper, R.; Jones, N.M.B.; O'Cathain, A.; Thomas, K.J.; Usherwood, T.; Westlake, L. Validating the SF-36 health survey questionnaire: New outcome measure for primary care. *Br. Med. J. Gen. Pract.* **1992**, *305*, 160–164. [CrossRef]

84.	Wittchen H-UU. Reliability and validity studies of the WHO—Composite International Diagnostic Interview (CIDI): A critical review. *J. Psychiatr. Res.* **1994**, *28*, 57–84.

85.	Weinreb, L.; Wehler, C.; Perloff, J.; Scott, R.; Hosmer, D.; Sagor, L.; Gundersen, C. Hunger: Its impact on children's health and mental health. *Pediatrics* **2002**, *110*, e41. [CrossRef] [PubMed]

86.	Seligman, H.K.; Schillinger, D. Hunger and socioeconomic disparities in chronic disease. *N. Engl. J. Med.* **2010**, *363*, 6–9. [CrossRef] [PubMed]

87.	Garner, A.S.; Shonkoff, J.P.; Siegel, B.S.; Dobbins, M.I.; Earls, M.F.; Garner, A.S.; Shonkoff, J.P. Early childhood adversity, toxic stress, and the role of the pediatrician: Translating developmental science into lifelong health. *Pediatrics* **2012**, *129*, e224–e231. [PubMed]

88.	Bruening, M.; van Woerden, I.; Todd, M.; Laska, M.N. Hungry to learn: The prevalence and effects of food insecurity on health behaviors and outcomes over time among a diverse sample of university freshmen. *Int. J. Behav. Nutr. Phys. Act.* **2018**, *15*. [CrossRef] [PubMed]

89.	Bruening, M.; Argo, K.; Payne-Sturges, D.; Laska, M.N. The struggle is real: A systematic review of food insecurity on postsecondary education campuses. *J. Acad. Nutr. Diet.* **2017**, *117*, 1767–1791. [CrossRef] [PubMed]

90.	Farahbakhsh, J.; Hanbazaza, M.; Ball, G.D.C.; Farmer, A.P.; Maximova, K.; Willows, N.D. Food insecure student clients of a university-based food bank have compromised health, dietary intake and academic quality. *Nutr. Diet.* **2017**, *74*, 67–73. [CrossRef] [PubMed]

91.	Bruening, M.; Brennhofer, S.; van Woerden, I.; Todd, M.; Laska, M. Factors related to the high rates of food insecurity among diverse, urban college freshmen. *J. Acad. Nutr. Diet.* **2016**, *116*, 1450–1457. [CrossRef] [PubMed]

92.	O'Connell, M.E.; Boat, T.; Warner, K. *Preventing Mental, Emotional, and Behavioral Disorders among Young People: Progress and Possibilities*; National Academies Press: Washington, DC, USA, 2009. Available online: https://www.ncbi.nlm.nih.gov/books/NBK32775/ (accessed on 27 June 2018).

93.	Kessler, R.C.; Berglund, P.; Demler, O.; Jin, R.; Merikangas, K.R.W.E. Lifetime prevalence and age-of-onset distributions of DSM-IV disorders in the National Comorbidity Survey replication. *Arch. Gen. Psychiatry* **2005**, *62*, 593–602. [CrossRef] [PubMed]

94.	Coates, J.; Swindale, A.; Bilinsky, P. *Household Food Insecurity Access Scale (HFIAS) for Measurement of Food Access: Indicator Guide*; FANTA III; Food and Nutrition Technical Assistance: Washington, DC, USA, 2007; Available online: https://www.fantaproject.org/monitoring-and-evaluation/household-food-insecurity-access-scale-hfias (accessed on 27 June 2018).

95.	Hamelin, A.-M.; Habicht, J.-P.; Beaudry, M. Food insecurity: Consequences for the household and broader social implications. *J. Nutr.* **1999**, *129*, 525S–528S. [CrossRef] [PubMed]

96.	Becker, C.B.; Middlemass, K.; Taylor, B.; Johnson, C.; Gomez, F. Food insecurity and eating disorder pathology. *Int. J. Eat. Disord.* **2017**, *50*, 1031–1040. [CrossRef] [PubMed]

97.	Vandenbroucke, J.P.; Von Elm, E.; Altman, D.G.; Gøtzsche, P.C.; Mulrow, C.D.; Pocock, S.J.; Poole, C.; Schlesselman, J.J.; Egger, M. Strengthening the Reporting of Observational Studies in Epidemiology (STROBE): Explanation and elaboration. *PLoS Med.* **2007**, *4*, 1628–1654. [CrossRef] [PubMed]

98.	Sterman, J.D. Learning from evidence in a complex world. *Am. J. Public Health* **2006**, *96*, 505–514. [CrossRef] [PubMed]

99.	Mabry, P.L.; Marcus, S.E.; Clark, P.I.; Leischow, S.J.; M'Endez, D. Systems science: A revolution in public health policy research. *Am. J. Public Health* **2010**, *100*, 1161–1163. [CrossRef] [PubMed]

100.	Friel, S.; Pescud, M.; Malbon, E.; Lee, A.; Carter, R.; Greenfield, J.; Cobcroft, M.; Potter, J.; Rychetnik, L.; Meertens, B. Using systems science to understand the determinants of inequities in healthy eating. *PLoS ONE* **2017**, *12*, e0188872. [CrossRef] [PubMed]

101. Tarasuk, V. Implications of a basic income guarantee for household food insecurity. In *Basic Income Guarantee Series*; Research Paper No. 24; Northern Policy Institute: Thunder Bay, ON, USA, 2017; Available online: http://proof.utoronto.ca/wp-content/uploads/2017/06/Paper-Tarasuk-BIG-EN-17.06.13-1712.pdf (accessed on 27 June 2018).

102. Public Policy and Food Insecurity Fact Sheet. *PROOF Food Insecurity Policy Research*; Public Policy and Food Insecurity Fact Sheet: Toronto, ON, USA, 2016; Volume 41, Available online: http://proof.utoronto.ca/wp-content/uploads/2016/06/public-policy-factsheet.pdf (accessed on 27 June 2018).

103. Forget, E.L. The town with no poverty: The health effects of a Canadian income guaranteed annual income field experiment. *Can. Public Policy* **2011**, *37*, 283–305. [CrossRef]

104. American Academy of Pediatrics Council on Community Pediatrics, Committee on Nutrition. Promoting food security for all children. *Pediatrics* **2015**, *136*, e1431–e1438.

105. Tarasuk, V.; Cheng, J.; de Oliveira, C.; Dachner, N.; Gundersen, C.; Kurdyak, P. Association between household food insecurity and annual health care costs. *Can. Med. Assoc. J.* **2015**, *187*, E429–E436. [CrossRef] [PubMed]

106. Holben, D.H.; Marshall, M.B. Position of the academy of nutrition and dietetics: Food Insecurity in the United States. *J. Acad. Nutr. Diet.* **2017**, *117*, 1991–2002. [CrossRef] [PubMed]

107. McGorry, P.; Tanti, C.; Stokes, R.E.A. Australia's national youth mental health foundation—Where young minds come first. *MJS* **2007**, *187*, 5–8.

108. Pinto, A.D.; Bloch, G.; Bloch, G. Framework for building primary care capacity to address the social determinants of health. *Can. Fam. Physician* **2017**, *63*, 476–482.

7

Walking the Food Security Tightrope—Exploring the Experiences of Low-to-Middle Income Melbourne Households

Sue Kleve [1,*], **Sue Booth** [2], **Zoe E. Davidson** [1] **and Claire Palermo** [1]

[1] Department of Nutrition, Dietetics and Food, School of Clinical Sciences, Faculty of Medicine, Nursing and Health Sciences, Monash University, Level 1, 264 Ferntree Gully Road, Notting Hill 3168, Australia; zoe.davidson@monash.edu (Z.E.D.); claire.palermo@monash.edu (C.P.)

[2] College of Medicine and Public Health, Flinders University, GPO Box 2100, Adelaide 5000, Australia; sue.booth@flinders.edu.au

* Correspondence: suzanne.kleve@monash.edu

Abstract: There is limited evidence of how Australian low-to-middle income (AUD $40,000–$80,000) households maintain food security. Using a sequential explanatory mixed methods methodology, this study explored and compared the food security (FS) and insecurity (FIS) experiences of these households. An initial quantitative survey categorised participants according to food security status (the 18-item United States Department of Agriculture Household Food Security Survey Module) and income level to identify and purposefully select participants to qualitatively explore food insecurity and security experiences. Of the total number of survey participants (n = 134), 42 were categorised as low-to-middle income. Of these, a subset of 16 participants (8 FIS and 8 FS) was selected, and each participant completed an in-depth interview. The interviews explored precursors, strategies to prevent or address food insecurity, and the implications of the experience. Interview data were analysed using a thematic analysis approach. Five themes emerged from the analysis: (i) food decision experiences, (ii) assets, (iii) triggers, (iv) activation of assets, and (v) consequences and emotion related to walking the food security tightrope. The leverage points across all themes were more volatile for FIS participants. Low-to-middle income Australians are facing the challenges of trying to maintain or improve their food security status, with similarities to those described in lower income groups, and should be included in approaches to prevent or address food insecurity.

Keywords: food insecurity; low-to-middle income; experience; mixed methodology research

1. Introduction

Food insecurity—the limited or uncertain availability of individuals' and households' physical, social, and economic access to sufficient, safe, nutritious, and culturally relevant food—is a complex, persistent, and multidimensional phenomenon [1]. Irrespective of an abundance of food and relative wealth, the issue of food insecurity is one experienced amongst high income countries, including Australia. The 2011–2012 National Health Survey, using a single-item tool, indicated that 4% of Australians, or approximately one million, were living in a household that was food insecure [2]. Utilising different valid multi-item tools, the prevalence of food insecurity in other high income countries was found to be 15% in New Zealand [3], 12.3% in Canada [4], 8% in England, Wales, and Northern Ireland (U.K.) [5], and 14% in the United States (U.S.) [6].

Food insecurity has a temporal dimension, and households may transition between episodic or chronic experiences [7]. The core characteristics of food insecurity have been described at both an individual and household level to include anxiety, concern, compromise to the quantity and nutritional quality of food, and social isolation [8,9]. The food insecurity experience may vary in severity along a continuum [10]. At one end of the continuum are initial indicators, such as anxiety and concern about an adequate food budget or food supply, and, at the other extreme end, the more severe indicators, perturbations in diet quality and quantity of food intake and hunger, become apparent [7,8,10,11]. Numerous negative implications of food insecurity have been reported, including physical, social, and emotional health impacts across the lifespan [12–16] and developmental and educational impacts in children [17]. Food insecurity is a serious public health issue.

Regardless of households' geographic location, food insecurity is influenced by the interactions of a range of factors as described by the four dimensions of food security—food availability, supply, utilisation, and stability [1]—and the socio-demographic characteristics of households [3,18–22]. The major predictor of food insecurity is a low income or limited available economic resources for purchasing food or general resources in a household [18,19,23–27]. Although an inverse relationship between income and food insecurity exists [19,24,28], not all very-low-income households are food insecure, nor are households progressing up the income gradient food secure [28–30]. While the prevalence of food insecurity is greater in very-low-income groups, evidence from high-income countries indicates that households beyond this income group are experiencing food insecurity [19,26,31–36]. Categorisation of food insecurity based on the static measure of annual income may be problematic as this measure is insensitive to sudden economic changes within a household [28].

Whilst the existence of food insecurity in higher-income groups has been reported, there has been limited research examining the factors that contribute to food insecurity in these groups. Additional factors for Canadian and U.S. higher-income households include a fluctuating income, a sudden change in employment, a change in household composition, illness, disability, increased housing costs, and housing tenure [34,36,37]. Further significant predictors reported from Victoria, Australia in low-to-middle income households include an inability to raise money in an emergency, housing tenure, support from friends, and the cost of food [32].

There is a limited understanding of the nature of the experience of food insecurity in low-to-middle income Australian households. This may hinder the development of approaches to address the determinants of food insecurity more broadly across income groups. Furthermore, the factors that protect people from food insecurity and the coping strategies of households need to be explored. Approaches to address food insecurity need to consider the complex range of determinants that trigger food insecurity in households; and, consequently, a measurement of food insecurity must capture these determinants.

This study had three aims. The first was to identify low-to-middle income Melbourne participants who are food secure and food insecure. The second was to explore and compare food security and insecurity experiences; specifically, the precursors to, and strategies for preventing or addressing, food insecurity. The third was to examine the implications of the experience of food insecurity for those experiencing it to inform policy and practice.

2. Materials and Methods

2.1. Study Design

The study employed a pragmatic approach and positioning. The researchers were interested in understanding the experience of food insecurity from the perspective of participants from low-to-middle income households and the implications of this on their lives for policy and practice. An explanatory sequential mixed methods research design approach of collecting, analysing, and integrating both quantitative and qualitative data in the research process was employed [38–40]. Typically, the emphasis in this design is on the quantitative phase; however, in this study, the research emphasis was on the qualitative phase to explore the experience of food security and food insecurity within low-to-middle income households. The initial quantitative results were used to identify and purposefully select participants to qualitatively examine the food insecurity phenomenon [38,41].

The study was conducted according to guidelines in the Declaration of Helsinki, and all procedures were approved by the Monash University Human Research Ethics Committee (CF14/1382-201400647). Informed consent was implied for the quantitative phase, and written informed consent was obtained for the qualitative phase.

2.2. Participants

A cross-sectional convenience sample was recruited from metropolitan Melbourne, Victoria. Suburbs were selected according to the 'Vulnerability Assessment for Mortgage, Petrol, and Inflation Risks and Expenditure' (VAMPIRE) 2008 Index [42]. The VAMPIRE index is based on Census data and calculates suburb vulnerability based on three socio economic stressors: mortgage, car, and income, providing a ranking from minimal to very high vulnerability. Those with high levels of car ownership, who journey to work by car, who have mortgage tenure, and/or who have low incomes are considered 'more vulnerable'. A higher vulnerability VAMPIRE rating is likely to impact on finances available for food [43]; thus, all Melbourne suburbs with medium to very high ratings were selected for inclusion. These suburbs provided a varied sample in which food insecurity is likely to occur in some households due to characteristic stressors [44].

The convenience sample aimed to identify information-rich participants to interview as part of the qualitative phase, rather than be representative of the population. Eligibility for study inclusion was conducted in two stages. In the quantitative phase, participants were over 18 years of age and residing in metropolitan Melbourne, living in or adjacent to VAMPIRE suburbs. In the qualitative phase, participants from the quantitative phase were included as low-to-middle income if they had a gross household income of AUD $40,000–$80,000 per annum before tax. This income categorisation was based on Australian Bureau of Statistics quintiles of gross Victorian household income [45]. Respondent anonymity was preserved by a unique code that was assigned for survey responses, and all interview participants were provided with a pseudonym. Figure 1 summarises the study design procedures.

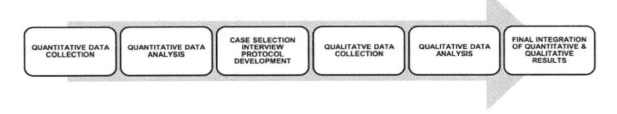

Figure 1. Summary of Sequential Explanatory Mixed Methods research design.

2.3. Quantitative Phase: Data Collection and Analysis

The quantitative survey, 'Food Security in Melbourne Households Survey' (FSiMH survey), was designed by the researchers using a mix of validated questions and instruments. Demographic questions were developed to gather information on factors that are associated with food insecurity in the literature and support categorisation based on income [19,32,46]. Food security status was determined using the validated 18-item United States Department of Agriculture Household Food Security Survey Module (USDA-HFSSM) [7]. The survey was promoted across a diverse range of community organisations and websites located in, or in close proximity to, the VAMPIRE suburbs. The main household shopper or food preparer was asked to complete the survey. The FSiMH survey was administered in both an electronic (Qualtrics, Provo UT, US platform) and paper format between September 2014 and February 2015.

The USDA-HFSSM was selected for determination of food security status because of its reliability across populations and population subgroups and its ability to capture the severity level and continuum of experience of food insecurity [7,47–49]. The USDA-HFSSM categorises households as food secure or food insecure with varying severity levels of experience. Households with affirmative scores of 0–2 are classified as food secure; those with an affirmative score of 0 are classified as food secure at the high food security (no reported indications of food-access limitations) severity level, whereas those with affirmative scores of 1 or 2 are classified as food secure at the marginal food security (anxiety over food sufficiency or a shortage of food in the house) severity level. Scores of 3 or greater are classified as food insecure at the low food security (reduced quality and variety of food with little or no indication of reduced intake) and very low food security (multiple indications of a disrupted eating pattern and reduced food intake) severity levels [7]. Studies from the United States and Canada report an increase in marginally food secure households that display greater health outcomes and similar characteristics to food insecure households [4,10,24,50]. Those who are marginally food secure may also be at greater risk of progressing to more severe forms of food insecurity. Consequently, using the philosophical pragmatic approach that guides this research, the modified Canadian food security categorisation was applied [4]. Respondents that were classified as experiencing marginal food security with a score of 1 or 2 were included in the food insecure category. The severity categorisations and scores are consistent with the USDA-HFSSM classifications [7,51].

Data were analysed using the statistical software package IBM SPSS Statistics for Windows, Version 22.0 (SPSS INC., Chicago, IL, USA). For the purpose of this analysis, respondents were dichotomised as food secure or food insecure, and demographic characteristics were explored descriptively and reported as counts and percentages.

2.4. Qualitative Phase: Data Collection and Analysis

The results from the quantitative phase supported the case selection and the interview protocol's development. The logic underpinning the interview protocol and questions was informed by both the existing literature [9,25,52–54] and the quantitative analysis, in particular the responses to the USDA-HFSSM items that described the experiences and consequences of food insecurity. The USDA-HFSSM assesses food security status based on an inability to access food due to a lack of financial resources; however, additional factors beyond this may impact upon food security status [47,55]. Consequently, the interviews allowed for elaboration and exploration beyond these economic factors and a deeper understanding and extension of the experiences of food insecurity that are measured by the USDA-HFSSM questions. The interviews explored low-to-middle income participants' experiences of accessing food (physical and economic), factors that influenced and impacted this, and the consequences of these factors. Four key areas were explored in the interviews: (i) accessing food and food choices for the household, (ii) factors impacting on food for the household, (iii) consequences when sufficient food quantity and preferred foods cannot be accessed, and (iv) coping and protective strategies: asset exploration (Supplementary Table S1). The researcher used a semi-structured interview format whereby the key areas were used to construct the main questions that were asked of participants and a series of prompting questions that were subsequently asked based on participants' initial response. The interviewer continued probing the participants until they were satisfied that responses of an adequate breadth and depth in each of the four interview areas were obtained.

All interviews were individually undertaken between June 2015 and September 2015 by the first author with each participant at a mutually suitable time in interview rooms at local community centres. The interviews were digitally recorded and transcribed, and field notes were kept after each interview. The interview duration ranged from 45 to 90 min. The NVivo qualitative software (QSR International, Version 10.3, Melbourne, Australia) was used to manage, store, and support the data analysis. A thematic data analysis was chosen, as the researchers acknowledged the complexities of food security and the need for more than one theoretical framework to explain the data and the emergence of new concepts. Braun and Clarke (2006) describe the benefits of a thematic analysis as 'providing a flexible and useful research tool, which can potentially provide a rich and detailed, yet complex account of data' [56]. The qualitative analysis approach included familiarisation with a transcript's content, open content coding with coding nodes, and inter-coder agreement. The codes were grouped into themes and subthemes in light of the research questions with the verification of themes amongst the researchers. A constant comparison approach to analysis was performed to describe patterns in the data to inform the initial formation of categories, where a content comparison within each category enabled the description of categories to evolve [57,58]. The constant comparison approach was implemented at three levels: for individual participants regardless of food security status; within food secure and food insecure groups; and between food secure and food insecure groups [57]. This analysis approach allowed for exploration of similarities and differences across and between groups.

3. Results

3.1. Quantitative Phase: Demographic Characteristics and Food Security Status

One hundred and thirty-four participants completed the FSiMH survey. Thirteen participants declined to indicate their income level, reducing the participant income data to $n = 121$. Forty-two participants were classified as low-to-middle income (food secure (FS), $n = 26$ and food insecure (FIS), $n = 16$), including 12 households with children.

The majority of participants were female and Australian-born. FIS participants $(n = 16)$ included participants that were homeowners with a mortgage $(n = 8)$, participants living with their spouse/partner and children $(n = 11)$, and participants that had some form of paid employment $(n = 11)$ (Table 1). In comparison, FS participants $(n = 26)$ included participants that were homeowners $(n = 19)$, of which nine were mortgage free, participants living with their spouse/partner and children $(n = 10)$, and participants that had some form of paid employment $(n = 10)$.

Table 1. Characteristics of low-to-middle income survey respondents $(n = 42)$ and in-depth interview participants $(n = 16)$ according to food security status.

Demographic Characteristics	Quantitative Survey Respondents $n = 42$		Respondents Selected for Qualitative Interview $n = 16$	
	Food Insecure $n = 16(\%)$	Food Secure $n = 26(\%)$	Food Insecure $n = 8(\%)$	Food Secure $n = 8(\%)$
Gender				
Male	1(6.2)	4(15.4)	0	1(12.5)
Female	15(93.8)	21(80.8)	8(100.0)	7(87.5)
Prefer not to say	0	1(3.9)	-	-
Age				
18–25	2(12.5)	2(7.7)	1(12.5)	1(12.5)
26–35	6(37.5)	4(15.4)	2(25.0)	2(25.0)
36–45	5(31.3)	7(26.9)	3(37.5)	1(12.5)
46–55	1(6.2)	6(23.0)	0	3(37.5)
56–65	2(12.5)	3(11.5)	2(25.0)	0
Over 65	0	4(15.4)	0	1(12.5)
Country of Birth				
Australia	11(69.0)	16(61.5)	5(62.5)	4(50.0)
Other	5(31.0)	10(38.5)	3(37.5)	4(50.0)
Housing Tenure				
Homeowner, mortgage	8(50.0)	10(38.5)	4(50.0)	3(37.5)
Homeowner, no mortgage	0	9(34.6)	1(12.5)	3(37.5)
Renting, privately	8(50.0)	4(15.4)	3(37.5)	1(12.5)
Other	0	3(11.5)	0	1(12.5)
Household Structure/Composition				
Living alone	1(6.2)	1(3.9)	2(25.0)	0
With parents/family	0	3(11.5)	1(12.5)	1(12.5)
With spouse/partner	1(6.2)	11(42.3)	1(12.5)	3(37.5)
With spouse/partner and children <18 years	10(62.5)	10(38.5)	4(50)	3(37.5)
With spouse/partner and children >18 years	1(6.2)	0	0	1(12.5)
With my children <18 years	2(12.5)	1(3.9)	0	0
Living in a share house	1(6.2)	0	0	0

Table 1. *Cont.*

Demographic Characteristics	Quantitative Survey Respondents $n = 42$		Respondents Selected for Qualitative Interview $n = 16$	
	Food Insecure $n = 16(\%)$	Food Secure $n = 26(\%)$	Food Insecure $n = 8(\%)$	Food Secure $n = 8(\%)$
Number of children in household				
0	4(25.0)	14(53.9)	3(37.5)	4(50.0)
1	3(18.8)	3(11.5)	1(12.5)	1(12.5)
2	8(50)	4(15.4)	3(37.5)	3(37.5)
3	1(6.2)	5(19.2)	1(12.5)	0
Education Level Attained				
Completed some school	4(25.0)	7(26.9)	2(25.0)	2(25.0)
Completed school	1(6.2)	2(7.7)	2(25.0)	1(12.5)
TAFE [1], diploma, or trade	6(37.5)	5(19.2)	0	1(12.5)
Any completed tertiary study	5(31.3)	12(46.2)	4(50.0)	4(50.0)
Employment				
Full-time paid work	4(25.0)	3(11.5)	2(25.0)	2(25.0)
Part-time paid work	3(18.8)	4(15.4)	0	1(12.5)
Casual paid work	3(18.8)	2(7.7)	1(12.5)	0
Work without pay (family business)	1(6.2)	1(3.9)	1(12.5)	3(37.5)
Home duties	3(18.8)	7(26.9)	1(12.5)	0
Unemployed	0	2(7.7)	0	0
Studying	2(12.5)	1(3.9)	0	0
Studying + casual/part time work	*	*	3(37.5)	1(12.5)
Studying + house duties	*	*	1(12.5)	0
Carer	0	1(3.9)	0	0
Retired	0	5(19.2)	0	1(12.5)
Income source				
Salary	*	*	5(62.5)	4(50)
Salary and Government benefit	*	*	3(37.5)	2(25.0)
Savings and Superannuation	*	*	0	1(12.5)
Savings and Government benefit	*	*	0	1(12.5)
Main Transport				
Car/Motor Bike	14(87.5)	24(92.3)	6(75.0)	8(100.0)
Walking/Bike	2(12.5)	0	1(12.5)	0
Public Transport	0	2(7.7)	1(12.5)	0

* Not collected in the Food Security in Melbourne Households (FSiMH) survey. [1] TAFE, Technical and Further Education.

Twenty-four low-to-middle-income participants, FS ($n = 12$) and FIS ($n = 12$), consented in the FSiMH survey to be contacted to participate in the qualitative phase. Eight participants declined due to an illness, a work commitment, or no longer being interested in further participation. Sixteen in-depth interviews, FS ($n = 8$) and FIS ($n = 8$), were completed, 13 face-to-face and 3 by telephone. A key emphasis of qualitative research is the focus on the quality and not the quantity of interviews; so, sampling for the qualitative interviews in this study continued until theoretical data saturation was achieved. Theoretical data saturation in this study meant that the researcher was satisfied with the quality of the information that was obtained to be able to answer the research questions [54]. The majority of interview participants were female ($n = 15$), and nine were living in households with children. The most common housing tenure included mortgage holders ($n = 11$), and four participants were privately renting.

The severity of food insecurity experienced by the qualitative interview participants ($n = 16$) varied: marginal food security ($n = 4$, two with children), low food security ($n = 2$, one with children), and very low food security ($n = 2$, both with children).

3.2. Qualitative Results

The qualitative interview data analysis yielded 5 interacting themes and 10 subthemes. Table 2 summarises the key similarities and differences between and across the food-secure and food-insecure participants. The five main themes are presented below.

Table 2. Summary of theme and subtheme comparison between and across the food-secure and food-insecure participants.

Themes and Sub Themes	Both Food-Secure & Food-Insecure Participants	Food-Secure Participants	Food-Insecure Participants
	Theme 1: Food decisions are complex, dynamic, and multi-factorial		
Roles and values that shape food decisions	Food provision is a priority especially if children are present but money available for food challenges this.	Greater freedom for social eating but less likely to eat out with children due to cost.	Food is the priority but this is a challenge when the budget is pressured
	Food provides a connection to a community.		Stress related to social eating; budget manipulation required. Dilemmas created and potential ramifications.
Other forces that shape household food decisions	Nutrition/health priority: Quality and variety	Cognisant of food ethics: supermarket duopoly. Some households' greater financial capacity: able to respond	Budget tightrope: constant compromises to food choices
	Time available to cook and shop		
	Theme 2: Multiple protective assets: financial, social, physical, human, natural		
Strength in food literacy capabilities and resources	Food literacy skills/resourcefulness		Amplification of resourcefulness and food literacy skills. Budget assets are highly refined, creative, time-consuming, and may be unique to the household but are in a constant state of play at greater intensity.
	Budgeting skills and strategies are defined but have a differing intensity level across all households		Food cost literacy: developed capabilities to monitor food costs; with product knowledge
	Highly refined planning, food preparation, shopping assets		
	Knowledge of food alternatives: supporting modifications to food for the household.	*	
	Resourcefulness present and developed based on life experiences.		
Strength in social capital capabilities and resources	Connection to community/agencies that is required to know what broader financial resources are possible.		Connections to the broader community and social support from family and friends; these relationship assets support other assets or may facilitate them to action.
	Communities look out for each other		Greater sense of resilience drawn from within based on personal experiences and at times less reliance on social relationships
	Relationships to support food literacy skills within and external to households: role models	*	
	Growing food facilitates relationships with neighbours/community		

Table 2. *Cont.*

Themes and Sub Themes	Both Food-Secure & Food-Insecure Participants	Food-Secure Participants	Food-Insecure Participants
	Theme 3: Food insecurity triggers act alone or are cumulative and may be beyond household control		
			Triggers/trigger risks are constantly in the background.
			Budget/financial/income triggers: shocks
			Cost of Living expenses and bill shocks: utilities and seasonal fluctuations. E.g., an increase in child care fees and unresponsive government support
Internal triggers	Time available to shop and cook can manifest in households in different ways	Episodic nature of triggers. Households may have experienced triggers in past life stages that increase the risk of food insecurity; these were recalled along with stress or anxiety. These triggers mirrored those described by food insecure (FIS) participants Financial resources may be available, but physical access is challenged e.g., moving to an area with limited public transport infrastructure/no car	Changes to household composition: these may be short or long-term but consequential impacts are felt. E.g., addition of a child or family member (adult child/sibling)
			Change in relationship status: divorce
			Budget stress of trying to shop in bulk or shop for specials: trying to plan ahead.
External triggers	Perceived fluctuations in cost of food	*	Households may not have the financial resources to weather food cost changes, especially when this is added to other internal triggers.
	Physical access to food shops, availability beyond the Coles/Woolworths-type supermarkets, the preference for local shopping		
	Theme 4: Assets amplified: juggling and applying management strategies as required		
Households transform	Assets are enacted in both households but at different levels (amplification effect)	Budget/shopping management assets are present, but are not or are rarely amplified to the extent of food insecure households.	Asset pooling and juggling across the households. Often, it is just the assets from the household gatekeeper wearing the stress and strain. Amplification of transformation of assets
assets into action			Assets used in all situations at home: day-to-day, entertaining at home, and eating out/purchase of takeaway food

Table 2. *Cont.*

Themes and Sub Themes	Both Food-Secure & Food-Insecure Participants	Food-Secure Participants	Food-Insecure Participants
Transform and adapt assets with external support	Both may receive financial support from Government benefits: Family Tax Benefit, Child Care Rebate, study assistance. Households attend community-based activities: gardens, farmers markets, or similar (food source, social) but often for a different purpose.	May have the social support assets but serve a different purpose than in FIS households. Not used as a food access means.	Households may require the assets that are transformed through social/financial support: community, family, or friends, and not through welfare/food relief agencies. Issues of inability to access, and pride; there are those who are in greater need. Households rely on grandparents to pay for activities, bring food, or 'shout' lunch in food court
Theme 5: The consequences and emotional rollercoaster of food access and provision			
Stress and strain matched with give and take	Attempts to protect children if food is scarce Frustrations in both households: cost of food, availability of food, marketing of food	Some food-secure households that have experienced food insecurity or have been at risk of food security in their lifetime reflected on the level of impact of the experience and the strain, and how this has shaped their desire to not experience this again: stress, embarrassment.	Often significant compromise on food quality, quantity, and nutrition: these are constantly amplified across households compared to food secure (FS) households. Compromises may be limited to one person in the household: the food gatekeeper. Guilt associated with compromises, especially if other household members (children) are affected. The relentless, constant stresses of making ends meet: the load of this, the potential for allostatic load, and impacts on physical, social, and emotional wellbeing. This is amplified in these households. Social consequences: the compromise that is made to these opportunities and potential repercussions to self and household budgets.
4R's: Resilience, Respect, Resourceful, and Responsible	Pride/respect in strategies and skills that a household may possess, especially relating to food procurement, cooking, and sharing. Resilience/Respect/Resourcefulness Responsibility present in all households, but greater in FIS households	Present and in action, but the intensity may vary across and within households	Present in FIS households, but is greatest for the food/household gatekeeper: amplification effect

* No additional difference noted.

3.2.1. Theme 1: Food Decisions are Complex, Dynamic, and Multi-Factorial

Irrespective of food security status, food decisions were complex, often interconnected, dynamic, and multifactorial in nature, with an array of influencing factors. The role and values that were associated with food, and internal factors, such as food budgets, were impacting factors. External factors, such as cost of food and food availability, also contributed to the dynamic nature of food decisions.

Food was a priority, as described by a FS participant, Amelia, who had experienced food insecurity growing up and stated that she *'would go without anything to make sure that food was on the table'* for her children. For those experiencing, or were at risk of, food insecurity, there were additional, often constant, pressures on food decisions for the household, where the complexity and interaction of deciding factors were magnified.

Both participant groups identified food as a social conduit that provided a connection to a community. However, this was described with some preoccupation by FIS participants, who detailed a more stressed approach to eating out or entertaining that impacted on their enjoyment of the social interaction when compared to FS participants:

> *'I try to avoid it. Most I'll have is a coffee from uni . . . if they (Uni friends) buy lunch . . . . you miss out, but—there are times when I was really hungry and I didn't have my lunch, so I had to buy it. That would mean . . . , 'what am I going to do about that money when I shop on the weekend?'*
> Ann (FIS)

In contrast, FS participants described food as a medium to socialise over, with a greater sense of 'freedom' that enables social situations. This in part was reported to be influenced by a greater available budget that provided flexibility, the participant's life stage, and the presence of children in the household.

Importance was placed on the quality and variety of nutritious foods. This value was often challenged for FIS participants, especially when the budget was tight, creating competing demands for the food dollar. Both groups of participants described a hierarchy of food decision drivers in which household bills were prioritised, impacting on the available food budget:

> *'meet my expenses first, and then what money I have left over is what I would do the shopping with. I think I've just stayed that way.'* Maureen (FIS)

Time was an important resource in food decisions for all participants, particularly when the main food gatekeeper worked, studied, and/or cared for children. Shopping and food preparation tasks were often time-consuming and labour-intensive. These tasks required high levels of organisation, and often impacted on decisions that were associated with foods that were purchased for convenience (for example, the use of pre-prepared vegetables) and the question of where to shop (for example, a supermarket versus a mix of shops). FIS participants reported investing a large amount of time and energy in shopping routines. A trade-off and compromise was described:

> *'one of the biggest things that I think a lot of people have trouble with; is time . . . So it might be saving a little bit of money, but then it's costing time, and time is probably more expensive now than that'* Ava (FS) and *'it's not easy to be able to spend money on whatever you want kind of thing, so I had to invest time to look around and shop around.'* Ann (FIS).

This highlights the difference in how each of the two participant types perceived time as a resource.

3.2.2. Theme 2: Multiple Protective Assets

The participants described an array of skills and strategies that were used to both protect and support food security. Food literacy and social connections were assets that could be enacted, especially in times of greater need. For FIS participants, assets (financial, human, social, physical, and natural) were of greater intensity, well-developed, and varied. All participants described these food literacy 'life skills' as invaluable, with their development varying over each participant's lifespan.

All participants described an array of financial management assets that were employed to manage food. The intensity of these skills was greatest for FIS participants. Some FS participants recalled life stages when fiscal resources were constrained. The management strategies that they used closely mirrored those that were used by FIS participants. FS participants described the importance of an overall budget to their household. However, how it was used varied significantly in FIS participants, where the budget was closely scrutinized, as Clara explains:

'depends on robbing Peter to pay Paul with the food budget . . . it goes down to the last $10 by the end of the week... what level of food we get for the week' Clara (FIS)

Both FS and FIS participants described a range of practical strategies; for example, planning for and organisation of food to support money saving and to have pantry staples. Aspects of Theme 1 overlay this range of practical strategies.

Broader connections to community were evident across both FIS and FS participants, and were reported to be protective against food insecurity. An example is neighbours looking out for each other and sharing home grown produce. Social support that was provided by family and friends was evident. This was often in the form of general groceries and food, including meals.

3.2.3. Theme 3: Food Insecurity Triggers Act Alone or Are Cumulative and May Be beyond Household Control

The food insecurity 'triggers' were often unforeseen events or experiences that impacted on food security status and were either internal or external to the participant's household. Internal triggers included income changes, expected and unexpected expenses, and household composition changes. External triggers often reflected the broader system, economic situation, and food supply. All participants reported that these triggers acted alone or in unison, magnifying their effect on each other. Triggers, real or potential, were perceived to hover in the background of day-to-day life for FIS participants and were commonly reported. Triggers impacting on the household budget and/or total finances were points of stress and heightened the risk of food insecurity. However, participants from FS households, especially those with children, said that they were often still 'walking a budget tightrope' Ava (FS). Those classified as food secure reported previous episodes where they had difficulties accessing food as a result of the reported food insecurity triggers. These experiences were detailed with evidence of anxiety and 'not wanting to go back there (being food insecure)' Amelia (FS).

The financial triggers described by both FS and FIS participants were reported to manifest in a number of forms, from a sudden and unexpected reduction in household income or a change in household composition (birth of a child) to unexpected household expenses, including an increase living and medical expenses. These impacted on the financial stability and well-being of households, and influenced decisions on the question of whether the main caregiver should return to employment to relieve the financial load:

'No longer did we have additional income, bills kept coming plus the mortgage things were very tight.' Ann (FIS) and 'When my wife stopped working, we nearly went broke. We were down to our last dollar.' Eric (FS)

Two FS participants without a car identified difficulties in easily accessing food due to limited public transport infrastructure in their area despite adequate financial resources.

3.2.4. Theme 4: Assets Amplified: Juggling and Applying Management Strategies as Required

Whilst the assets described in Theme 2 were ever-present for all participants, it was not until one or more of the triggers (Theme 3) occurred that the assets were transformed and amplified into coping strategies. For FIS participants, there was a distinct difference in the rate and urgency of transformation of these assets. Often, these management strategies did not occur in isolation but in unison or in a staged format. This process of putting these assets into action could occur with or without support from the participant's immediate household.

Saving money was recognised as an important strategy for all participants. For FIS participants, this was invariably difficult; it meant that there was never a reserve or buffer to draw upon. In contrast, most FS participants had at least one option as a backup plan if finances were limited, including savings, credit cards, and loan redraws. This was a key point of difference when compared to FIS participants who did not have these options:

'There are times when we have had to redraw on our home loan to have more money to live off... to buy food but sometimes the usual savings account may be down so we use Visa—that's how we manage our money—then pay the card off at the end of the month so we never have to pay interest.' Rowena (FS)

When finances were limited, alternative funding for shopping was enacted, including supermarket reward and loyalty schemes that allow cash/credit for shopping, by both FS and FIS participants:

'We have [Loyalty scheme name], quite often, it will be, 'Do I need to convert my [Loyalty] points to [Loyalty] dollars, and can we go to [named Supermarket] and spend $10 getting what we need?' I always leave that as my backup of the backup plan.' Clara (FIS)

Both participant types discussed how such strategies often meant spending more on food or other household items that impact on food budgets in the short term. However, the long-term benefit of credit towards future shopping outweighed this short-term risk.

3.2.5. Theme 5: The Consequences and Emotional Rollercoaster of Food Access and Provision

The consequences and emotions that were associated with food access and provision varied considerably. For FIS participants, the experience was often fraught with relentless emotional lows. The reported consequences of not being able to access food ranged from worry to compromises on food choices and amounts. Food-secure participants reflected on a significant past experience that was related to financial difficulties that impacted on food access and provision and instigated a range of emotions. Whilst stress and anxiety were evident for some FS participants, it was not to the extent described by FIS participants. However, the impact of these past experiences was significant enough for FS participants to reflect and articulate why they wanted things to be different:

'The juggle and stress to make ends meet was too much I deferred for a year, worked fulltime, earnt money, then went back the following year and completed my degree. I don't want to go back to that stress.' Lucy (FS)

Whilst the stress of food provision often dominated participants' stories, there were also elements of triumph that were centred on respect, resilience, responsibility, and resourcefulness.
For both FIS and FS participants, respect, resilience, and resourcefulness grew from difficult experiences during childhood and adolescence:

'I'm a ... stronger person because of my childhood: a person with a different upbringing may look at things differently.' Clara (FIS) and

'It was really hard growing up and moving around all the time. Family is everything to me; it means stability, and I'm the rock for the family now ... having them over for a meal helps this ... ' Amelia (FS)

These experiences often shaped their current food access and provision life skills.

4. Discussion

The purpose of this study was to identify low-to-middle income food secure and food insecure households from Melbourne and explore and compare food security and insecurity experiences and implications. The results highlight the precarious nature of achieving food security in lower-income groups and the resourcefulness, resilience, and array of assets or strengths that participants use when facing triggers that threaten their food security. Furthermore, they indicate that those who were categorised as food secure using the USDA-HFSSM may be at risk due to the existence of additional factors beyond those of a financial origin, such as a lack of physical access to, or a limited supply of, culturally appropriate foods. To our knowledge, this is the first study to explore the experience of food insecurity of low-to-middle income households in Australia.

4.1. Low-to-Middle Income Households' Experiences: Assets, Resourcefulness, Resilience, and Emotions

The food insecurity triggers that were described by both groups of participants, such as a change in income, increased cost of living expenses, and changes in household composition, are consistent with those reported for low-to-middle income households in Canada and the U.S. [34,36] and lower-income U.S. and Australian households [25,59,60]. The key differences between food-secure and food-insecure participants were the number and complexity of factors and the cumulative and relentless nature of the triggers.

The interviews allowed for the exploration of the range of assets possessed by both FS and FIS low-to middle income participants. At the core of these assets was food literacy and social connection, which supported both the capabilities and resources of the household. The existence of assets and skills inclusive of, but not limited to, budgeting and planning for food, and purchasing and preparing food, have been reported in food-insecure, lower-income households [52,61–63]. A key difference between FS and FIS participants in this study was the amplification of these assets and their ability to provide a crucial buffer to the food insecurity experience, but only up to a certain point. This is consistent with the limited capacity of food literacy skills to ameliorate the food insecurity experience because of the complex range of food insecurity determinants [64,65]. The range of assets was found to support the high degree of resourcefulness with food acquisition and (food and financial) management that was demonstrated by FS and FIS participants. The resourcefulness of individuals facing food insecurity has been reported previously, and should be considered in approaches to prevent or address food insecurity [63,64].

The asset of support was important to both FS and FIS participants. Social support in the food security literature has been described in the contexts of emotional, instrumental (child care, food, or material items), and informational support (advice and factual information) [66]. Consistent with this literature, the social support that is reported in this study was described as arising from two sources: (1) networks of family and friends, and (2) networks in the broader environment, such as community agencies and government benefits systems. Both FS and FIS participants described sourcing support predominately from friends and family and limited interaction with community welfare. This was driven by the potential shame and stigma, and confirms that reported in some low-income groups [63].

The associated emotions and experiences of trying to achieve or maintain food security were evident in both participant groups. Despite previous and current food insecurity experiences, its impacts were felt both psychologically and physically. Participants detailed the stress, shame, embarrassment, and concern due to the stigma of not being able to pay for food and/or feed children. The emotional experiences of these low-to-middle income participants are consistent with those reported principally by women in Australian and Canadian low-income, food-insecure households [9,25,63]. Often, counteracting these emotions was the high degree of resilience present in many participants. Resilience is a dynamic concept influenced by life-course events, and has been believed to contain two key elements: adversity and positive adaptation [67,68]. The level of resilience evident in both FS and FIS participants was shaped through life experiences that were often adverse in nature [69].

4.2. Categorisation of Food Security and Examining Etiology

The USDA HFSSM classification of food insecurity is based on a lack of money available to purchase food, and the interviews confirmed that financial factors/stressors were the main food insecurity trigger in the participant groups. While this finding supports the association with financial factors that has been described in the literature, it is important to reflect upon this trigger more broadly in the context of both financial constraints and assets [52,70]. The finding provides a rationale for examining the financial causes of food insecurity beyond household annual income, which is a static, insensitive measure and may not reflect sudden household economic changes that can temporarily lead to bouts of food insecurity [28,71]. Of note is that all low-to-middle income participants' main income sources were from salaries alone, in some cases supplemented with Government assistance payments, such as the Family Tax Benefit. This is supported by previous studies that found that those who are employed also experience food insecurity [24,50,72,73]. Employment status, in particular having multiple part-time jobs rather than full-time work, has been associated with an increased risk of food insecurity [73]. Additionally, having more than one income earner in a household has been shown to reduce the odds of experiencing food insecurity [72]. In this study, 12 of the 16 interviewed participants indicated that the primary income earner in the household was employed at a full-time or near full-time level. Furthermore, in seven of these households, another member was employed full-time, part-time, or casually.

The participants discussed the need for sufficient income or financial resources to meet the rising cost of living expenses. The capacity to have savings available when needed was described by both FS and FIS participants as a crucial strategy to buffer against the impact of unexpected expenses, but one that some FIS participants described as being difficult to implement. The evidence for savings as a protective factor against food insecurity is recognised both internationally [74] and nationally [22,75]. Australian evidence on the association between the capacity to save and food insecurity is limited. Foley (2010) reported that those Australians who were unable to save were 6.5 times more likely to have experienced food insecurity in the last 12 months [75].

This research highlights two points related to food security status classification that warrant further consideration.

4.2.1. Marginal Food Security Severity Categorisation

This study modified the food security classification from that of the original USDA-HFSSM protocol, where one or two affirmative responses were classified as food insecure at the severity level of marginally food secure, and allowed for exploration of their experience [10,14,24]. Understanding the marginally food secure experience has importance from epidemiological, public health, and public policy perspectives [14]. The decision to categorise those participants that were experiencing marginal food security as food insecure was supported by the findings, particularly by those stories that portrayed the experience of anxiety and stress regarding food provision. Despite two FIS participants being classified as marginally food insecure, their stories revealed a history of more severe forms of food insecurity over their lifetime and described rapid transitions between severity levels. As suggested by Loopstra (2013), those experiencing marginal food security may experience poorer health outcomes and increased forms of material hardship when compared to food-secure individuals [50].

4.2.2. Classification of Food Security Status beyond Financial Resource Constraints

Whilst financial resource challenges may be the primary determinant of food security status, there may be circumstances where other determinants beyond this are challenged. The USDA-HFSSM is based on economic access to food; it does not take into consideration other reasons for the existence of food insecurity. A recent systematic literature review indicated that there is an absence of multi-item tools that can assess food security beyond the one dimension of financial access [47]. Both FS and FIS participants described additional experiences beyond those of financial resources that challenged their food security status and constituted limitations in their physical access to a food supply. For FS participants, this was despite having adequate financial resources. One FS participant described her recent move from interstate to an area that had poor public transport infrastructure, and, as she did not have a car, this resulted in a limited capacity to source culturally relevant foods. Despite being able to access some food in a small but more expensive food outlet, her food choices were compromised. A lack of access to a car has been associated with an increased difficulty of accessing food outlets [19,76]. This experience highlights the importance of all dimensions of food security, including an adequate supply, physical and economic access, and the resources to utilise food, to achieve and maintain food security [1], and supports the need for a food security measurement tool that is inclusive of these dimensions. Such a measurement tool, the Household Food and Nutrition Security Survey (HFNSS), which is based on the USDA-HFSSM, has been developed and undergone preliminary validation in Australia [77,78].

4.3. Strengths, Limitations, and Further Research

This study is the first Australian study to examine the existence and experience of FS and FIS in low-to-middle income Australian households. Additionally, the focus of the research in the qualitative phase provides an important contribution to the literature, particularly in Australia, as it provides the first exploration of the experience of food insecurity within this income group. The mixed-methods approach allowed for detailed exploration of the experiences of food insecurity and food security. The methodology supported the understanding of the construct and experience of food insecurity in this income group more than a quantitative or qualitative methodology alone. The constant comparison approach to the analysis supported the interpretation of the findings. An additional strength was the case selection method for the interviews, which supported the transferability of the qualitative findings. Selecting participants from those that had participated in the quantitative survey allowed for further interpretation of the findings when supported by the stories of participants.

A potential limitation is the gender-biased nature of the recruitment. This resulted from the main food provider completing the survey, which resulted in a higher number of women participants (88%). Fifteen women and one male were interviewed, which potentially may impact on the credibility and dependability of the interview data. The inclusion of only one male voice provided a narrow view of how men may perceive food insecurity. However, this response rate is reflective of gender food provision roles, where women predominantly have the responsibility of being the principal food provider [79], which may subsequently affect how they report these experiences. While a theoretical gender lens was not applied in this study, the findings on the physical, social, and emotional food insecurity experiences of women have been previously described in food-insecure households [80].

Further exploration of the experiences of, and the role of the extensive range of assets in, these low-to-middle income participants can better inform responses to food insecurity. In addition, more research is needed to explore the experience of food insecurity in different contexts, including: geographic locations of rural and metropolitan areas of Australia, sub-population groups, and both lower- and higher-income groups. This should include the exploration of determinants inclusive of a range of financial indicators, such as capacity to save, but also additional determinants of food insecurity. The use of mixed methods in future research efforts is crucial to provide a more detailed and rich understanding of the true and precarious nature of this phenomenon.

5. Conclusions

This study reveals novel and important findings on the existence of food insecurity amongst low-to-middle income Melbourne households, an income group that would not necessarily be considered food insecure within the context of a high-income country. Additionally, these findings support the precarious nature and balancing act of achieving food security for some low-to-middle income households. The experiences of those classified as marginally food secure confirm the need for further research within this severity-level group regardless of income.

While limited financial resources are a primary determinant of food security status, this research confirmed that there are multiple additional determinants that must be considered to maintain food security.. The results revealed the constant balancing act, especially of a range of financial, social, physical, and personal assets, that must be undertaken to prevent or alleviate the experiences of food insecurity. The findings of this work may be used to support policies and practices to prevent or alleviate food insecurity in low-to-middle income groups in urban Australia.

Author Contributions: Conceptualization, S.K., S.B., Z.E.D., and C.P.; Methodology, S.K., S.B., Z.E.D., and C.P.; Software, S.K.; Formal Analysis, S.K.; Investigation, S.K.; Data Curation, S.K.; Writing (Original Draft Manuscript Preparation), S.K.; Writing (Review & Editing), all authors.

Acknowledgments: The authors thank the Department of Nutrition, Dietetics, and Food vacation scholarship students Emma Chappell and Tracey Nau for their support in identifying community agencies in VAMPIRE suburbs. The authors also thank Steph Ashby, dietitian and honours student, for her assistance with the implementation of the 'Food Security in Melbourne Households' survey.

References

1.   Food and Agriculture Organization. An Introduction to the Basic Concepts of Food Security. Available online: www.fao.org/docrep/013/al936e/al936e00.pdf (accessed on 2 August 2018).

2.   Australian Bureau of Statistics. Australian Health Survey: Nutrition State and Territory Results 2011–2012 Cat No. 4364.0.55.009. Available online: http://www.abs.gov.au/AUSSTATS/abs@.nsf/DetailsPage/4364.0.55.0092011-12?OpenDocument (accessed on 10 August 2018).

3.   Carter, K.N.; Lanumata, T.; Kruse, K.; Gorton, D. What are the determinants of food insecurity in New Zealand and does this differ for males and females? *Aust. N. Z. J. Public Health* **2010**, *34*, 602–608. [CrossRef] [PubMed]

4.   Tarasuk, V.; Mitchell, A.; Dachner, N. Household Food Insecurity in Canada, 2012. Available online: http://nutritionalsciences.lamp.utoronto.ca/Research (accessed on 19 August 2018).

5.   Bates, B.; Roberts, C.; Lepps, H.; Porter, L. *The Food and Your Survey Wave 4. Combined Report for England, Wales and Northern Ireland*; Food Standards Agency: London, UK, 2017; pp. 26–29.

6.   United States Department of Agriculture. Food Security Status of U.S. Households in 2014. Available online: http://www.ers.usda.gov/topics/food-nutrition-assistance/food-security-in-the-us.aspx (accessed on 1 September 2018).

7.   Bickel, G.; Nord, M.; Price, C.; Hamilton, W.; Cook, J. *Guide to Measuring Household Food Security, Revised 2000*; U.S. Department of Agriculture: Alexandria, VA, USA, 2013; pp. 1–75.

8.   Radimer, K.L.; Olson, C.M.; Campbell, C.C. Development of Indicators to Assess Hunger. *J. Nutr.* **1990**, *120*, 1544–1548. [CrossRef] [PubMed]

9.   Hamelin, A.-M.; Beaudry, M.; Habicht, J.-P. Characterization of household food insecurity in Québec: Food and feelings. *Soc. Sci. Med.* **2002**, *54*, 119–132. [CrossRef]

10.   Coleman-Jensen, A.U.S. Food Insecurity Status: Toward a Refined Definition. *Soc. Indic. Res.* **2010**, *95*, 215–230. [CrossRef]

11.   Radimer, K.L. Measurement of household food security in the USA and other industrialised countries. *Public Health Nutr.* **2002**, *5*, 859–864. [CrossRef] [PubMed]

12.   Vozoris, N.T.; Tarasuk, V.S. Household food insufficiency is associated with poorer health. *J. Nutr.* **2003**, *133*, 120–126. [CrossRef] [PubMed]

13.   Stuff, J.E.; Casey, P.H.; Szeto, K.L.; Gossett, J.M.; Robbins, J.M.; Simpson, P.M.; Connell, C.; Bogle, M.L. Household food insecurity is associated with adult health status. *J. Nutr.* **2004**, *134*, 2330–2335. [CrossRef] [PubMed]

14. Cook, J.T.; Black, M.; Chilton, M.; Cutts, D.; Ettinger de Cuba, S.; Heeren, T.C.; Rose-Jacobs, R.; Sandel, M.; Casey, P.H.; Coleman, S.; et al. Are food insecurity's health impacts underestimated in the U.S. population? Marginal food security also predicts adverse health outcomes in young U.S. children and mothers. *Adv. Nutr.* **2013**, *4*, 51–61. [CrossRef] [PubMed]

15. Tarasuk, V.; Cheng, J.; de Oliveira, C.; Dachner, N.; Gundersen, C.; Kurdyak, P. Association between household food insecurity and annual health care costs. *Can. Med. Assoc. J.* **2015**, *187*, E429–E436. [CrossRef] [PubMed]

16. Adams, D.; Galvin, L. *Institutional Capability. Food Security and Local Government in Tasmania*; Heart Foundation: Tasmania, Australia, 2015; pp. 1–29.

17. Winicki, J.; Jemison, K. Food insecurity and hunger in the kindergarten classroom: Its effect on learning and growth. *Contemp. Econ. Policy* **2003**, *21*, 145–157. [CrossRef]

18. Bartfeld, J.; Dunifon, R. State-level predictors of food insecurity among households with children. *J. Policy Anal. Manag.* **2006**, *25*, 921–942. [CrossRef]

19. Gorton, D.; Bullen, C.R.; Mhurchu, C.N. Environmental influences on food security in high-income countries. *Nutr. Rev.* **2010**, *68*, 1–29. [CrossRef] [PubMed]

20. Chilton, M.M.; Rabinowich, J.R.; Woolf, N.H. Very low food security in the USA is linked with exposure to violence. *Public Health Nutr.* **2014**, *17*, 73–82. [CrossRef] [PubMed]

21. McIntyre, L.; Wu, X.; Fleisch, V.C.; Emery, H.J.C. Homeowner versus non-homeowner differences in household food insecurity in Canada. *J. Hous. Built Environ.* **2016**, *31*, 349–366. [CrossRef]

22. Nolan, M.; Williams, M.; Rikard-Bell, G.; Mohsin, M. Food insecurity in three socially disadvantaged localities in Sydney, Australia. *Health Promot. J. Aust.* **2006**, *17*, 247–254. [CrossRef]

23. Kirkpatrick, S.I.; Tarasuk, V. Assessing the relevance of neighbourhood characteristics to the household food security of low-income Toronto families. *Public Health Nutr.* **2010**, *13*, 1139–1148. [CrossRef] [PubMed]

24. Gunderson, C.; Kreider, B.; Pepper, J. The economics of food insecurity in the United States. *AEPP* **2011**, *33*, 281–303. [CrossRef]

25. King, S.; Moffitt, A.; Bellamy, J.; Carter, S.; McDowell, C.; Mollenhauser, J. *When There's Not Enough to Eat. A National Study of Food Insecurity among Emergency Relief Clients*; Anglicare, Diocese of Sydney: Sydney, Australia, 2012; pp. 1–138.

26. Ramsey, R.; Giskes, K.; Turrell, G.; Gallegos, D. Food insecurity among adults residing in disadvantaged urban areas: Potential health and dietary consequences. *Public Health Nutr.* **2012**, *15*, 227–237. [CrossRef] [PubMed]

27. Langellier, B.A.; Chaparro, M.P.; Sharp, M.; Birnbach, K.; Brown, E.R.; Harrison, G.G. Trends and Determinants of Food Insecurity among Adults in Low-Income Households in California. *J. Hunger Environ. Nutr.* **2012**, *7*, 401–413. [CrossRef]

28. Rose, D. Economic determinants and dietary consequences of food insecurity in the United States. *J. Nutr.* **1999**, *129* (Suppl. 2), S517–S520. [CrossRef] [PubMed]

29. Tarasuk, V. Household food insecurity in Canada. *Top. Clin. Nutr.* **2005**, *20*, 299–312. [CrossRef]

30. Guo, B. Household Assets and Food Security: Evidence from the Survey of Program Dynamics. *J. Fam. Econ. Issues* **2011**, *32*, 98–110. [CrossRef]

31. Martin-Fernandez, J.; Grillo, F.; Parizot, I.; Caillavet, F.; Chauvin, P. Prevalence and socioeconomic and geographical inequalities of household food insecurity in the Paris region, France, 2010. *BMC Public Health* **2013**, *13*, 486. [CrossRef] [PubMed]

32. Kleve, S.; Davidson, Z.E.; Gearon, E.; Booth, S.; Palermo, C. Are low-to-middle-income households experiencing food insecurity in Victoria, Australia? An examination of the Victorian Population Health Survey, 2006–2009. *Aust. J. Prim. Health* **2017**, *23*, 249–256. [CrossRef] [PubMed]

33. Tarasuk, V.; Vogt, J. Household food insecurity in Ontario. *Can. J. Public Health* **2009**, *100*, 184–188. [PubMed]

34. Olabiyi, O.M.; McIntyre, L. Determinants of Food Insecurity in Higher-Income Households in Canada. *J. Hunger Environ. Nutr.* **2014**, *9*, 433–448. [CrossRef]

35. Nord, M. *Food Spending Declined and Food Insecurity Increased for Middle-Income and Low-Income Households from 2000 to 2007*; 61; United States Department of Agriculture: Washington, DC, USA, 2009; pp. 1–25.

36. Nord, M.; Brent, C. *Food Insecurity in Higher Income Households*; United States Department of Agriculture: Washington, DC, USA, 2002.

37. Huang, J.; Guo, B.; Kim, Y. Food insecurity and disability: Do economic resources matter? *Soc. Sci. Res.* **2010**, *39*, 111–124. [CrossRef]

38. Creswell, J.W.; Piano Clark, V.L. *Designing and Conducting Mixed Methods Research*, 2nd ed.; Sage Publications Inc.: Thousand Oaks, CA, USA, 2011; pp. 1–443.

39. Tashakkori, A.; Teddlie, C. *Handbook of Mixed Methods in Social & Behavioral Research*, 1st ed.; Sage Publciations: Thousand Oak, CA, USA, 2003; pp. 1–768.

40. Tashakkori, A.; Teddlie, C. *Handbook of Mixed Methods in Social & Behavioral Research*, 2nd ed.; Sage: Thousand Oak, CA, USA, 2010.

41. Morgan, D. Practical strategies for combining qualitatve and quantitative methods. Applications in health research. *Qual. Health Res.* **1998**, *8*, 362–376. [CrossRef] [PubMed]

42. Dodson, J.; Sipe, N. *Unsettling Suburbia the New Landscape of Oil and Mortgage Vulnerability in Australian Cities*; 17; Griffith University: Queensland, Australia, 2008; pp. 1–42.

43. Webber, C.B.; Rojhani, A. Rise In Gasoline Price Affects Food Buying Habits of Low-Income, Ethnically-Diverse Families Enrolled In Southwest Michigan WIC Program. *J. Nutr. Educ. Behav.* **2009**, *41* (Suppl. 4), S1. [CrossRef]

44. Rossimel, A.; Han, S.S.; Larsen, K.; Palermo, C. Access and affordability of nutritious food in metropolitan Melbourne. *Nutr. Diet.* **2016**, *73*, 13–18. [CrossRef]

45. Australian Bureau of Statistics. Household Income and Income Distribution Australia Detailed Tables Table 2011 Table 2012. Available online: www.abs.gov.au?AUSSTATS/abs@.nsf/DetailsPage/6523.02011-12? OpenDocument (accessed on 25 August 2018).

46. Victorian Department of Health. Victorian Population Health Survey 2008. Available online: www.health. vic.gov.au/healthstatus/vphs.htm (accessed on 3 February 2014).

47. Ashby, S.; Kleve, S.; McKechnie, R.; Palermo, C. Measurement of the dimensions of food insecurity in developed countries: A systematic literature review. *Public Health Nutr.* **2016**, *19*, 2887–2896. [CrossRef] [PubMed]

48. Ramsey, R.; Giskes, K.; Turrell, G.; Gallegos, D. Food insecurity among Australian children: Potential determinants, health and developmental consequences. *J. Child Health Care* **2011**, *15*, 401–416. [CrossRef] [PubMed]

49. Marques, E.S.; Reichenheim, M.E.; de Moraes, C.L.; Antunes, M.M.; Salles-Costa, R. Household food insecurity: A systematic review of the measuring instruments used in epidemiological studies. *Public Health Nutr.* **2015**, *18*, 877–892. [CrossRef] [PubMed]

50. Loopstra, R.; Tarasuk, V. What does increasing severity of food insecurity indicate for food insecure families? Relationships between severity of food insecurity and indicators of material hardship and constrained food purchasing. *J. Hunger Environ. Nutr.* **2013**, *8*, 337–349. [CrossRef]

51. Economic Research Service. Ranges of Food Security and Food Insecurity. USDA Labels Describe Range of Food Security. 2006. Available online: www.ers.usda.gov/topics/food-nutrition-assistance/food-security-in-the-us/definitions-of-food-security/#ranges (accessed on 1 September 2017).

52. Hamelin, A.-M.; Mercier, C.; Bédard, A. Discrepancies in households and other stakeholders viewpoints on the food security experience: A gap to address. *Health Educ. Res.* **2010**, *25*, 401–412. [CrossRef] [PubMed]

53. Hamelin, A.-M.; Mercier, C.; Bédard, A. Needs for food security from the standpoint of Canadian households participating and not participating in community food programmes. *Int. J. Consum. Stud.* **2011**, *35*, 58–68. [CrossRef]

54. Liamputtong, P. *Qualitative Research Methods*, 4th ed.; Oxford University Press: Melbourne, Australia, 2013; pp. 1–379.

55. Committee on World Food Security. *Coming to Terms with Terminology*; CFS 2012/39/4; Food and Agriculture Organisation: Rome, Italy, 2012; pp. 1–33.

56. Braun, V.; Clarke, V. Using thematic analysis in psychology. *Qual. Res. Psychol.* **2006**, *3*, 77–101. [CrossRef]

57. Boeije, H. A Purposeful Approach to the Constant Comparative Method in the Analysis of Qualitative Interviews. *Qual. Quant.* **2002**, *36*, 391–409. [CrossRef]

58. Liamputtong, P. *Research Methods in Health. Foundations for Evidence-Based Practice*, 2nd ed.; Oxford University Press: Melbourne, Australia, 2013.

59. De Marco, M.; Thorburn, S.; Kue, J. "In a Country as Affluent as America, People Should be Eating": Experiences With and Perceptions of Food Insecurity Among Rural and Urban Oregonians. *Qual. Health Res.* **2009**, *19*, 1010–1024. [CrossRef] [PubMed]

60. King, S.; Bellamy, J.; Kemp, B.; Mollenhauer, J. *Hard Choices. Going Without in a Time of Plenty a Study of Food Insecurity in NSW and the ACT*; Prepared on behalf of ANGLICARE Sydney, the Samaritans Foundation and Anglicare NSW South, NSW West & ACT; ANGLICARE Diocese of Sydney Social Policy & Research Unit: Parramatta, Australia, 2013.

61. Loopstra, R.; Tarasuk, V. Perspectives on community gardens, community kitchens and the good food box program in a community-based sample of low-income families. *Can. J. Public Health* **2013**, *104*, e55–e59. [PubMed]

62. Tarasuk, V. A Critical Examination of Community-Based Responses to Household Food Insecurity in Canada. *Health Educ. Behav.* **2001**, *28*, 487–499. [CrossRef] [PubMed]

63. Buck-McFadyen, E. Rural food insecurity: When cooking skills, homegrown food, and perseverance aren't enough to feed a family. *Can. J. Public Health* **2015**, *106*, 140–146. [CrossRef] [PubMed]

64. Gallegos, D. The nexus between food literacy. Food security and disadvantage. In *Food Literacy: Key Concepts for Health and Education*, 1st ed.; Vidgen, H., Ed.; Routledge: London, UK, 2016; pp. 134–150.

65. Collins, P.A.; Power, E.M.; Little, M.H. Municipal-level responses to household food insecurity in Canada: A call for critical, evaluative research. *Can. J. Public Health* **2014**, *105*, e138–e141. [CrossRef] [PubMed]

66. Davis, B.L.; Grutzmacher, S.K.; Munger, A.L. Utilization of Social Support among Food Insecure Individuals: A Qualitative Examination of Network Strategies and Appraisals. *J. Hunger Environ. Nutr.* **2016**, *11*, 162–179. [CrossRef]

67. Fletcher, D.; Sarkar, M. Psychological Resilience: A Review and Critique of Definitions, Concepts, and Theory. *Eur. Psychol.* **2013**, *18*, 12–23. [CrossRef]

68. Rutter, M. Resilience as a dynamic concept. *Dev. Psychopathol.* **2012**, *24*, 335–344. [CrossRef] [PubMed]

69. Younginer, N.A.; Blake, C.E.; Draper, C.L.; Jones, S.J. Resilience and Hope: Identifying Trajectories and Contexts of Household Food Insecurity. *J. Hunger Environ. Nutr.* **2015**, *10*, 230–258. [CrossRef]

70. Coleman-Jensen, A.; Gregory, C.; Singh, A. *Household Food Security in the United States in 2013*; United States Department of Agriculture, Economic Research Service: Washington, DC, USA, 2014.

71. Chang, Y.; Chatterjee, S.; Kim, J. Household Finance and Food Insecurity. *J. Fam. Econ. Issues* **2014**, *35*, 499–515. [CrossRef]

72. McIntyre, L.; Bartoo, A.C.; Emery, J.H. When working is not enough: Food insecurity in the Canadian labour force. *Public Health Nutr.* **2012**, *17*, 49–57. [CrossRef] [PubMed]

73. Coleman-Jensen, A.J. Working for Peanuts: Nonstandard Work and Food Insecurity across Household Structure. *J. Fam. Econ. Issues* **2011**, *32*, 84–97. [CrossRef]

74. Olson, C.M.; Rauschenbach, B.S.; Frongillo, E.A., Jr.; Kendall, A. Factors contributing to household food insecurity in a rural upstate New York county. *Fam. Econ. Nutr. Rev.* **1997**, *10*, 2–17.

75. Foley, W.; Ward, P.; Carter, P.; Coveney, J.; Tsourtos, G.; Taylor, A. An ecological analysis of factors associated with food insecurity in South Australia, 2002–2007. *Public Health Nutr.* **2010**, *13*, 215–221. [CrossRef] [PubMed]

76. Burns, C.; Bentley, R.; Thornton, L.; Kavanagh, A. Reduced food access due to a lack of money, inability to lift and lack of access to a car for food shopping: A multilevel study in Melbourne, Victoria. *Public Health Nutr.* **2011**, *14*, 1017–1023. [CrossRef] [PubMed]

77. Archer, C.; Gallegos, D.; McKechnie, R. Developing measures of food and nutrition security within an Australian context. *Public Health Nutr.* **2017**, *20*, 2513–2522. [CrossRef] [PubMed]

78. Kleve, S.; Gallegos, D.; Ashby, S.; Palermo, C.E.; McKechnie, R. Preliminary validation and piloting of a comprehensive measure of household food security in Australia. *Public Health Nutr.* **2018**, *21*, 526–534. [CrossRef] [PubMed]

79. DeVault, M.L. *Feeding the Family: The Social Organization of Caring as Gendered Work*; University of Chicago Press: Chicago, IL, USA, 1991.

80. Matheson, J.; McIntyre, L. Women respondents report higher household food insecurity than do men in similar Canadian households. *Public Health Nutr.* **2014**, *17*, 40–48. [CrossRef] [PubMed]

8

Re-Evaluating Expertise: Principles for Food and Nutrition Security Research, Advocacy and Solutions in High-Income Countries

Danielle Gallegos [1,2,*] and Mariana M. Chilton [3]

[1] School of Exercise and Nutrition Sciences, Queensland University of Technology; Brisbane 4059, Australia
[2] Center for Children's Health Research, Institute of Health and Biomedical Innovation, Queensland University of Technology, Brisbane 4101, Australia
[3] Department of Health Management and Policy, Dornsife School of Public Health, Drexel University, Philadelphia, PA 19104, USA; mmc33@drexel.edu
[*] Correspondence: danielle.gallegos@qut.edu.au

Abstract: Drawing on examples from Australia and the United States, we outline the benefits of sharing expertise to identify new approaches to food and nutrition security. While there are many challenges to sharing expertise such as discrimination, academic expectations, siloed thinking, and cultural differences, we identify principles and values that can help food insecurity researchers to improve solutions. These principles are critical consciousness, undoing white privilege, adopting a rights framework, and engaging in co-creation processes. These changes demand a commitment to the following values: acceptance of multiple knowledges, caring relationships, humility, empathy, reciprocity, trust, transparency, accountability, and courage.

Keywords: food and nutrition security; research; values; co-creation; trauma-informed

1. Introduction

Food insecurity is a symptom of our social, economic, political, and ecological systems in crisis. Hunger is not due to a lack of food production or availability but rather to the unequal and unjust distribution of people's entitlements to social and economic support [1]. The economically, politically, and socially powerful also control access to food and conditions under which food is available, effectively limiting the capabilities of others. These crises have at their root the continued legacy of colonization and the overarching neoliberal principles of the market economy and personal responsibility. These conditions perpetuate the structural and social institutions that undermine individual and collective agency. The result for people who are low-income is limited access to healthy food and other basic needs such as safe and affordable housing, utilities, gainful employment, and opportunities for political and civic participation.

Rising obesity rates across all social strata, overall low breastfeeding rates, and continued disparities in food insecurity point to systems failures and to inadequate approaches to improve nutrition and food security. Included in these failures is the lack of engagement with appropriate experts with lived experience. Experts from dominant classes have become adept at aligning with powerful authorities in order to interpret and translate complex issues into "health-speak" while viewing people who lack income as passive recipients of expert nutrition and financial knowledge. In high-income countries a primary response to food and nutrition insecurity has been the growth of the charitable food sector, while government and public support for adequate wages and entitlements to basic needs, adequate means for earning money, and a publicly funded safety net have been receding or are under threat [2–4]. The lack of success in addressing food and nutrition insecurity indicates that there is a serious gap between supposed knowledge sitting with the "experts" from academia, law, non-governmental organizations (NGOs), corporations, and other arenas of social and political power, and the realities of people who struggle with food insecurity. This gap is an indication that experts with financial resources and power do not truly understand the causes and experiences of food insecurity, and thereby promote solutions that are misplaced or inadequate.

While there are many examples of people with lived experiences with poverty and food insecurity that are active in academia in a way that informs their work and strengthens their approaches, the academic research community overall has failed to effectively work with and learn from people who have lived experience in a manner that can promote lasting change [5,6]. Though there are several inspiring exceptions such as The Food Action Research Centre (FoodArc) in Nova Scotia, Canada and the Poverty and the Social Exclusion Program in the United Kingdom, the tendency in the academic study of food insecurity is to drown out, exclude, or marginalize the experiences of people with lived experience [7–9]. Additionally, those with lived experience with food insecurity within academia can help to lead the way for researchers and others, yet due to potential stigma and structural barriers, they may not be willing to do so [10]. As there are growing numbers of people who have experienced poverty and also report food insecurity during college years [11,12], engaging with people with lived experiencing in food insecurity in all arenas will strengthen and inform solutions that have otherwise been lacking.

We encourage researchers, policy makers and non-profit organizations to ensure that the lived experience and wisdom of those who experience food and nutrition insecurity, including those in academia and other professional occupations, are central in the conceptualization of food and nutrition security challenges and solutions. We identify some challenges for doing so. Focusing our efforts on governments, social services agencies, NGO's, and civil society (rather than on public private partnerships that engage the corporate sector) we characterize ways in which experts of all kinds can work together to identify the local, regional and national solutions that lead to effective nutrition and food security.

This paper emerges from research undertaken by the authors working in different paradigms (nutrition and anthropology) with individuals and communities that are economically oppressed which include but are not limited to; indigenous peoples, migrants and refugees, and those experiencing hunger, poverty, and trauma. We acknowledge that we are both white and privileged; and that we are products of and operate within the colonialist structures of education, health and welfare. Our context likely limits our viewpoints and clouds our own understanding of what we have learned so far about solutions to food insecurity. We outline here what we hope can be the beginning of a dialogue about our own limitations and the limitations of the research community. We start with our experiences in addressing poverty and food insecurity through our lenses as people who have had the privilege to work with families and communities that have experienced food and nutrition insecurity. Gallegos has worked as a public health nutritionist among Torres Strait and Pacific Islander communities, migrant and refugee communities, and marginalized youth in Australia. Chilton has worked with the Southern Cheyenne and Arapaho tribes in the United States and with caregivers of young children participating in public assistance in the United States who are primarily African American and Latinx.

First, we identify the significance of working in partnership with experts with lived experience of food insecurity, we then address the challenges to collaboration and co-creation, and finally we describe the necessary principles and values that can help to drive potential solutions.

2. Examples and Insights on Benefits of Shared Expertise

We are aware that there are many types of programs that have partnered with people who know food insecurity and hunger first-hand with indigenous groups, farmers and community activists [13,14]. However, in the interest of utilizing our own experiences as grounding for our conviction that partnership is key, we focus on specific examples from Australia and the United States. The Australian example provides insight into how co-creation of solutions can be developed in programs already prescribed by health and political structures. It could be argued that the solutions developed in this program were expedient and immediate, framed by the structures in which the program was embedded. The U.S. example demonstrates the additional step around developing capacity for political action that go to root causes of food insecurity such as violence and discrimination, and the systems that perpetuate these dynamics.

2.1. Australia

Good Food for New Arrivals (GFNA) was a nutrition intervention program funded by the Commonwealth Department of Health through the national child nutrition program and the Department of Family and Community Services from 2001 to 2008 [15,16]. The original aim of GFNA was not to address food and nutrition security but rather to develop nutrition resources to "educate" newly arrived refugee families about nutrition within the western context. Originally the program set out to change what were unhealthy food choices as determined by nutrition and health promotion professionals. Rather than rely on this second-hand knowledge, the program undertook a community participatory approach that engaged members of identified communities (South Sudanese, Hazara Afghani, African 'Grand Lacs' (Democratic Republic of Congo, Rwanda, Burundi), Iraqi and Iranian [17]. Community members identified iron deficiency, poor appetite in children, food safety and foods appropriate for school as key issues. GFNA was also the first program to identify that food and nutrition insecurity was an issue for refugees settling in Australia with 70% of households running out of money for food [18]. Over the program's duration GFNA developed a set of resources that addressed multiple issues identified by both communities and health professionals. However, an evaluability assessment of the program identified that the underlying funding premise was that refugees were "doing something wrong". After engagement with communities GFNA identified that the deficits lay within the infrastructural constraints of the system and with health professionals [19]. This realization led to the identification of a broader range of activities including the development of nutrition champions from within communities and influencing system changes such as the speed at which welfare payments were processed on arrival. The examples of the reasons for running out of food clearly demonstrated a link to trauma and adverse childhood events and included: high medical costs associated with amputation due to a landmine, having family back in the country of origin and feeling guilty about eating, and also moving from having no food to having some food [18].

2.2. United States

Witnesses to Hunger (Witnesses) is an ongoing participatory action program that works with women who know hunger first-hand to increase their meaningful participation in the national dialogue on poverty. Witnesses began in Philadelphia in 2008 with 42 mothers of young children that then expanded to multiple cities to reach over 100 participants. Most members of Witnesses were eager to share their experiences of poverty, their ideas on ways to overcome it, and to inform key decision-makers about the importance of improving labor laws, neighborhood zoning codes, education, tax and labor policies, and to recognize the true value of each person, of motherhood, childhood, and family struggle. Utilizing a human rights approach where the rights-holders participate in shaping the problem, challenges, and solutions, members of Witnesses to Hunger have not only contributed to ethnographic and qualitative research, but also mounted over 30 exhibits of their photographs in locations such as the US Senate, the US House of Representatives, city halls and state houses for audiences that include elected officials, federal, city and state agency administrators, community leaders, the press and the lay public [20,21]. Exhibits also include public forums, hearings and formal testimonies with elected officials. In addition to exhibits, policy briefs, individual and group visits to elected officials, members of Witnesses launched their own blog series and developed a social media presence. They speak at conferences and have co-authored scholarly publications and newspaper opinion essays that demand focus on root causes of food insecurity such as violence (institutional racism, community violence, interpersonal violence, and policy violence), discrimination, and inadequate health and welfare systems.

2.3. Benefits and Insights

From these two case studies of co-creation and mutual engagement, there emerged four significant insights: (1) solutions should recognize personal and collective agency and seek to promote freedom and opportunity; (2) complex issues are dependent on policy change across interlocking systems, and solutions therefore need to be broadly conceptualized across and not within systems (e.g., political, health, economic, welfare); (3) root causes as identified by experts with lived experience should inform the solutions; (4) and co-creation efforts require building trust and transparency.

First, the immediate solutions usually generated by researchers and advocates alike are those that are "top-down" that view the food insecure person, family or community as passive recipients of assistance. For example, many researchers suggest that if we improve public nutrition assistance programming, or seek to improve other aspects of the safety net such as improving access to housing vouchers or healthcare, people's lives will improve [22–24]. This was the case for GFNA, although there was an intent to build capacity in developing "nutrition champions", the onus was on improving access to the elements of the current "broken" system. This system was filled with delays in getting access to income and food resulting in an increased reliance on individuals and organizations to fill the gap. The engagement with Witnesses identified that policy solutions needed to go beyond simply "improving the safety net." Members of Witnesses viewed the safety net as an untrustworthy system that remains broken, inadequate, and undesirable. Members of Witnesses did not want to receive more government assistance; rather, they had a strong desire for freedom and opportunity in developing more entrepreneurship, improving access to education for themselves and their children, and to safe neighborhoods which included ridding their neighborhoods of drug dealers and users, and greater investment in public services such as improved playgrounds, blight alleviation, garbage pickup, and other opportunities for neighborhood improvements.

Secondly, GFNA and Witnesses identified that food and nutrition security was not just the remit of a single system but involved policy change across systems. Food and nutrition security are not simply about lack of food but are an indication of a failure of income, housing and health systems to deliver. Members of Witnesses were eager to learn about how to shape policy. Yet, as training was provided to those who were interested in advocating for solutions, the members quickly discovered that available policy solutions were too siloed. They preferred approaches to be more holistic. For instance, they saw a direct relationship between the trade-offs of paying for food and housing, and therefore, they wanted to advocate for programs that incentivized higher paying jobs and entrepreneurship, so people could pay for their own food and market rate rents. Their frustration with the official policy process was tangible, and they have mostly abandoned standard policy-related solutions and turned their attention to more home-grown solutions that involve neighborhood clean-ups, clothing exchanges, and improved access to local housing.

Thirdly, members of Witnesses have insisted that food insecurity was *not* their most significant issue; whereas, exposure to violence and lack of safety were the central problems that tied all other problems together [21,25]. This was also evident for GFNA. But despite the program being sponsored by a torture and trauma agency, food and nutrition was effectively compartmentalized away from these issues. For Witnesses however, the insistence on the importance of safety led the research team into a new area of research and policy focus on exposure to violence and trauma [26,27]. With this new knowledge about the centrality of trauma and adversity, and the need for individual and collective resilience and, holistic, group-oriented approaches to social services, the research team developed a new intervention effort called the Building Wealth and Health Network (The Network). The Network works with caregivers of young children through a trauma-informed peer support approach (to address exposure to violence), financial empowerment education and new savings accounts, where people's savings are doubled (to address economic insecurity) [28,29]. The Network has reduced the odds of economic insecurity and improved mental health and income. Without that intentional and long-term engagement and magnanimous expertise of members of Witnesses, they would never have been able to develop effective solutions.

Finally, while GFNA undertook a participatory approach and there was recognition of individual and collective agency, the capabilities of community members were not fully realized. On reflection, part of this was a failure of those in power to fully trust experts with lived experience and their conceptualization of the issues and the solutions. This lack of trust often masqueraded as lack of time to develop partnerships, difficulty in engaging individuals and communities, as well as empathy regarding the overwhelming number of issues community members faced. The project officers undertook a wide range of activities and advocacy on behalf of the community members [15,16]. On the flip-side, GFNA was one of the first projects to employ members of the community as project consultants in order to provide cultural and experiential expertise (previously community members were expected to volunteer their services). In Witnesses to Hunger, the long-standing nature of the relationship between members of Witnesses (primarily Black and Latinx women) and the research team (racially diverse, with majority white leadership in terms of funding and decision-making) engendered some feelings of mutual trust and accountability, especially as all engagement by members of Witnesses was treated as professional work for which members were paid market-rate wages and honoraria. However, partnering across racial barriers and the spoken memory of generations of mistrust, misunderstanding, and oppression among black women by white women has generated ongoing challenges that bring to light questions about racism, leadership, and misaligned priorities, mission and goals.

Throughout both of these examples of partnered research it is clear that the best solutions are not simply based in science and standard empirical evidence, but also in what Maria Miess asserts is the wisdom that comes from experience and struggle [30].

3. Challenges of Sharing Expertise and Co-Creation of Solutions

There are many challenges to sharing expertise among traditional, highly educated and well-resourced experts (this includes those with lived experience that adopt a traditional scientific approach) and experts who have lived experience and who do not share the tools, resources and power of academia. These include the refusal to look at food insecurity as related to social factors such as (1) historical and contemporary racism and discrimination, (2) the culture of academia, (3) siloed thinking, and (4) marginalization and cultural differences in meaning.

3.1. Historical and Contemporary Racism and Discrimination

Our first challenge to overcome is our lack of willingness to identify the discriminatory social structures that cause poverty, deprivation, and trauma. As a single example among so many for African Americans, in 1898 with the publication of the Philadelphia Negro, sociologist William Edward Burghardt Du Bois identified how the struggles within the black community—poor health, unemployment and deplorable living conditions—are due to racial segregation. These directly stem from a socially constructed racial hierarchy that isolates, segregates and disenfranchises black people. He asserted that segregation and discrimination results in devastating poverty. The 1968 Kerner Commission Report described that the single most important issue for the struggles of African American people in terms of housing, poor nutrition, poor health, and low educational attainment in the United States is that whites systematically discriminate against and marginalize people of color [31], for example in its municipal, city, state and regional housing policies, in media coverage, and in general American society. Yet nutrition and food security researchers in the United States continuously ignore the dynamics of racism and discrimination that underlie poverty. Against this backdrop, it is only in the past few years that researchers in nutrition are beginning to call out discrimination and lack of equity as significant to the experience of food insecurity, obesity, and other nutrition-related conditions. The multiple forms of discrimination and oppression (systemic, interpersonal, structural, historical, etc.) are difficult to measure, and often do not fit in a simple model, yet researchers have begun to identify how lifetime, historical and systemic exposure to racism as associated with food and nutrition insecurity [32–34].

Australia has also demonstrated repeated failure to significantly address the blatant harms caused by discrimination. The same year as the Kerner Commission, William Edward Hanley Stanner delivered the nationally acclaimed Boyer Lecture "The Great Australian Silence" which argued that the history of invasion and the theft of lands and the genocide of Aboriginal and Torres Strait Islanders has been ignored [35]. Since this time, the Australian state has generally continued to ignore harms committed against Indigenous peoples [36]. In 2008 the Closing the Gap initiative was launched following a Social Justice report identifying serious inequity in health and life expectancy between Indigenous and white people. For instance, there are much higher mortality rates among Indigenous infants, and Indigenous men are dying more than 10 years earlier than their white counterparts [37]. Clearly, Australian health professionals failed to address the underlying structural power imbalances, intergenerational trauma and racism contributing to poor health [38,39]. Over time, nutrition researchers have all highlighted the inequalities related to food and nutrition for Aboriginal and Torres Strait Islander peoples and have identified the role of colonialism on the quantity and quality of food for Indigenous communities [40–43]. However, most are still describing the problem rather than identifying the root causes, that is, institutionalized racism, discrimination, poverty and marginalization.

3.2. Culture of Academia

The culture of academia and the legacy of western European influences in scientific investigation creates blind spots that allow for scientists to ignore or obfuscate how discrimination shapes economic insecurity, illness and health. The definition of food insecurity itself—the lack of access to enough food for an active and healthy life due to economic circumstances [44]—lacks connection to social and political circumstances such as lack of access to living wages, lack of political power of people who are low-income, and to discrimination and exclusion. An improved definition would draw attention to context behind "economic circumstances" to include concepts of "economic exploitation" and "marginalization" that demonstrate how food insecurity is a concept that is in relationship to societal dynamics. Despite Krieger's 1994 call to action for epidemiologists to move beyond biomedical individualism to acknowledge how health and disease have their roots in history, social relationships and political structures [45], food insecurity research published in English language research journals has been mired in the risk-exposure binary that still dominates health research. As Zuberi and Bonilla-Silva assert, researchers continue to ignore the large societal conditions that drive poor health and poor nutrition, and ignore their own place in perpetuating those conditions [46].

Most research and funding for research emanates from universities, well-resourced public policy centers, and from government sources, where a majority of people who are carrying out the research, making funding decisions, and generating research questions and methods are people without lived experience, and who do not see how the systems in which they are involved (i.e., education and government) are perpetuating poverty. While it is common knowledge in research circles that among food insecurity and poverty researchers there are people who have lived experiences with poverty, it is unclear how many there are, as this has not been previously studied or counted, and it is possible that such researchers would not readily describe these experiences due to real and perceived stigma as mentioned above. The culture of academia could also improve to be more accepting and inclusive of research scientists with lived experiences to help deepen understanding of the experiences and emphasize the importance of innovative approaches grounded in experience. Class, race and gender inequities are not solely among individual researchers, but are also built into institutional practices. As an example, universities and health systems have a long history of causing gentrification that further isolates people of color and people who are poor from mainstream resources [47]. Additionally, scientific methods demand strict definition of measurable problems, and center around testing of hypotheses of limited measures of covariates and outcomes. The pressures of producing peer reviewed research to establish academic credibility, and incentives for promotion in academia that utilize metrics unrelated to impact or how much engagement and authentic collaboration there is with research participants both work to devalue, isolate or discourage participatory research. Additionally, there is little to no incentive or recognition of the intensive time and trust building processes necessary for effective participatory research [48]. Overall the glorification of mainstream science and the pressures of academia to publish scientific research prioritize only one way of knowing about social problems such as food insecurity. This has led to a lack of appreciation for lived experience and wisdom from the streets, the farm, the reservation, and the neighborhood.

Qualitative researchers may view themselves as less engaged in research that ignores broader contexts of discrimination and inequality. However, we argue that most qualitative research still relies on a one-way process that extracts stories and experience from people who have lived experience, that generally enhances the investigator's career through publishing books and articles, while those studied remain unseen, without political power, economic security, and legal recourse. We suggest that research move beyond the relatively simple process of gathering insight and stories from individuals and groups, and move into the co-creation of understanding and move to mutual problem solving in partnership. There are strong traditions from which to draw, such as action research by Sol Tax, applied anthropology, critical participatory action research [49–51], and indigenous methodologies where knowing and knowledge is built through relationality via yarning circles (Australian) [52], *talanoa* (Pacific/Maori) [53]. These methodologies are conversational techniques that involve the sharing of stories. They have at their core equal respectful engagement and the co-creation of knowledge [54].

3.3. Siloed Thinking

Reducing health inequalities and addressing social determinants of health requires greater integration across government and civil society. Sir Michael Marmot and colleagues have identified that action however is limited by organizational boundaries and "siloes" [55] (p. 86). Additionally, in most neoliberal high-income countries, funding streams are aligned with discrete government agencies that are based on outdated systems. In the US, it is well known that funding streams cannot be easily merged or braided together without acts of Congress. Even when federal agencies seek to work together, there becomes a territoriality of concern regarding programs where agency leaders are afraid of losing funding if they share some of their funding with other programs [22,56]. In Australia and the UK there is strong rhetoric about "whole-of-government" approaches for persistent social and environmental challenges. However, the three primary barriers for horizontal governance or "joined-up" government are identified as: a deeply entrenched program focus based on funding streams that remain siloed, centralized decision-making that undermine devolved decision-making, and the reliance on co-locating services rather than adjusting the underlying operating systems [57,58]. Overall, this siloed thinking is what Rebecca Costa refers to as a "super meme"—a way of thinking that is simply accepted despite the fact that it is irrational—that stymies innovative action to solve society's most intractable problems such as hunger [59].

3.4. Marginalization and Cultural Differences in Meaning

The poor are marginalized or excluded by multiple systems such as zoning laws, school funding laws (as in the US), higher education discrimination, housing discrimination, as well as the systems of academic inquiry. An example of this is how from the perspective of academic researchers, sex workers, people who are homeless, or people who are "disconnected" from public welfare programs are considered "hard to reach" because of recruitment methods that have limited timeframes during the day, extensive costs to the individuals, and inadequate community engagement [60]. Additionally, food insecurity researchers tend to look at food insecurity over a short period of time, usually in cross-sectional studies, or in a one-two year time frame, with a few exceptions. Yet some groups have a very different view. Indigenous peoples may view their experiences with hunger and ill-health as stemming from times of genocide of their peoples and through ongoing injustices of broken treaty rights (where treaties exist) or failure to recognize sovereignty through constitutional reform [61,62]. Additionally, they may consider hunger to be an issue consistent with the violation of their sovereignty and the rights of nature [63].

4. New Principles for Food and Nutrition Security Research

While the challenges mentioned above are serious, they can be overcome through new ways of thinking about our work, and through adopting core principles and values. Developing solutions for food and nutrition insecurity, particularly when the issue involves marginalized groups in high-income countries. New approaches require a change in mindset and in our ways of working. We argue here for a set of core principles and values that should underpin and inform our actions in research and in devising evidence-based solutions. These principles draw from a variety of traditions such as civic agriculture and civic dietetics, trauma-theory, emancipatory education, and indigenous worldviews. Learning from these frameworks we propose four core principles that should guide our work in alleviating household food insecurity: (1) a critical consciousness that requires individuals to constantly question their own and others' positions; (2) working to deconstruct white supremacy; (3) a rights-based approach that ensures engagement with people with lived experience, and (4) actively engaging in co-creation processes where power is shared and all expertise is regarded as meaningful.

4.1. Use Critical Consciousness and Emancipatory Processes That Transgress Boundaries

Critical consciousness lies at the heart of working "inside out" to question perceptions of ourselves, of privilege and of the social and structural institutions that seek to maintain divisions in society. Critical consciousness highlights the need for a reflexive approach (that is not just thinking but also acting) to understand and change inequities in power and privilege. It requires reorientation to a commitment to love for humanity and social justice [64,65]. This raising of consciousness leads to what Freire described as engaged discourse, collaborative problem-solving and a re-humanization of our social relationships. Critical consciousness is required to understand that marginalization is not inherent within an individual but is rather a result of the structural and social forces that create that lived experience [66]. For example, just focusing on the food insecure individual or household locates the marginalized person as "the problem," whereas the problem is located within the social and political context.

While Freire's original conceptualization was focused on those who were experiencing oppression and or marginalization, increasingly it is being applied to all types of participants in social programs including the researcher or those involved in developing and delivering programs [67]. Critical consciousness therefore has three essential elements: critical reflection—an analysis and rejection of the social inequities that limit agency and contribute to poor health and wellbeing; political efficacy—the perceived capacity to effect social and political change individually or collectively; and critical action—the actions taken to change aspects of society that are unjust [68]. Integrating feminist and intersectional approaches is also important to integrate attention to multiple, intersecting identities such as race, gender and sexuality, that consider a whole person approach, and that puts the authority of lived experiences at the center of inquiry. This approach helps all experts involved to transgress boundaries of race, gender, age, class, sexuality and beyond to resist and subvert patriarchal oppression and white supremacy [69]. These practices can be put into action in ongoing nutrition education efforts, participatory action endeavors, and other types of qualitative research efforts. In Witnesses to Hunger, these principles were utilized in every group meeting, where members were invited to explore from their own experiences how policies fell short, and worked together to identify their ideas for solutions that were then crafted into the exhibits, information booklets, and postcards for bringing along to meetings with legislators. This community self-empowerment education approach is also utilized by the Poverty Truth Commissions that were first established in Scotland and spread to other cities in the UK, currently hosted and promoted by Church Action on Poverty [70,71].

4.2. Utilize an Anti-Oppression Framework and a Trauma-Informed Lens

An anti-oppression framework is one that seeks to undo the effects of oppression, oppose the roots of all forms of oppression, and to adopt an emancipatory approach to social change. Anti-oppressive practice has penetrated a variety of fields, and became most highly developed in social work practice and psychology, where attention to breaking down status quo definitions of identity, eliminating boundaries of social division based on gender, race, ethnicity, age, and other identities can help to improve the therapeutic relationship as well as bring about societal change. The approach also seeks to call attention to power differentials in our relationships. An anti-oppressive approach demands not only the practice of actively seeking to ensure we do not oppress others, but also to continuously recognize our own roles in perpetuating our privilege and power that can lead to oppression. This means actively taking a decolonization stance, employing approaches and methodologies that disrupt and reverse the ongoing exploitation and subjugation of people who have been marginalized, excluded and oppressed [9,53].

The intergenerational and interpersonal trauma associated with colonialism and imperialism and the vast arrays of "isms" and phobias such as racism, sexism, ableism, classism, homophobia, and xenophobia, can be acknowledged and addressed in our everyday actions and in our policy proposals. Trauma informed practice realizes the widespread impact of trauma, and pathways to recovery, recognizes symptoms of trauma in clients, participants, families, staff, systems, and in ourselves, responds to fully integrate trauma-knowledge to improve and inform policies procedures and practices, and actively resists re-traumatization [72]. Given decades of evidence that exposure to violence such as intimate partner violence, child abuse, neglect and other adverse childhood experiences, suicide attempts and ideation, and post-traumatic stress disorder are strongly associated with household food insecurity [26], taking a trauma-informed lens to co-creating solutions is fundamentally important.

A trauma-informed approach to self-organization was essential in the methods of Witnesses to Hunger [21], and later created the foundation of The Building Wealth and Health Network [73], which significantly reduced food insecurity. Other trauma-informed approaches are being integrated throughout many school districts across the United States [74,75], and there are more calls for trauma-informed policy-making [76,77].

4.3. Utilize a Human Rights Approach

The right to food and to be free from hunger are fundamental human rights in the Universal Declaration of Human Rights and in the International Covenant on Economic, Social and Cultural Rights (ICESCR). It incorporates being able to have access to culturally appropriate and healthy food in order to live a healthy and fulfilling life without fear. Viewing food security as a human rights issue means that good nutrition should not be left to benevolence or charity, relegated to the remit of the charitable food sector. Instead food security should be respected, protected, and fulfilled by governments and NGOs to promote the health, security, and wellbeing of all people [78,79]. In order to advance the right to food, it is necessary to ensure that there is a national plan to respect, protect, and fulfil the right to food, and a comprehensive approach to ensure participation of many stakeholders (especially those who are most affected by food insecurity), in the development of solutions, as well as for redress and repair when the right to food is violated. Having a national measurement mechanism for monitoring and accountability is essential. The governments of Australia, UK and New Zealand (among others) fail to regularly monitor food insecurity and issues related to access and provision of food. This keeps comprehensive solutions to food and nutrition insecurity unknown or ad hoc. While national monitoring is not the only way to get started with a human rights approach, it can help to provide information and empirical evidence for monitoring and evaluation of interventions.

Adopting a rights framework is a key tenet of the recommended approach to ensure:

-       Solutions ensure equitable access to nutritious food regardless of one's circumstances;

- Solutions move beyond charitable approaches to those that address capabilities and enhance individual freedoms to achieve health and wellbeing;
- Trauma and stigma are not inflicted or exacerbated and healing opportunities that build resilience are integrated into food-related programming;
- Food sovereignty is respected and promoted;
- Policy development does not exacerbate inequalities or contravene other human rights in recognition that all human rights are universal, inalienable, indivisible, interdependent and interconnected;
- Rights holders have a central role in bringing about solutions.

Advancing human rights, and the right to food is very challenging. This is especially true in high income countries such as Australia and the United States, where there are major cultural assumptions by a powerful elite that trivialize and downplay the importance of economic and social rights [3,78,80]. Additionally, the focus on food, rather than on the social, economic and political conditions that cause food insecurity limit the understanding and adoption of the rights framework. The emphasis on charitable food provision, the slow dismantling of an already inadequate social security safety net, and reliance on "trickle-down" economics to alleviate poverty are serious obstacles to helping civil society adopt a rights framework and to demand right to food [78,81,82]. Despite these challenges, if the research and advocacy communities in high income countries could begin to adopt a broader justice framework, and promote such solutions among advocates, the press, and policy-makers, it can help support the current efforts of civil society to ensure people can be empowered to demand their right to food, and to health and wellbeing. Efforts such as the Participation and the Practice of Rights (PPR) in Northern Ireland, Detroit Black Community Food Security Network and the Southern Rural Black Women's Initiative for Economic and Social Justice (SRBWI) and other organizations of the US Human Rights Network, the international campaign La Via Campesina which advocates for food sovereignty, and the Right to Food Coalition in Australia, are just a few of many examples where economic social and cultural rights are being advanced by civil society despite the above-listed challenges. The research community has much to learn from these ongoing efforts.

4.4. Seek Co-Creation of Problems and Solutions

There is growing recognition in research circles that there needs to be a different paradigm of knowledge production [83] and a fundamental shift from privileging experimental expertise to experiential expertise [84]. Characterizing problems from the perspective of the scientific "expert" is using knowledge as a form of "discursive power in ways that privilege some definitions of health and social problems and marginalize others" [85]. If change is to occur, those in positions of knowledge "expert" status need to reorient their inquiries from describing the problem to research that seeks to understand the effectiveness of interventions [85].

In undertaking collective processes of inquiry, empowerment and action, the experimental and experiential experts need to work to remove power differentials and utilize their respective strengths to co-create a mutual understanding of: the life-world, the dispositions and aspirations of those who live in that life-world, the problem as socially-constructed and the solutions that will be best fit in that context [86]. In taking this approach we agree with other scholars that it is no longer possible or ethical to separate the "research" from the ensuing policy discussion. In the case of food and nutrition security the understanding of the problem and the solutions requires both experimental and experiential experts to lend their voices to ongoing policy discussions [49,85]. Indeed as Fine indicates, "it is the obligation of the scholar to not only expose social injustice but to transform unjust conditions" [49] (p. 116). Examples of such co-creation are efforts by Witnesses to Hunger, and the Poverty and the Social Exclusion in the United Kingdom research project funded by the Economic and Social Research Council consisting of collaboration between the University of Bristol (lead), Heriot-Watt

University, The Open University, Queen's University Belfast, University of Glasgow and the University of York [8,87].

5. Values for Sharing Expertise and Co-Creation

Underpinning the principles are a set of underlying values informing approaches to researching and programming for food security. Table 1 characterizes the values that inform this process and help to create an ethos of action that questions the status quo, empowers partnership development and makes use of different forms of expertise. These qualities require self and political awareness.

Table 1. Underlying Values for Sharing Expertise.

Value	Description
Knowledges	Recognize that knowledge comes in a variety of forms and is not limited to book learning and the scientific method. Different forms of knowledge extend to different forms of expertise. Each participant brings a unique set of expertise to problem identification and solution creation that can be brought together to construct new knowledge.
Relationships	Build relationships that are genuine and long-lasting. These relationships need to be built on trust, reciprocity and an understanding of and explicit attention to differences that create power inequities.
Humility	For those with the power, education and privilege it is essential that we express an understanding of how our unearned privilege and societal rank limits our skill sets, and that these skills are not necessarily better than those of others. Coming to the work with humility and a beginner's mind helps to undo power differentials based on education, gender, sexual orientation, economic resources, race, class, cultural background and spiritual beliefs.
Empathy	Build a powerful imagination in order to understand the life situations of others in order to be able to respond to social inequities. Empathy requires an understanding of the differences between self and other and an ability to understand and relate to another's perspective, emotion and experience.
Reciprocity	Exchange material resources, ideas, social obligations and power for mutual benefit. Reciprocity is fundamentally steeped in conceptualizing balance and an interconnectedness across time and space. Reciprocity requires giving and receiving.
Trust	Trust is premised on respect, transparency, accountability and reciprocity. There needs to be mutual trust in the process and outcomes of the co-creation of knowledge and solutions.
Transparency and accountability	Recognize that there are mutual accountabilities for individuals and organizations. There may be accountabilities to education institutions, funders and donors, political ideologies, families, communities, and cultural traditions. There will be tensions between these accountabilities but in order for trust to develop transactions and encounters need to be transparent. In this way the primary accountability is to social change and to the disruption of institutional and social structures that maintain inequity.
Courage	Understand that to work in a different way, to be politically active and to challenge the status quo takes self-knowledge, fearlessness and a willingness to be vulnerable and uncomfortable.

These values transcend any one field of study and action and can provide some grounding to to continue to address the challenges of racism and discrimination, the limited culture of academia, siloed thinking, and marginalization and cultural differences in meaning and time horizons.

6. Conclusions

Co-creation of solutions and sharing expertise across boundaries of race, class, education level, gender and age are beneficial and necessary for devising meaningful, effective and lasting changes in food and nutrition insecurity. The co-creation of solutions on food and nutrition insecurity will however not come easily. The challenges of racism and discrimination, the culture of academia, our siloed thinking, and cultural differences will consistently be in the backdrop of our efforts, and may actively get in the way of creating and then implementing solutions. We propose here some organizing principles and values to help overcome these challenges. Without actively engaging with these, researchers may be perpetuating inequality and injustices that drive poor nutrition and health. Embracing multiple forms of knowledge, humility and courage, among many other values, may be difficult and unrewarded currently in our own spheres. Yet we suggest that the rewards of improving food and nutrition insecurity for millions far outweighs the discomfort many of us might have with shaking up and altering our ways of doing. We invite the rest of the food insecurity research community, especially those with lived experience, to weigh in on these principles and values, and we hope they will join us in establishing a shared international consensus for co-creating solutions that promote the right to food, and promote health and wellbeing for all.

Author Contributions: D.G. and M.M.C. contributed equally to this manuscript.

References

1. Sen, A. Ingredients of famine analysis: Availability and entitlements. *Q. J. Econ.* **1981**, *96*, 433–464. [CrossRef] [PubMed]
2. Fisher, A. *Big Hunger: The Unholy Alliance Between Corporate America and Anti-Hunger Groups*; MIT Press: Cambridge, MA, USA, 2017.
3. Riches, G. *Food Bank Nations: Poverty, Corporate Charity and the Right to Food*; Routledge: London, UK, 2018.
4. Caraher, M.; Furey, S. Growth of food banks in the UK (and Europe): Leftover food for leftover people. In *The Economics of Emergency Food Aid Provision: A Financial, Social and Cultural Perspective*; Palgrave Pivot: London, UK, 2018; pp. 25–48.
5. Cale, G. Confessions Of A Poverty-Class Academic-In-Training. Available online: https:// conditionallyaccepted.com/2015/09/01/workingclass-pt1/ (accessed on 15 January 2019).
6. Sarcozona, Poverty in the Ivory Tower, in Tenure, She Wrote. Available online: https://tenureshewrote. wordpress.com/2014/01/16/succeeding-in-graduate-school-despite-poverty/ (accessed on 15 January 2019).
7. Food Action Resource Center. Food ARC: Research Inspiring Change. Available online: https://foodarc.ca/ (accessed on 17 January 2019).
8. Poverty and Social Exclusion. PSE: Poverty and Social Exclusion, Reporting Research, Examining Policy, Stimulating Debate. Available online: http://www.poverty.ac.uk/ (accessed on 15 January 2019).
9. Smith, L.T. *Decolonizing Methodologies: Research and Indigenous Peoples*; Zed Books Ltd.: New York, NY, USA, 2013.
10. Heller, J.L. The enduring problem of social class stigma experienced by upwardly mobile white academics. *McGill Sociol. Rev.* **2011**, *2*, 19–38.
11. Goldrick-Rab, S.; Richardson, J.; Schneider, J.; Hernandez, A.; Cady, C. *Still Hungry and Homeless in College*; Wisconsin Hope Lab, 2018. Available online: https://hope4college.com/wp-content/uploads/2018/09/ Wisconsin-HOPE-Lab-Still-Hungry-and-Homeless.pdf (accessed on 14 February 2019).
12. Gallegos, D.; Ramsey, R.; Ong, K.W. Food insecurity: Is it an issue among tertiary students? *High. Educ.* **2014**, *67*, 497–510. [CrossRef]
13. Activating Change Together for Community Food Security: Knowledge Mobilization Working Group. Knowledge Mobilization in Participatory Action Research: A Synthesis of the Literature. 2014. Available online: https://foodarc.ca/wp-content/uploads/2014/09/ACT-for-CFS-Knowledge-Mobilization-in-PAR-Jan-2014.pdf (accessed on 5 December 2018).
14. White, M. Environmental reviews & case studies: D-town farm: African American resistance to food insecurity and the transformation of Detroit. *Environ. Pract.* **2011**, *13*. [CrossRef]
15. Ellies, P.; Gallegos, D. *Good Food for New Arrivals: Final Report*; Association for Services to Torture and Trauma Survivors and East Metropolitan Population Health Unit: Perth, Australia, 2004.

16.   Vicca, N.; Straton, R.; Gallegos, D. *Good Food for New Arrivals: Final Evaluation Report*; Association for Services to Torture and Trauma Survivors and Centre for Social and Community Research, Murdoch University: Perth, Australia, 2009.

17.   Gallegos, D.; Ellies, P. Good Food for New Arrivals: A case study of inclusive health practice. In *Settling in Australia: The Social Inclusion of Refugees*; Colic-Peisker, V., Tilbury, F., Eds.; Centre for Social and Community Research, Murdoch University: Perth, Australia, 2007; pp. 97–107.

18.   Gallegos, D.; Ellies, P.; Wright, J. Still there's no food! Food in a refugee population in Perth, Western Australia. *Nutr. Diet.* **2008**, *65*, 78–83. [CrossRef]

19.   Durham, J.; Gillieatt, S.; Ellies, P. An evaluability assessment of a nutrition promotion project for newly arrived refugees. *Health Promot. J. Aust.* **2007**, *18*, 43–49. [CrossRef]

20.   Chilton, M.; Rabinowich, J.; Council, C.; Breaux, J. Witnesses to Hunger: Participation through photovoice to ensure the right to food. *Health Human Rights* **2009**, *11*, 73–86. [CrossRef] [PubMed]

21.   Knowles, M.; Rabinowich, J.; Gaines-Turner, T.; Chilton, M. *Witnesses to Hunger: Methods for Photovoice and Participatory Action Research in Public Health*; Human Organization: Oklahoma City, OK, USA, 2015; Volume 74.

22.   Bartfeld, J.; Gundersen, C.; Smeeding, T.; Ziliak, J.P. (Eds.) *SNAP Matters: How Food Stamps Affect Health and Well-Being*; Stanford University Press: Stanford, CA, USA, 2015.

23.   Sandel, M.C.D.; Meyers, A.; Ettinger de Cuba, S.; Coleman, S.; Black, M.; Casey, P.; Chilton, M.; Cook, J.; Shortell, A.; Heeren, T.; et al. Co-enrollment for child health: How receipt and loss of food and housing subsidies relate to housing security and statutes for streamlined, multi-subsidy application. *J. Appl. Res. Child. Informing Policy Child. Risk* **2014**, *5*, 2.

24.   Seligman, H.K.; Berkowitz, S.A. Aligning programs and policies to support food security and public health goals in the United States. *Annu. Rev. Public Health* **2019**, *40*, 2.1–2.19. [CrossRef] [PubMed]

25.   Chilton, M.M.; Rabinowich, J.R.; Woolf, N.H. Very low food security in the USA is linked with exposure to violence. *Public Health Nutr.* **2014**, *17*, 73–82. [CrossRef] [PubMed]

26.   Sun, J.; Knowles, M.; Patel, F.; Frank, D.A.; Heeren, T.C.; Chilton, M. Childhood adversity and adult reports of food insecurity among households with children. *Am. J. Prevent. Med.* **2016**, *50*, 561–572. [CrossRef] [PubMed]

27.   Chilton, M.; Knowles, M.; Bloom, S.L. The intergenerational circumstances of household food insecurity and adversity. *J. Hunger Environ. Nutr.* **2017**, *12*, 269–297. [CrossRef] [PubMed]

28.   Booshehri, L.; Dugan, J.; Patel, F.; Bloom, S.; Chilton, M.M. Trauma-informed Temporary Assistance for Needy Families (TANF): A Randomized Controlled Trial with a Two-Generation Impact. *J. Child Family Stud.* **2018**, *27*, 1594–1604. [CrossRef] [PubMed]

29.   Sun, J.; Patel, F.; Kirzner, R.; Newton-Famous, N.; Owens, C.; Welles, S.L.; Chilton, M. The Building Wealth and Health Network: Methods and baseline characteristics from a randomized controlled trial for families with young children participating in temporary assistance for needy families (TANF). *BMC Public Health* **2016**, *16*, 583. [CrossRef] [PubMed]

30.   Mies, M.; Shiva, V. *Ecofeminism*; Zed Books: London, UK, 2014; 328p.

31.   Gillon, S.M. *Separate and Unequal: The Kerner Commission and the Unraveling of American Liberalism*, 1st ed.; Basic Books: New York, NY, USA, 2018; 374p.

32.   Kumanyika, S. *Getting to Equity in Obesity Prevention: A New Framework*; National Academy of Medicine: Washington, DC, USA, 2017.

33.   Odoms-Young, A.; Bruce, M.A. Examining the impact of structural racism on food insecurity: Implications for addressing racial/ethnic disparities. *Family Community Health* **2018**, *41* (Suppl. 2), S3–S6. [CrossRef] [PubMed]

34.   Burke, M.P.; Jones, S.J.; Frongillo, E.A.; Fram, M.S.; Blake, C.E.; Freedman, D.A. Severity of household food insecurity and lifetime racial discrimination among African-American households in South Carolina. *Ethn. Health* **2018**, *23*, 276–292. [CrossRef] [PubMed]

35.   Collins, J.; Thompson, W.K. Reconciliation in Australia? Dreaming beyond the cult of forgetfulness. In *Reconciliation in Conflict-Affected Communities: Practices and Insights from the Asia-Pacific*; Jenkins, B., Subedi, D.B., Jenkins, K., Eds.; Springer: Singapore, 2018; pp. 185–206.

36.   McMillan, M.; Rigney, S. Race, reconciliation, and justice in Australia: From denial to acknowledgment. *Ethn. Racial Stud.* **2018**, *41*, 759–777. [CrossRef]

37. Deravin, L.; Francis, K.; Anderson, J. Closing the gap in Indigenous health inequity—Is it making a difference? *Int. Nurs. Rev.* **2018**, *4*, 477–483. [CrossRef]

38. Pholi, K. Is' Close the Gap'a useful approach to improving the health and wellbeing of Indigenous Australians? *Aust. Rev. Public Aff.* **2009**, *9*, 1–13.

39. Gannon, M. Indigenous health: Closing the gap-10 year review. *Aust. Med.* **2018**, *30*, 25.

40. Gracey, M. Historical, cultural, political, and social influences on dietary patterns and nutrition in Australian Aboriginal children. *Am. J. Clin. Nutr.* **2000**, *72*, 1361S–1367S. [CrossRef] [PubMed]

41. McDermott, R.; O'Dea, K.; Rowley, K.; Knight, S.; Burgess, P. Beneficial impact of the Homelands Movement on health outcomes in Central Australian Aborigines. *Aust. N. Z. J. Public Health* **1998**, *22*, 653–658. [CrossRef] [PubMed]

42. Brimblecombe, J.; Maypilama, E.; Colles, S.; Scarlett, M.; Dhurrkay, J.G.; Ritchie, J.; O'Dea, K. Factors influencing food choice in an Australian Aboriginal community. *Qual. Health Res.* **2014**, *24*, 387–400. [CrossRef] [PubMed]

43. Lee, A.J.; Leonard, D.; Moloney, A.A.; Minniecon, D.L. Improving Aboriginal and Torres strait islander nutrition and health. *Med. J. Aust.* **2009**, *190*, 547–548. [PubMed]

44. Bickel, G.; Nord, M.; Price, C.; Hamilton, W.; Cook, J. *Measuring Food Security in the United States: Guide to Measuring Household Food Security*; US Department of Agriculture, Food and Nutrition Service, Office of Analysis and Evaluation: Alexandria, VA, USA, 2000.

45. Krieger, N. Epidemiology and the web of causation: Has anyone seen the spider? *Soc. Sci. Med.* **1994**, *39*, 887–903. [CrossRef]

46. Zuberi, T.; Bonilla-Silva, E. *White Logic, White Methods: Racism and Methodology*; Rowman & Littlefield Publishers: Lanham, ML, USA, 2008; 416p.

47. Gomez, M.B. *Race, Class, Power, and Organizing in East Baltimore: Rebuilding Abandoned Communities in America*; Lexington Books: Lanham, ML, USA, 2013; 271p.

48. Minkler, M.; Wallerstein, N. *Community-Based Participatory Research for Health: From Process to Outcomes*, 2nd ed.; Jossey-Bass: San Francisco, CA, USA, 2008; 508p.

49. Fine, M. *Just Research in Contentious Times: Widening the Methodological Imagination*; Teachers College Press: New York, NY, USA, 2017.

50. Daubenmier, J.M. *The Meskwaki and Anthropologists: Action Anthropology Reconsidered*; Critical Studies in the History of Anthropology; University of Nebraska Press: Lincoln, RI, USA, 2008; 416p.

51. Bennett, L.A.; Whiteford, L.M.; National Association for the Practice of Anthropology (U.S.). *Anthropology and the Engaged University: New Vision for the Discipline Within Higher Education*; Annals of Anthropological Practice; Wiley Subscription Services, Inc.: Hoboken, NJ, USA, 2013; 204p.

52. Martin, B. Methodology is content: Indigenous approaches to research and knowledge. *Educ. Philos. Theory* **2017**, *49*, 1392–1400. [CrossRef]

53. Suaalii-Sauni, T.; Fulu-Aiolupotea, S.M. Decolonising Pacific research, building Pacific research communities and developing Pacific research tools: The case of the talanoa and the faafaletui in Samoa. *Asia Pac. Viewpoint* **2014**, *55*, 331–344. [CrossRef]

54. Walker, M.; Fredericks, B.; Mills, K.; Anderson, D. "Yarning" as a method for community-based health research with Indigenous women: The Indigenous Women's Wellness Research Program. *Health Care Women Int.* **2014**, *35*, 1216–1226. [CrossRef]

55. Marmot, M. Social determinants of health inequalities. *Lancet* **2005**, *365*, 1099–1104. [CrossRef]

56. Dean, S. Testimony of Stacy Dean, Vice President for Food Assistance Policy Before the House Committee on Agriculture's Subcommittee on Department Operations, Oversight, and Nutrition, O. House Committee on Agriculture's Subcommittee on Department Operations, and Nutrition, Editor. 2014. Available online: https://www.cbpp.org/testimony-of-stacy-dean-vice-president-for-food-assistance-policy-before-the-house-committee-on-0 (accessed on 14 February 2019).

57. O'Flynn, J.; Buick, F.; Blackman, D.; Halligan, J. You win some, you lose some: Experiments with joined-up government. *Int. J. Public Adm.* **2011**, *34*, 244–254. [CrossRef]

58. Carey, G.; Crammond, B.; Keast, R. Creating change in government to address the social determinants of health: How can efforts be improved? *BMC Public Health* **2014**, *14*, 1087. [CrossRef] [PubMed]

59. Costa, R.D. *The Watchman's Rattle: Thinking Our Way Out of Extinction*; Vanguard Press: Philadelphia, PA, USA, 2010; 346p.

60. Bonevski, B.; Randell, M.; Paul, C.; Chapman, K.; Twyman, L.; Bryant, J.; Brozek, I.; Hughes, C. Reaching the hard-to-reach: A systematic review of strategies for improving health and medical research with socially disadvantaged groups. *BMC Med. Res. Methodol.* **2014**, *14*, 42. [CrossRef] [PubMed]

61. Pickering, K.; McShane-Jewell, B.; Brydge, M.; Gilbert, M.; Black Elk, L. *National Commission on Hunger: Invited Written Testimony on Food Insecurity, Plains Indian Tribes, Pine Ridge and Rosebud Indian Reservations, U*; National Commission on Hunger: Washington, DC, USA, 2015. Available online: https://cybercemetery.unt.edu/archive/hungercommission/20151217003520/https://hungercommission.rti.org/Portals/0/SiteHtml/Activities/WrittenTestimony/InvitedWritten/NCH_Invited_Written_Testimony_Kathleen_Pickering.pdf (accessed on 10 November 2018).

62. Jalata, A. The impacts of English colonial terrorism and genocide on Indigenous/black Australians. *SAGE Open* **2013**, *3*, 2158244013499143. [CrossRef]

63. Wittman, H. Food sovereignty: A new rights framework for food and nature? *Environ. Soc. Adv. Res.* **2011**, *2*, 87–105.

64. Freire, P. *Pedagogy of the Oppressed*; Continuum: New York, NY, USA, 2007.

65. Freire, P. *Education for Critical Consciousness*; Bloomsbury Publishing: London, UK; New York, NY, USA, 1974.

66. Godfrey, E.B.; Burson, E. Interrogating the intersections: How intersectional perspectives can inform developmental scholarship on critical consciousness. In *Envisioning the Integration of an Intersectional Lens in Developmental Science. New Directions for Child and Adolescent Development*; Santos, C.E., Toomey, R.B., Eds.; Jossey-Bass: San Francisco, CA, USA, 2018; pp. 17–38.

67. Kumagai, A.K.; Lypson, M.L. Beyond cultural competence: Critical consciousness, social justice, and multicultural education. *Acad. Med.* **2009**, *84*, 782–787. [CrossRef] [PubMed]

68. Watts, R.J.; Diemer, M.A.; Voight, A.M. Critical consciousness: Current status and future directions. *New Dir. Child Adolesc. Dev.* **2011**, *134*, 43–57. [CrossRef] [PubMed]

69. Hooks, B. *Teaching to Transgress: Education as the Practice of Freedom*; Routledge: New York, NY, USA, 1994; 216p.

70. Church Action on Poverty. Poverty Truth Commissions. Available online: http://www.church-poverty.org.uk/povertytruth (accessed on 15 January 2019).

71. Faith in Community Scotland. Poverty Truth Commission. 2019. Available online: https://www.faithincommunityscotland.org/ (accessed on 15 January 2019).

72. Substance Abuse and Mental Health Services Administration. *SAMHSA's Concept of Trauma and Guidance for a Trauma-Informed Approach*; In HHS Publication No. (SMA) 14-4884; Office of Policy, Planning and Innovation, Substance Abuse and Mental Health Services Administration, HHS.: Rockville, MD, USA, 2014.

73. Booshehri, L.G.; Dugan, J.; Patel, F.; Bloom, S.; Chilton, M. Trauma-informed Temporary Assistance for Needy Families (TANF): A randomized controlled trial with a two-generation impact. *J. Child Family Stud.* **2018**, *27*, 1594–1604. [CrossRef] [PubMed]

74. Walkley, M.; Cox, T.L. Building trauma-informed schools and communities. *Child. Schools* **2013**, *35*, 123–126. [CrossRef]

75. Substance Abuse and Mental Health Services Administration. Trauma-Informed Care in Behavioral Health Services. In *Treatment Improvement Protocol (TIP) Series*; Health and Human Services, Ed.; Substance Abuse and Mental Health Services Administration: Rockville, MD, USA, 2014.

76. Hecht, A.A.; Biehl, E.; Buzogany, S.; Neff, R.A. Using a trauma-informed policy approach to create a resilient urban food system. *Public Health Nutr.* **2018**, 1–10. [CrossRef] [PubMed]

77. Prewitt, E. State, Federal Lawmakers Take Action on Trauma-Informed Policies, Programs. 2014. Available online: http://acestoohigh.com/2014/04/30/state-federal-lawmakers-take-action/ (accessed on 21 September 2014).

78. Chilton, M.; Rose, D. A rights-based approach to food insecurity in the United States. *Am. J. Public Health* **2009**, *99*, 1203–1211. [CrossRef] [PubMed]

79. Gallegos, D.; Booth, S.; Kleve, S.; McKechnie, R.; Lindberg, R. Food insecurity in Australian households: From charity to entitlement. In *A Sociology of Food and Nutrition: The Social Appetite*; Germov, J., Williams, L., Eds.; Oxford University Press: Oxford, UK, 2017; pp. 55–74.

80. Booth, S. Food. In *First World Hunger Revisited*; Riches, G., Silvasti, T., Eds.; Palgrave Macmillan: London, UK, 2014.

81. Dowler, E.A.; O'Connor, D. Rights-based approaches to addressing food poverty and food insecurity in Ireland and UK. *Soc. Sci. Med.* **2012**, *74*, 44–51. [CrossRef] [PubMed]

82. Poppendieck, J. *Sweet Charity? Emergency Food and the End of Entitlement*; Viking Press: New York, NY, USA, 1998.

83. Popay, J. What will it take to get the evidential value of lay knowledge recognised? *Int. J. Public Health* **2018**, *63*, 1013–1014. [CrossRef] [PubMed]

84. El Ansari, W.; Phillips, C.J.; Zwi, A.B. Narrowing the gap between academic professional wisdom and community lay knowledge: Perceptions from partnerships. *Public Health* **2002**, *116*, 151–159. [CrossRef] [PubMed]

85. Murphy, K.; Fafard, P. Knowledge translation and social epidemiology: Taking power, politics and values seriously. In *Rethinking Social Epidemiology: Towards a Science of Change*; O'Campo, P., Dunn, J.R., Eds.; Springer: Dordrecht, The Netherlands, 2012; pp. 267–283.

86. Popay, J.; Williams, G.; Thomas, C.; Gatrell, T. Theorising inequalities in health: The place of lay knowledge. *Sociol. Health Ill.* **1998**, *20*, 619–644. [CrossRef]

87. Kent, G. Community Engagement in Challenging Times, Poverty and Social Exclusion in the UK, in Working Paper—Methods Series No. 25. 2013. Available online: http://www.poverty.ac.uk/editorial/community-engagement-challenging-times (accessed on 14 February 2019).

9

Testing the Price of Healthy and Current Diets in Remote Aboriginal Communities to Improve Food Security: Development of the Aboriginal and Torres Strait Islander Healthy Diets ASAP (Australian Standardised Affordability and Pricing) Methods

Amanda Lee [1,2,*] and **Meron Lewis** [1]

[1] School of Public Health, Faculty of Medicine, The University of Queensland, Herston, Queensland 4006, Australia; m.lewis@uq.edu.au

[2] The Australian Prevention Partnership Centre, The Sax Institute, Ultimo 2007, New South Wales, Australia

* Correspondence: amanda.lee@uq.edu.au

Abstract: Aboriginal and Torres Strait Islander peoples suffer higher rates of food insecurity and diet-related disease than other Australians. However, assessment of food insecurity in specific population groups is sub-optimal, as in many developed countries. This study tailors the Healthy Diets ASAP (Australian Standardised Affordability and Pricing) methods protocol to be more relevant to Indigenous groups in assessing one important component of food security. The resultant Aboriginal and Torres Strait Islander Healthy Diets ASAP methods were used to assess the price, price differential, and affordability of healthy (recommended) and current (unhealthy) diets in five remote Aboriginal communities. The results show that the tailored approach is more sensitive than the original protocol in revealing the high degree of food insecurity in these communities, where the current diet costs nearly 50% of disposable household income compared to the international benchmark of 30%. Sixty-two percent of the current food budget appears to be spent on discretionary foods and drinks. Aided by community store pricing policies, healthy (recommended) diets are around 20% more affordable than current diets in these communities, but at 38.7% of disposable household income still unaffordable for most households. Further studies in urban communities, and on other socioeconomic, political and commercial determinants of food security in Aboriginal and Torres Strait Islander communities appear warranted. The development of the tailored method provides an example of how national tools can be adapted to better inform policy actions to improve food security and help reduce rates of diet-related chronic disease more equitably in developed countries.

Keywords: food security; diet price; food price; affordability; food policy; nutrition policy; fiscal policy; obesity prevention; non-communicable disease; monitoring and surveillance; INFORMAS

1. Introduction

1.1. Background

Poor diet is now the major preventable risk factor contributing to the burden of disease globally [1]. In Australia, Aboriginal and Torres Strait Islander peoples suffer the poorest health of all population groups and have a lower life expectancy [2]. At least 75% of the mortality gap between Aboriginal and Torres Strait Islanders and other Australians is attributed to diet-related chronic diseases such as cardiovascular disease, chronic kidney disease, and type 2 diabetes [3]. Malnutrition is a major problem in Aboriginal and Torres Strait Islander communities. This includes both over-nutrition, particularly the consumption of too many 'discretionary' food and drinks (those not necessary for health, that are high in saturated fat, added sugar, salt and/or alcohol), and under-nutrition, particularly dietary deficiencies related to inadequate intake of healthy foods in the five food groups and unsaturated spreads and oils allowance, as recommended by the Australian Dietary Guidelines [3,4]. Forty-one percent of the energy intake reported by Aboriginal and Torres Strait Islanders in the Australian Health Survey (AHS) 2011–2013 was derived from 'discretionary' food and drinks [5]. This was higher than reported by non-Indigenous Australians, for whom 35% of the energy intake of adults and 39% of the energy intake of children was derived from discretionary choices [6].

Few Australians (<4%) consume diets consistent with the Australian Dietary Guidelines (ADGs) [4,7]. The contribution of poor diets to the rising rates of overweight and obesity associated with chronic disease is of particular concern. Twenty-five percent of all Australian children aged two to 17 years and 63% of Australian adults aged 18 years and over are overweight or obese [8]. These proportions are even higher for Aboriginal and Torres Strait Islander groups, with 30% of children aged two to 17 years and 66% of adults being overweight or obese [3]. Nutrition policy actions are needed urgently to improve the current diet of the whole Australian population and particularly of Aboriginal and Torres Strait Islander groups.

Good nutrition is underscored by food security. This is when "all people, at all times, have physical, social and economic access to sufficient, safe and nutritious food that meets their dietary needs and food preferences for an active and healthy life" [9]. Food security has been deemed to be a fundamental human right [10]. The Universal Declaration of Human Rights affirms that "everyone has the right to a standard of living adequate for the health and well-being of himself and of his family, including food" [11]. The right to adequate food has been seen as "a right of people to be given a fair opportunity to feed themselves, now and in the future" [12] rather than a right to be fed. In this way, food security is impacted by the availability, accessibility, affordability and acceptability (appropriateness) of the food supply. The experience of these determinants of food security can vary greatly amongst different groups of the population in developed economies like Australia [3,4].

One specific barrier to food security in Australia is believed to be the relative expense of healthy foods. This is particularly the case, among low socioeconomic groups [13–17] in which Aboriginal and Torres Strait Islanders are over-represented. More than one in five Aboriginal and Torres Strait Islanders reported living in a household that had run out of food in the past year and had not been able to afford to buy more in 2011–2013 [18]. This proportion was much higher than in the non-Indigenous population (3.7%) [6]. The affordability of healthy food is believed to be a key aspect of the inequitable distribution of household food security in developed economies such as Australia [13] and a major challenge to food security in remote Aboriginal and Torres Strait Islander communities particularly [3,19]. For over twenty years food prices have been shown consistently to be around 30% higher in remote Aboriginal and Torres Strait Islander communities than in urban centres [20], yet median household incomes are lower in remote areas than in urban areas [3].

However, past food price surveys in Australia have applied a wide variety of 'food basket' costing tools and methods [20] and results are not comparable across different locations or times due to dissimilarity of metrics in the different approaches [20]. These include: number and type of foods surveyed; application of availability and/or quality measures; definition of reference households; estimated household income calculation methods; food store sampling frameworks; data collection methods; and analysis [20]. Until recently, standardised methods to assess and compare the price and affordability of healthy diets with currently consumed, unhealthy diets were lacking in Australia [20] and globally [21]. Such methods are essential to provide robust, meaningful data to inform health and fiscal policy actions, for example, decisions around exemption of basic, healthy foods from Goods and Services Tax (GST) and introduction of health levies on sugary drinks [17,22].

The Healthy Diets ASAP methods protocol was developed to assess, compare and monitor the price and affordability of healthy and current diets among the general population in Australia [22,23]. The method was based on the 'optimal' approach to monitor food price and affordability globally proposed by the International Network for Food and Obesity/non-communicable Diseases Research, Monitoring and Action Support (INFORMAS) [21]. Surprisingly, testing of the Healthy Diets ASAP methods protocol demonstrated that the price of healthy diets recommended by the Australian Dietary Guidelines were 12–15% less expensive than reported current (unhealthy) diets in Australia [22,24]. The results also suggested that Australians were spending 49–64% of their household food budget on discretionary foods and drinks [22,24].

In addition to application at international and national levels, the 'optimal' approach of the INFORMAS diet price and affordability framework [21] has the potential to be modified for use in specific populations and localities. This allows for comparison of diet price and affordability in specific population groups and locations with that of the general population, to inform the development of targeted health and fiscal policies. For example, in Australia, the Healthy Diets ASAP approach has been applied in country Victoria, as reported elsewhere in this special edition [25]. As another example, the INFORMAS 'optimal' approach to assessing diet price and affordability has been tailored to different population groups in New Zealand [26]; results showed that a healthy diet would be more affordable than the current diet for both the total New Zealand population (3.5% difference) and Pacific households (4.5% difference) but the cost of both diets would be similar for Māori households (0.57% difference). However, while previous surveys have used market baskets to estimate the price of 'healthy' basic foods in remote Aboriginal and Torres Strait Island communities [3,20,27], the 'optimal' approach in the INFORMAS step-wise framework to monitor food price data [20] had not been adapted for use in Aboriginal and Torres Strait Islander groups in Australia to enable generation of policy-relevant data.

1.2. The Healthy Diets ASAP Methods Protocol

The Healthy Diets ASAP methods protocol for application with the Australian population as a whole has been reported in detail elsewhere [23]. The protocol consists of five parts; (i) construction of the healthy (recommended) and current (unhealthy) diet pricing tools, (ii) calculation of both median and low-income household incomes; (iii) store location and sampling, (iv) price data collection, and (v) analysis and reporting. To modify the protocol for Aboriginal and Torres Strait Islander groups only the first and second parts of the protocol required adjustment. The remaining three parts of the protocol were retained exactly to optimise comparability of results.

Part one of the Healthy Diets ASAP methods protocol covers the development of two diet pricing survey tools. These are the current (unhealthy) diet pricing tool and the healthy (recommended) diet pricing tool. The current (unhealthy) diet pricing tool comprises the mean fortnightly intake of specific foods and drinks reported in the AHS 2011–2013, expressed in grams or millilitres, by each age/gender group corresponding to the four individuals comprising a reference household (an adult male 31–50 years old, an adult female 31–50 years old, a 14-year-old boy and an eight-year-old girl) in the AHS 2011–2013 [28]. The amounts of foods and drinks consumed per day were derived from the AHS 2011–2013 Confidentialised Unit Record Files (CURFs) of reported dietary intake at 5-digit code level [28]. The mean reported daily dietary intakes for the four individuals were multiplied by 14 to produce the quantities consumed per household per fortnight. The healthy (recommended) diet pricing tool reflects the types and amounts of corresponding foods and drinks for the reference household for a fortnight consistent with the ADGs [4]. In both diet pricing tools, an allowance for edible portion foods/as cooked, as specified in AUSNUT 2011-13 [28], was included; however, post-plate wastage was not estimated or included.

In the second part of the Healthy Diets ASAP methods protocol pertaining to household income, median household income is sourced from national Australian census data which provide a total (gross) amount per household per week (i.e. before taxation). To estimate household income at time points between the five-yearly census, national wage price indexes (published quarterly) are applied [29].

The indicative low (minimum) income for the household is calculated from minimum wage and welfare payments provided by the Department of Human Services [30,31]. A set of assumptions relating to employment, housing type, education attendance, disability status, savings and investments and children's immunisation status are used to determine the appropriate welfare payments and taxation payable. As taxation payable is included, the indicative low (minimum) income is considered disposable income.

Affordability of the healthy and current diets for the reference household is determined by comparing the cost of each diet with the median (gross) household income and with the indicative low (minimum) disposable income of low income households per fortnight. Internationally, a benchmark of 30% of income has been used as a cut-off point to indicate affordability of a diet [16,21].

1.3. Aim

The aim of this study was to modify and test the Healthy Diets ASAP methods protocol to be more relevant to the Aboriginal and Torres Strait Islander population. It developed methods and tools to assist others to apply the approach in order to compare the price, price differential and affordability of healthy (recommended) and current (unhealthy) diets of Aboriginal and Torres Strait Islanders living in different locations with other population groups in Australia.

2. Methods

2.1. Development of the Aboriginal and Torres Strait Islander Healthy Diets ASAP Methods

It was not necessary to amend the Healthy Diets ASAP healthy (recommended) diet pricing tool to adapt the Healthy Diets ASAP methods protocol for application with Aboriginal and Torres Strait Islander groups as the Australian Dietary Guidelines already include culturally-appropriate and commonly available food and drink options and are similar at broad food group level for both Aboriginal and Torres Strait Islanders and non-Indigenous people [4].

However, the Healthy Diets ASAP current (unhealthy) diet pricing tool required modification to reflect the mean intake of each relevant Aboriginal and Torres Strait Islander age and gender group in the National Aboriginal and Torres Strait Islander Nutrition and Physical Activity Survey component of the AHS 2011–2013 [5]. This was compared with the mean dietary intake of each relevant age and gender group of the whole Australian population reported in the AHS 2011–2013 [5,6] to calculate a reported consumption ratio for each food group or, where data were available, for component food and drinks in each food group. This ratio was applied to derive estimates of the current dietary intake of all foods and drinks included in the current diet pricing tool in Aboriginal and Torres Strait Islander groups.

In relation to assessment of household income, it was not necessary to adapt the Healthy Diets ASAP methods protocol to determine the median (gross) household income in Aboriginal and Torres Strait Islander communities in remote areas as census data is reported for relevant Statistical Areas (SA2).

However, assumptions regarding characteristics of the household members were reviewed in relation to any welfare and taxation policies specific to Aboriginal and Torres Strait Islander people and/or to those people living in remote locations in order to better reflect Aboriginal and Torres Strait Islander households living in remote areas for the calculation of indicative low (minimum) disposable income [30,32]. The current quantums of relevant welfare and taxation payments were applied to calculate the indicative low (minimum) disposable household income.

2.2. Testing of the Aboriginal and Torres Strait Islander Healthy Diets ASAP Methods

Prices of food and drinks were collected in five community stores on the Anangu Pitjantjatjara Yankunytjatjara (APY) Lands of South Australia (Figure 1) using the Healthy Diets ASAP food price data collection sheet as per the Healthy Diets ASAP methods protocol [23] by AL in June 2017 as part of ongoing Nganampa Health Council service delivery. In each location, a single store is the main source of food in the community. Further information about the communities is available elsewhere [27].

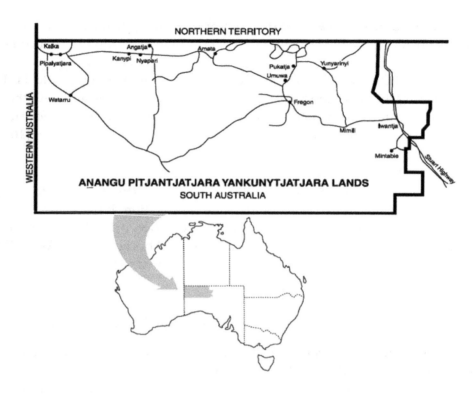

Figure 1. Map showing the Anangu Pitjantjatjara Yankunytjatjara (APY) Lands of South Australia.

Under the Healthy Diets ASAP pricing collection methods protocol, several discretionary food prices are collected from commercial premises outside of a supermarket, including for pizza, hamburger, beef pie and hot chips. As such premises were not available in the remote communities, relevant prices were collected from the store's hot takeaway section, or if not available, for frozen pizza, frozen hamburger and frozen pies, as these items were commonly heated by the purchaser in a microwave at the store for immediate consumption. Frozen potato chip prices were not collected however, due to the large price differential between a single serve of hot chips and the significantly larger bag of frozen chips, and the requirement for more complex cooking methods than microwaving. Alcohol prices were not collected as the communities are 'dry' and alcohol was not available for sale.

Price data were double entered by ML into data entry and analysis Excel© spreadsheets developed for the Healthy Diets ASAP methods protocol [23,33]. If the price of a specific food item was unavailable, the average price for that item in the other four stores was used. If an item was out of stock, the shelf price was collected. The mean prices for each diet and component food groups were calculated. The data were analysed according to both the Healthy Diets ASAP methods protocol and the Aboriginal and Torres Strait Islander Healthy Diets ASAP methods, and results were compared.

Median (gross) household income data from the Community Profile for the APY Lands SA2 [34] was transcribed directly and adjusted by the Wage Price Index percentage increase from June 2016 (at census data collection) to June 2017 (when the food price data were collected) [29].

2.3. Ethical Standards Disclosure

The QUT University Human Research Ethics Committee assessed this study as meeting the conditions for exemption from Human Research Ethics Committee review and approval in accordance with section 5.1.22 of the National Statement on Ethical Conduct in Human Research (2007); the exemption numbers are 1500000161 and 1800000151. All data were obtained from publicly available sources and did not involve human participants.

3. Results

3.1. Developing the Aboriginal and Torres Strait Healthy Diets ASAP Methods Part One: Construct of the Diet Pricing Tools

3.1.1. The Aboriginal and Torres Strait Islander Healthy Diets ASAP Current (Unhealthy) Diet Pricing Tool

The reported consumption ratio calculated by comparing the reported dietary intakes of each food group, and relevant components, by Aboriginal and Torres Strait Islanders [5] with the whole Australian population [7] in the AHS 2011–2013 is presented in Table 1.

Table 1. Reported consumption ratios of each food group and food group component for Aboriginal and Torres Strait Islanders [5] compared with the broader Australian population [7].

Food Group and Food Group Component	Reported Consumption Ratio
Vegetables & legumes	0.67
Fruit	0.8
Grain (cereal) foods—wholegrains	0.74
Grain (cereal) foods—others	1
Meat, poultry, fish & alternatives—red meat & poultry	1.14
Meat, poultry, fish & alternatives—others	0.94
Milk, yoghurt, cheese & alternatives	0.8
Unsaturated oils & spreads	0.7
Discretionary foods—sugar-sweetened drinks	1.8
Discretionary foods—others	1.1
Water	1
Alcohol	1

The reported consumption ratios were applied to calculate the amounts of foods and drinks comprising the Aboriginal and Torres Strait Islander Healthy Diets ASAP current (unhealthy) diet pricing tool as presented in Table 2. The composition of the original Healthy Diets ASAP current (unhealthy) diet pricing tool for the whole population is also presented in Table 2.

Table 2. Composition of the Healthy Diets ASAP and Aboriginal and Torres Strait Islander Healthy Diets ASAP current (unhealthy) diet and healthy (recommended) diet pricing tools (pertaining to the diet of a reference household per fortnight [1]).

Current (Unhealthy) Diet Pricing Tool			Healthy (Recommended) Diet Pricing Tool	
Food or Drink	Healthy Diets ASAP Quantity	Aboriginal and Torres Strait Islander Healthy Diets ASAP Quantity	Food or Drink	Healthy Diets ASAP and Aboriginal and Torres Strait Islander Healthy Diets ASAP Quantity
Bottled water, still (mL)	5296	5296	Bottled water, still (mL)	5296
Artificially sweetened 'diet' soft drink (mL)	2391	2630		
Fruit			*Fruit*	
Apples, red, loose (g)	3497	2797	Apples, red, loose (g)	5460
Bananas, Cavendish, loose (g)	899	719	Bananas, Cavendish, loose (g)	5460
Oranges, loose (g)	1664	1331	Oranges, loose (g)	5460
Fruit salad, canned in juice (g)	2046	1637		
Fruit juice	3026	3329		
Vegetables			*Vegetables*	
Potato, white, loose (g)	1460	978	Potato, white, loose (g)	2320
Sweetcorn, canned, no added salt (g)	206	138	Sweetcorn, canned, no added salt (g)	1160
Broccoli, loose (g)	422	282	Broccoli, loose (g)	1470
White cabbage, loose (g)	235	157	White cabbage, loose (g)	1470
Iceberg lettuce, whole (g)	795	533	Iceberg lettuce, whole (g)	1470
Carrot, loose (g)	753	505	Carrot, loose (g)	2205
Pumpkin (g)	240	161	Pumpkin (g)	2205
Four bean mix, canned (g)	74	50	Four bean mix, canned (g)	1005
Diced tomatoes, canned, in tomato juice (g)	234	157	Diced tomatoes, canned, in tomato juice (g)	1638
Onion, brown, loose (g)	84	57	Onion, brown, loose (g)	1638
Tomatoes, loose (g)	488	327	Tomatoes, loose (g)	1638

Table 2. *Cont.*

Current (Unhealthy) Diet Pricing Tool			Healthy (Recommended) Diet Pricing Tool	
Food or Drink	Healthy Diets ASAP Quantity	Aboriginal and Torres Strait Islander Healthy Diets ASAP Quantity	Food or Drink	Healthy Diets ASAP and Aboriginal and Torres Strait Islander Healthy Diets ASAP Quantity
Frozen mixed vegetables, pre-packaged (g)	1184	793	Frozen mixed vegetables, pre-packaged (g)	1638
Frozen peas, pre-packaged (g)	273	183	Frozen peas, pre-packaged (g)	1638
Baked beans, canned (g)	369	247	Baked beans, canned (g)	1005
Salad vegs in sandwich	120	120	Salad vegs in sandwich	120
Veg in tinned meat and vegetable casserole (g)	646	736		
Grain (cereal) foods			*Grain (cereal) foods*	
Wholegrain cereal biscuits Weet-bix™ (g)	430	319	Wholegrain cereal biscuits Weet-bix™ (g)	2216
Wholemeal bread, pre-packaged (g)	1054	780	Wholemeal bread, pre-packaged (g)	4272
Rolled oats, whole (g)	870	870	Rolled oats, whole (g)	6648
White bread, pre-packaged (g)	3033	3033	White bread, pre-packaged (g)	893
Cornflakes (g)	680	680	Cornflakes (g)	670
White pasta, spaghetti (g)	1326	1326	White pasta, spaghetti (g)	2042
White rice, medium grain (g)	1622	1622	White rice, medium grain (g)	2042
Dry water cracker biscuit (g)	258	258	Dry water cracker biscuit (g)	781
Bread in sandwich	120	120	Bread in sandwich	120
Meats, poultry, fish, eggs, nuts and seeds			*Meats, poultry, fish, eggs, nuts and seeds*	
Beef mince, lean (g)	267	305	Beef mince, lean (g)	1168
Lamb loin chops (g)	257	293	Lamb loin chops (g)	1169
Beef rump steak (g)	1056	1204	Beef rump steak (g)	1172
Tuna, canned in vegetable oil (g)	1052	989	Tuna, canned in vegetable oil (g)	1841
Whole barbeque chicken, cooked (g)	1661	1893	Whole barbeque chicken, cooked (g)	1471
Eggs (g)	872	820	Eggs (g)	2208
Meat in tinned meat and vegetable casserole (g)	646	736	Peanuts, roasted, unsalted (g)	780
Chicken in sandwiches	120	120	Chicken in sandwiches	120
Milk, yoghurt, cheese and alternatives			*Milk, yoghurt, cheese and alternatives*	
Cheddar cheese, full fat (g)	624	499	Cheddar cheese, full fat (g)	704
Cheddar cheese, reduced fat (g)	44	35	Cheddar cheese, reduced fat (g)	516
Milk, full fat (mL)	5961	4769	Milk, full cream (mL)	6438
Milk, reduced fat (mL)	2929	2344	Milk, reduced fat (mL)	12000
Yoghurt, full fat plain (g)	204	163	Yoghurt, full fat plain (g)	2576
Yoghurt, reduced fat, flavoured (vanilla) (g)	676	541	Yoghurt, reduced fat, flavoured (vanilla) (g)	5100
Flavoured milk (mL)	2416	2658		
Unsaturated oils				
Canola margarine (g)	170	119	Canola margarine (g)	412
Sunflower oil (mL)	7	5	Sunflower oil (mL)	291
Olive oil (mL)	7	5	Olive oil (mL)	291
Discretionary choices				
Beer, full strength (mL)	4661	4661		
White wine, sparkling (mL)	863	863		
Whisky (mL)	266	266		
Red wine (mL)	1078	1078		
Butter (g)	280	308		
Muffin, commercial (g)	1455	1601		
Cream-filled sweet biscuit, pre-packaged (g)	496	546		
Muesli bar, pre-packaged (g)	373	410		
Mixed nuts, salted (g)	255	281		
Pizza, commercial (g)	1182	1300		
Savoury flavoured biscuits (g)	222	244		
Confectionary (g)	418	460		
Chocolate (g)	441	485		
Sugar-sweetened beverages (Coca Cola) (mL)	12012	21621		
Meat pie, commercial (g)	1638	1802		
Frozen lasagne, pre-packaged (g)	4322	4754		
Hamburger, commercial (g)	2413	2654		
Beef sausages (g)	1048	1152		
Ham (g)	189	208		
Potato crisps, pre-packaged (g)	518	570		
Potato chips, hot, commercial (g)	670	737		
Ice cream (g)	1830	2013		
White sugar (g)	564	621		
Salad dressing (mL)	277	305		
Tomato sauce (mL)	569	626		
Chicken soup, canned (g)	1340	1474		
Orange juice (mL)	3027	3330		
Fish fillet crumbed, pre-packaged (g)	302	332		
Instant noodles, wheat-based (g)	381	419		

[1] The reference household comprises four people: adult male 19–50 years old; adult female 19–50 years old; boy 14 years old; girl 8 years old.

3.1.2. The Aboriginal and Torres Strait Islander Healthy Diets ASAP Healthy (Recommended) Diet Pricing Tool

The amounts of foods and drinks comprising the Aboriginal and Torres Strait Islander Healthy Diets ASAP healthy (recommended) diet pricing tool (unchanged from the original protocol [23]) are presented in Table 2.

3.2. Developing the Aboriginal and Torres Strait Healthy Diets ASAP Methods Part Two: Determination of Median and Low-Income Household Income

The Community Profile for the APY Lands SA2 states that the median weekly household income in 2016 was $AUD1150 and the average household contained 3.8 people [34]. The Australian Wage Price Index [29] increased from June 2016 (at census data collection) to June 2017 (when the food price data was collected) by 1.9%. Applying this index gave an estimated median weekly household income on the APY Lands in June 2017 of $AUD1171. Thus, the fortnightly median (gross) household income for the reference household in the APY Lands in June 2017 was $AUD2342.

The method to determine the indicative low (minimum) disposable household income was modified to include in the underlying assumptions (Table 3) that the reference family is comprised of people identifying as Aboriginal and/or Torres Strait Islanders and that they live in a remote location as determined by the Australian Tax Office [32]. Compared with the Healthy Diets ASAP methods protocol, the assumptions included an AbStudy school term allowance for the 14-year-old boy [30] and a remote area tax offset amount applied in assessment of taxation for the adult male, as shown in Table 4. All other assumptions were the same as those for non-Indigenous households and those living in non-remote areas [30].

Table 3. Assumptions used to determine the indicative low (minimum) disposable household income of the reference household.

Assumptions for the Reference Household Consisting of an Adult Male, an Adult Female, a 14-Year-Old Boy and an 8-Year-Old Girl
• The family is privately renting a house at $AUD75/week [34]
• The adult male works on a permanent basis at the national minimum wage ($AUD17.29 per hour [31]) for 38 h a week
• The adult female works on a part-time basis at the national minimum wage ($AUD17.29 per hour) for 6 h a week
• Both children attend school and are fully immunised
• None of the family are disabled
• The family has some emergency savings that earn negligible interest
• The family are Aboriginal and/or Torres Strait Islanders
• The family live in a remote location

Table 4. Calculation of the indicative low (minimum) disposable household income of the reference Aboriginal and Torres Strait Islander household.

Income Type	Amount Per Fortnight ($AUD)
Paid employment–adult male	1345.20
Paid employment–adult female	212.40
Family Tax Benefit A	420.70
Family Tax Benefit A Supplement	55.87
Family Tax Benefit B	108.64
Family Tax Benefit B Supplement	13.62
Clean Energy Supplement (across all payments)	9.94
Rent Assistance	nil
AbStudy School term allowance–14 yr old boy	20.80
Income tax paid (tax owing on employment income of adult male, less low income tax offset, less remote area tax offset	−48.09
Total Fortnightly Income	**2139.08**

3.3. Testing the Aboriginal and Torres Strait Islander Healthy Diets ASAP Methods: The Cost of The Diets and Component Food Groups

The mean (± standard deviation) cost of the healthy diet was $AUD827.63 (± $42.24) in the five remote Aboriginal communities surveyed.

The cost of the current diet in the five remote Aboriginal communities using the Healthy Diets ASAP methods protocol and Aboriginal and Torres Strait Islander Healthy Diets ASAP methods, and the difference between the two, are presented in Table 5. Application of the Aboriginal and Torres Strait Islander Healthy Diets ASAP methods assessed the cost of the current diet at $AUD1023.16 (± $40.90) which was 7% higher than the cost of $AUD956.18 (± $39.60) assessed by application of the original Healthy Diets ASAP methods protocol.

Table 5. Mean cost of the current (unhealthy) diet in five remote Aboriginal communities using the Healthy Diets Australian Standardised Affordability and Pricing (ASAP) methods protocol and Aboriginal and Torres Strait Islander Healthy Diets ASAP methods.

Diet Component	Healthy Diets ASAP (Whole Population) Methods Protocol		Aboriginal and Torres Strait Islander Healthy Diets ASAP Methods		Cost Difference between Using Aboriginal and Torres Strait Islander Healthy Diets ASAP Methods and Healthy Diets ASAP Methods Protocol
	Mean Cost ($AUD)	Std Dev ($AUD)	Mean Cost ($AUD)	Std Dev ($AUD)	Difference $AUD (% Change)
Water	8.83	—	8.83	—	—
Fruit	80.66	8.70	68.13	6.93	−12.54 (−15%)
Vegetables & Legumes	56.31	3.21	43.48	2.15	−12.83 (−23%)
Grains & Cereals	66.42	2.35	63.37	2.29	−3.05 (−5%)
Meats, nuts, seeds, eggs	110.65	3.33	119.95	3.16	9.30 (+8%)
Milk, yoghurt, cheese	80.66	13.72	71.93	14.08	−8.73 (−11%)
Unsaturated oils & spreads	2.03	0.01	1.42	0.01	−0.61 (−30%)
Artificially sweetened soft drink	10.52	—	11.57	—	1.05 (+10%)
Take-away foods	181.32	17.53	199.45	19.28	18.13 (+10%)
Sugar-sweetened drinks	68.18	—	115.35	—	47.18 (+69%)
Discretionary choices-other	290.62	13.36	319.68	14.70	29.06 (+10%)
Total cost	**956.18**	**39.60**	**1023.16**	**40.90**	**66.97 (+7%)**

[1] The current diet for a fortnight for the reference household comprising four people: adult male 19–50 years old; adult female 19–50 years old; boy 14 years old; girl 8 years old.

Using the Aboriginal and Torres Strait Islander Healthy Diets ASAP methods, the cost of a healthy diet was 24% less than the cost of the current diet. If the original Healthy Diets ASAP methods protocol was used, the cost of the healthy diet was 16% less than the current diet.

Using the Healthy Diets ASAP methods protocol, the proportion of the total cost of the current diet derived from discretionary foods and drinks was 56.5%. This figure was 62.0% when the Aboriginal and Torres Strait Islander Healthy Diets ASAP methods were used.

The total cost of the current (unhealthy) diet was $AUD66.97 per fortnight (7%) more expensive when the Aboriginal and Torres Strait Islander specific methods were used rather than the original Healthy Diets ASAP methods protocol for the whole population (Table 5). The main source of difference for healthy foods was that the cost of all fruit and vegetables included in the current diet was $AUD25.37 per fortnight (19%) less when assessed by the Aboriginal and Torres Strait Islander Healthy Diets ASAP methods than by the Healthy Diet ASAP methods protocol. The healthy unsaturated oils and spreads were cost 30% less using the Aboriginal and Torres Strait Islander specific methods; however, this was a difference of only $AUD0.61 per fortnight, given the low quantities of these foods consumed. Conversely, the cost of all unhealthy discretionary foods and drinks included in the current diet was $AUD94.37 (17%) more expensive per fortnight when assessed by the Aboriginal and Torres Strait Islander Healthy Diets ASAP methods than by the Healthy Diets ASAP methods protocol. The major source of this variance was the cost of sugar-sweetened drinks which were $AUD47.18 per fortnight (69%) more expensive when assessed by the Aboriginal and Torres Strait Islander specific methods.

3.4. Testing of the Aboriginal and Torres Strait Islander Healthy Diets ASAP Methods: Affordability of Healthy Diets

The affordability of healthy diet and the current diets determined by both the Healthy Diets ASAP methods protocol and the Aboriginal and Torres Strait Islander Healthy Diets ASAP methods in five remote Aboriginal communities are shown in Table 6. When determined by the Aboriginal and Torres Strait Islander Healthy Diets ASAP methods, the affordability of the current diet was around 7% poorer than when assessed by the original Healthy Diets ASAP methods protocol. When assessed by the Aboriginal and Torres Strait Islander Healthy Diets ASAP methods, the affordability of the current diet as a proportion of both the median (gross) household income (35.3%) and indicative low (minimum) disposable household income (38.7%) respectively was above the internationally acceptable benchmark of 30% [16,21]. As assessed by the Aboriginal and Torres Strait Islander Healthy Diets ASAP methods, the healthy diet would be around 20% more affordable than the current diet, but at 35.3% of the median (gross) household income and 38.7% of the indicative low (minimum) disposable household income, would still be unaffordable compared to the internally acceptable benchmark of 30% [16,21].

Table 6. Affordability of current diets and healthy diets in remote Aboriginal communities on the APY Lands.

Diet	Mean Diet Cost (±Std Dev) ($AUD)	Affordability with Median (Gross) Household Income ($AUD2342)	Affordability with Indicative Low (Minimum) Disposable Household Income ($AUD2139.08)
Healthy (recommended) diet	827.63 (42.24)	35.3%	38.7%
Current (unhealthy) diet determined by the Healthy Diets ASAP methods protocol	956.18 (39.60)	40.8%	44.7%
Current (unhealthy) diet determined by the Aboriginal and Torres Strait Islander Healthy Diets ASAP methods	1023.16 (40.90)	43.7%	47.8%

4. Discussion

4.1. Discussion of Approach

Food insecurity is a key factor contributing to the high double-burden of malnutrition experienced by Indigenous Australians [3]. However, as in many developed nations, food security is poorly assessed in Australia, where, for over twenty years irregular national dietary surveys have included a single question on individual food security around running out of food and not being able to afford to buy more [3]. This measure, while a useful indicator, is likely to underestimate the full extent of the problem. There is a pressing need to better understand food insecurity from an Aboriginal and Torres Strait Islander perspective in order to develop Indigenous-specific tools for assessment of availability, affordability, accessibility and acceptability of healthy food and drinks and other determinants of food security, particularly at household and community level [3,35]. This paper attempted to do this in the area of food price and affordability, in order to provide relevant data to inform the development of tailored fiscal and nutrition policy actions with Aboriginal and Torres Strait Islander communities.

Adjustment of the whole-of-population Healthy Diets ASAP current (unhealthy) diet pricing tool by the reported consumption ratio method, proved to be a simple, expedient method to customise the tool for application in remote Aboriginal and Torres Strait Islander communities, particularly as it did not require redevelopment of the original data collection tools. However, this method does rely on the availability of quality dietary (food and drink) intake survey data for both the whole population at the national level and for specific population groups, which may not always be available, even in developed countries [21].

The total cost of the current diet was 7% more expensive when the Aboriginal and Torres Strait Islander specific methods were used rather than the original Healthy Diets ASAP methods protocol for the whole population. This was due to differences in the reported intakes of foods and drinks that contributed substantially to the current diet in Aboriginal and Torres Strait Islander groups compared with the broader Australian population. Major differences were seen for sugar-sweetened drinks (with reported intakes nearly double that of broader Australia) contributing most (69%) of the additional expense, and reported intakes of fruit and vegetables (which were 30% less than the broader population) reducing the current diet costs by 19%, when determined by the Aboriginal and Torres Strait Islander Healthy Diets ASAP methods.

While data on median (gross) household income of Aboriginal and Torres Strait Islanders specifically are not readily available, the use of median (gross) household income from the relevant 2016 Census data Community Profiles [34] did provide meaningful information once updated with the wage price index [29], and at $AUD2342 per household per fortnight (gross), was consistent with expectations given the low (minimum) disposable household income of $AUD2139 estimated in the test communities using different methods. This study demonstrated that determination of the indicative low (minimum) disposable household income for Aboriginal and Torres Strait Islander households living in remote areas was feasible. This figure for Aboriginal and Torre Strait Islander households living in non-remote areas would be slightly less, due to the non-applicability of the remote area tax offset.

Testing demonstrated that it is feasible to apply the Aboriginal and Torres Strait Islander Healthy Diets ASAP methods stores in remote communities. However, further studies would be required to test utility of the approach in urban centres. Among other differences, remote community stores, stock a much smaller range of items than supermarkets in urban areas. In this study there were four instances where the listed food item in the pricing tool was unavailable in any size or brand. Each store outlet surveyed in the five remote communities operates as a general store selling fresh fruit, vegetables, meat, bread, frozen foods, pantry items, and other goods. Four of the stores also sold a range of hot takeaway food items. Some food items were available only in sizes much smaller than stated on the price collection data sheet; for example, plain yoghurt is listed as 1kg on the Healthy Diets ASAP food price data collection sheet, but was only available in 200g tubs in three of the five stores. This contributed to the high standard deviation in the cost of the food groups observed where larger items were missing, particularly the milk, yoghurt and cheese food group. Conversely, as part of the nutrition policy in place in the five stores surveyed, the price of 600mL bottled water is mandated at $AUD1.00, so that for this item the standard deviation of prices across the five stores was zero.

Testing of the Aboriginal and Torres Strait Islander Healthy Diets ASAP methods supported the notion that the approach has acceptable face validity in providing assessment of the price, price differential and affordability of current (unhealthy) and healthy (recommended) diets of Aboriginal and Torres Strait Islander groups living in remote communities. The results were consistent with expectations arising from consideration of the reported dietary intake data of the two different populations [5,7] and the relative prices of foods in the remote Aboriginal community stores [27].

Consistent with similar surveys, particularly in Australia where the GST of 10% is not applied to basic, healthy foods [22–25], application of the Aboriginal and Torres Strait Islander Healthy Diets ASAP methods in remote Aboriginal communities showed that a healthy diet ($AUD827.63) was less expensive than the current diet ($AUD1,023.16) per household per fortnight. However, at 76% of the cost of the current diet, a healthy diet was potentially more affordable in the remote Aboriginal communities studied than in other places, where the cost of the healthy diet ranges between 80–85% [22–25]. Surprisingly, this price differential between the current and healthy diets was larger than in other studies even though alcohol was not included in the current diet, as the communities are 'dry' and alcohol is not available for sale. One likely reason for this is that the five community stores surveyed on the APY Lands have in place a prescribed nutrition policy which mandates, among other potential benefits, that fruit and vegetables are sold at cost price, that 600mL bottled water is priced at $AUD1.00, and that low mark ups on the wholesale price of other healthy foods, such as lean meat and wholemeal bread, are standard. Previous studies have found that this nutrition policy contributes to relative affordability of healthy foods, particularly fruit and vegetables, compared to unhealthy, discretionary choices [27].

Despite these promising findings, further scrutiny showed that healthy diets would be unaffordable due to the low household incomes in the communities surveyed. When assessed by the Aboriginal and Torres Strait Islander Healthy Diets ASAP methods, healthy diets would cost over 35% of median (gross) household income and nearly 39% of indicative low (minimum) disposable household incomes in these communities, compared to the international affordability benchmark of 30% of disposable household income [16,21].

The high level of food insecurity and food stress in these communities was confirmed, as the current diet cost over 43% of median (gross) household income and nearly 48% of indicative low (minimum) disposable household incomes when assessed by the Aboriginal and Torres Strait Islander Healthy Diets ASAP methods.

The tailored Aboriginal and Torres Strait Islander Healthy Diets ASAP methods were more sensitive than the original Healthy Diets ASAP methods protocol in revealing the current degree of food security in the communities surveyed. If the tailored methods developed and tested in this study had not been used, the severity of food security issues in the remote Aboriginal communities surveyed would have been partially masked, and valuable data relevant to potential policy actions would have remained undetected.

Worryingly, while 41% of the energy intake of the diet was derived from discretionary choices [5], application of the Aboriginal and Torres Strait Islander Healthy Diets ASAP methods showed that 62% of the current food budget in the remote communities surveyed was spent on discretionary food and drinks; of this over 18% was spent on sugary drinks and over 30% on take-away foods. This high reliance on discretionary food and drinks has been described previously and appears to be driven by the increasing availability, range and variety of unhealthy discretionary foods and drinks in community stores over the last three decades [27]. Such changes in the food supply reflect those seen more broadly in Australia, and globally [27].

These results highlight that, given the high proportion of food insecurity and diet-related disease in Aboriginal and Torres Strait Islander groups, nothing should be done to risk increasing the price differential of healthy to discretionary food and drinks in remote Aboriginal communities, as this could act as a further barrier to healthy diets. While better understanding of price elasticities and access to income entitlements in remote communities would be useful, the findings also suggest that investigation into the nature and effect of drivers of food choice other than price, such as housing, access to educational and employment opportunities, availability and functionality of food preparation/cooking facilities, transport, convenience, product placement in stores, promotion, advertising and food preferences appears warranted.

4.2. Limitations

Similar to the original Healthy Diets ASAP methods protocol, there are several inherent limitations in the Aboriginal and Torres Strait Islander Healthy Diets ASAP methods. Given that the approach is based on the reported mean dietary intakes of select age and gender groups of Aboriginal and Torres Strait Islanders at the national level, the diet pricing tools should be considered as reference instruments and the cost of the current diet is unlikely to be the same as actual expenditure on food and drinks by all Aboriginal and Torres Strait Islander people or households currently [36].

All diet pricing tools should ideally include foods that are culturally acceptable, commonly consumed and widely available. Whilst the amounts of the foods included in the diet survey pricing tools are reflective of the respective food and food group consumption of Aboriginal and Torres Strait Islander groups reported in the AHS 2011-13 [5] at the three digit-level, the Healthy Diet ASAP methods protocol includes foods and drinks reported in the AHS 2011-13 [6] at the five-digit level.

Therefore, a very small number of the specific foods and drinks included tend to reflect reported consumption of the Australian population as a whole, rather than Aboriginal and Torres Strait Islander peoples specifically. While all foods in the pricing tools were generally available and accessible in the remote community stores surveyed, formal assessment of their cultural acceptability has not been undertaken as yet. Subsequent modifications may be required to accommodate specific food preferences; for example, further reduction of the quantities of plain yoghurt included as this item was frequently out of stock and was considered by store managers to be a low demand item.

No adjustments were made to account for the marked under-reporting in the AHS 2011-13 [5,6]. Nor were adjustments made for the greater proportion of 'convenience' items in the current (unhealthy) diet pricing tool compared with the healthy (recommended) diet pricing tool. Given the high rates of overweight/obesity in Aboriginal and Torres Strait Islander groups, and that the Foundation Diets of the modelling used to inform the Australian Guide to Healthy Eating component of the Australian Dietary Guidelines were prescribed for the shortest and least active in each age group [37], the healthy (recommended) diet tool under-estimates the requirements of taller, more active and healthy weight individuals.

5. Conclusions

The Aboriginal and Torres Strait Islander Healthy Diets ASAP methods tailor nationally-standardised diet price and affordability method protocols to improve applicability to Indigenous Australians. The method incorporates relevant household income data and reported dietary intakes of Aboriginal and Torres Strait Islander groups to more appropriately assess, compare, monitor and benchmark the price, price differential and affordability of current (unhealthy) and healthy (recommended) diets in different communities.

The development of the tailored Aboriginal and Torres Strait Islander Healthy Diets ASAP methods provides an example of how standardised national tools can be adapted at sub-population and regional levels to provide better data to inform policy actions to improve food security and help reduce rates of diet-related disease more equitably in developed countries.

Author Contributions: Conceptualisation, A.L.; Methodology, A.L.; Formal Analysis, M.L.; Investigation, A.L.; Writing—Original Draft Preparation, M.L. and A.L.; Writing—Review & Editing, A.L.; Project Administration, A.L.

Acknowledgments: We acknowledge the support and assistance of the Nganampa Health Council, the Ngaanyatjarra Pitjantjatjara Yankunytjatjara Women's Council (NPYWC), and the Mai Wiru Regional Stores Council Aboriginal Corporation.

References

1.   Institute for Health Metrics and Evaluation. Global Burden of Disease Country Profile Australia. Available online: http://www.healthdata.org/sites/default/files/files/country_profiles/GBD/ihme_gbd_country_report_australia.pdf (accessed on 12 November 2017).
2.   Australian Institute of Health and Welfare. *Australian Burden of Disease Study: Impact and Causes of Illness and Death in Aboriginal and Torres Strait Islander People 2011*; Series No. 6; Australian Burden of Disease Stufy: Canberra, Australia, 2015.
3.   Lee, A.; Ride, K. *Review of Nutrition among Aboriginal and Torres Strait Islander People*; Australian Indigenous HealthInfoNet: Perth, Australia, 2018.
4.   National Health and Medical Research Council. *Australian Dietary Guidelines—Providing the Scientific Evidence for Healthier Australian Diets*; National Health and Medical Research Council: Australia, Canberra, 2013. Available online: https://www.eatforhealth.gov.au/sites/default/files/content/n55_australian_dietary_guidelines.pdf (accessed on 9 February 2016).

5. Australian Bureau of Statistics. 4727.0.55.008—Australian Aboriginal and Torres Strait Islander Health Survey: Consumption of Food Groups from the Australian Dietary Guidelines, 2012–2013. Available online: http://www.abs.gov.au/ausstats/abs@.nsf/PrimaryMainFeatures/4727.0.55.008?OpenDocument (accessed on 20 September 2018).

6. Australian Bureau of Statistics. 4364.0.55.007—Australian Health Survey: Nutrition First Results—Foods and Nutrients, 2011–2012. Available online: http://www.abs.gov.au/AUSSTATS/abs@.nsf/DetailsPage/4364.0.55.0072011-12?OpenDocument (accessed on 12 November 2017).

7. Australian Bureau of Statistics. 4364.0.55.012—Australian Health Survey: Consumption of Food Groups from the Australian Dietary Guidelines, 2011–2012. Available online: http://www.abs.gov.au/ausstats/abs@.nsf/mf/4364.0.55.012 (accessed on 12 November 2017).

8. Australian Bureau of Statistics. 4364.0.55.003—Australian Health Survey: Updated Results, 2011–2012—Overweight and Obesity. Available online: http://www.abs.gov.au/ausstats/abs@.nsf/lookup/33C64022ABB5ECD5CA257B8200179437?opendocument (accessed on 12 November 2017).

9. FAO. *The State of Food Insecurity in the World 2001*; Food and Agriculture Organization of the United Nations: Rome, Italy, 2002.

10. Davy, D. Australian's efforts to improve food security for Aboriginal and Torres Strait Islander peoples. *Health Hum. Rights* **2016**, *18*, 209. [PubMed]

11. United Nations. *Universal Declaration of Human Rights*; Unated Nations: Geneva, Switzerland, 1948.

12. Eide, W.B.; Kracht, U. Towards a definition of the right to food and nutrition: Reflections on General Comment No. 12. *SCN News* **1999**, *18*, 39–40.

13. Kettings, C.; Sinclair, A.J.; Voevodin, M. A healthy diet consistent with Australian health recommendations is too expensive for welfare-dependent families. *Aust. N. Z. J. Public Health* **2009**, *33*, 566–572. [CrossRef] [PubMed]

14. Williams, P.G. Can the poor in Australia afford healthy food? *Nutr. Diet.* **2011**, *68*, 6–7. [CrossRef]

15. Ward, P.R.; Verty, F.; Cartrer, P.; Tsurtos, G.; Conveney, J.; Wong, C.K. Food Stress in Adelaide: The Relationship between Low Income and the Affordability of Healthy Food. *J. Environ. Public Health* **2013**, *2013*, 10. [CrossRef] [PubMed]

16. Barosh, L.; Friel, S.; Engelhardt, K.; Chan, L. The cost of a healthy and sustainable diet—Who can afford it? *Aust. N. Z. J. Public Health* **2014**, *38*, 7–12. [CrossRef] [PubMed]

17. Landrigan, T.J.; Kerr, D.A.; Dhaliwal, S.S.; Pollard, C.M. Removing the Australian tax exemption on healthy food adds food stress to families vulnerable to poor nutrition. *Aust. N. Z. J. Public Health* **2017**, *41*. [CrossRef] [PubMed]

18. Australian Bureau of Statistics. 4727.0.55.005—Australian Aboriginal and Torres Strait Islander Health Survey: Nutrition Results—Food and Nutrients, 2012–2013. Available online: http://www.abs.gov.au/ausstats/abs@.nsf/PrimaryMainFeatures/4727.0.55.005?OpenDocument (accessed on 20 September 2018).

19. Queensland Health. 2014 Healthy Food Access Basket Survey. Available online: https://www.health.qld.gov.au/research-reports/reports/public-health/food-nutrition/access/overview (accessed on 8 February 2016).

20. Lewis, M.; Lee, A. Costing 'healthy' food baskets in Australia—A systematic review of food price and affordability monitoring tools, protocols and methods. *Public Health Nutr.* **2016**, *19*, 2872–2886. [CrossRef] [PubMed]

21. Lee, A.; Murchu, C.N.; Sacks, G.; Swinburn, B.A.; Snowdon, W.; Vandevijvre, S.; Hawkes, C.; L Abbe, M.; Rayner, M.; Sandres, D. Monitoring the price and affordability of foods and diets globally. *Obes. Rev.* **2013**, *14* (Suppl. S1), 82–95. [CrossRef] [PubMed]

22. Lee, A.J.; Kane, S.; Ramsey, R.; Good, E.; Dick, M. Testing the price and affordability of healthy and current (unhealthy) diets and the potential impacts of policy change in Australia. *BMC Public Health* **2016**, *16*, 315. [CrossRef] [PubMed]

23. Lee, A.J.; Kane, S.; Lewis, M.; Good, E.; Pollard, C.M.; Landrigan, J.T.; Dick, M. Healthy diets ASAP—Australian Standardised Affordability and Pricing methods protocol. *Nutr. J.* **2018**, *17*, 88. [CrossRef] [PubMed]

24. Lee, A.; Lewis, M.; Kane, S. Are Healthy Diets really More Expensive? Findings Brief. The Australian Prevention Partnership Centre. Available online: https://preventioncentre.org.au/our-work/research-projects/are-healthy-diets-really-more-expensive/ (accessed on 18 November 2018).

25.   Love, P.; Wheland, J.; Bell, C.; Garinger, F.; Russell, C.; Lewis, M.; Lee, M. Healthy diets in rural Victoria—Cheaper than unhealthy alternative, yet affordable. *Int. J. Environ. Res. Public Health* **2018**, *15*, 2469. [CrossRef] [PubMed]

26.   Mackay, S.; Buch, T.; Vandevijvere, S.; Goodwin, R.; Korohina, E.; Tahifote, M.F.; Lee, A.J.; Swinburn, B.A. Cost and Affordability of Diets Modelled on Current Eating Patterns and on Dietary Guidelines, for New Zealand Total Population, Māori and Pacific Households. *Int. J. Environ. Res. Public Health* **2018**, *15*, 1255. [CrossRef] [PubMed]

27.   Lee, A.; Rainow, S.; Tregenza, J.; Tregenza, L. Nutrition in remote Aboriginal communities: Lessons from Mai Wiru and the Anangu Pitjantjatjara Yankunytjatjara Lands. *Aust. N. Z. J. Public Health* **2016**, *40*, S81–S88. [CrossRef] [PubMed]

28.   Australian Bureau of Statistics. 4324.0.55.002 Microdata: Australian Health Survey: Nutrition and Physical Activity, 2011–2012. Available online: http://www.abs.gov.au/ausstats/abs@.nsf/PrimaryMainFeatures/4324.0.55.002?OpenDocument (accessed on 12 November 2017).

29.   Australian Bureau of Statistics. 6345.0—Wage Price Index, Australia, June 2017. Available online: http://www.abs.gov.au/AUSSTATS/abs@.nsf/allprimarymainfeatures/A52F591B2454B045CA2581D8000E926D?opendocument (accessed on 29 September 2018).

30.   Department of Human Services. Online Estimators. Available online: http://www.humanservices.gov.au/customer/enablers/online-estimators (accessed on 22 October 2015).

31.   Fair Work Ombudsman. Minimum Wages. Available online: https://www.fairwork.gov.au/how-we-will-help/templates-and-guides/fact-sheets/minimum-workplace-entitlements/minimum-wages (accessed on 22 October 2015).

32.   Australian Taxation Office. Individual Offsets and Rebates: Zone and Overseas Forces. Available online: https://www.ato.gov.au/Individuals/Income-and-deductions/Offsets-and-rebates/Zones-and-overseas-forces/ (accessed on 27 January 2018).

33.   Microsoft Corporation. *Microsoft Office*, Version 2007; Microsoft Corporation: Washington, WA, USA, 2007.

34.   Australian Bureau of Statistics. QuickStats. 2016. Available online: http://quickstats.censusdata.abs.gov.au/census_services/getproduct/census/2016/quickstat/406021138 (accessed on 29 September 2018).

35.   Lee, A.; Ride, K. *Review of Programs and Services to Improve Aboriginal and Torres Strait Islander Nutrition and Food Security*; Australian Indigenous HealthInfoNet: Perth, Australia, 2018.

36.   Mhurchu, C.N.; Eyles, H.; Schilling, C.; Yang, Q.; Kaye-Blake, W.; Genc, M.; Blakely, T. Food prices and consumer demand: Differences across income levels and ethnic groups. *PLoS ONE* **2013**, *8*, e75934. [CrossRef] [PubMed]

37.   National Health and Medical Research Council. *A Modelling System to Inform the Revision of the Australian Guide to Healthy Eating*; National Health and Medical Research Council: Canberra, Australia, 2011. Available online: https://www.eatforhealth.gov.au/sites/default/files/files/the_guidelines/n55c_australian_dietary_guidelines_food_modelling_140121.pdf (accessed on 11 February 2016).

10

Social Assistance Payments and Food Insecurity in Australia: Evidence from the Household Expenditure Survey

Jeromey B. Temple [1,*], Sue Booth [2] and Christina M. Pollard [3]

[1] Demography and Ageing Unit, Melbourne School of Population and Global Health, University of Melbourne, Melbourne 3010, Australia

[2] College of Medicine and Public Health, Flinders University, Adelaide 5000, Australia; sue.booth@flinders.edu.au

[3] Faculty of Health Sciences, School of Public Health, Curtin University, Perth 6102, Australia; C.Pollard@curtin.edu.au

* Correspondence: Jeromey.Temple@unimelb.edu.au

Abstract: It is widely understood that households with low economic resources and poor labour market attachment are at considerable risk of food insecurity in Australia. However, little is known about variations in food insecurity by receipt of specific classes of social assistance payments that are made through the social security system. Using newly released data from the 2016 Household Expenditure Survey, this paper reports on variations in food insecurity prevalence across a range of payment types. We further investigated measures of financial wellbeing reported by food-insecure households in receipt of social assistance payments. Results showed that individuals in receipt of Newstart allowance (11%), Austudy/Abstudy (14%), the Disability Support Pension (12%), the Carer Payment (11%) and the Parenting Payment (9%) were at significantly higher risk of food insecurity compared to those in receipt of the Age Pension (<1%) or no payment at all (1.3%). Results further indicated that food-insecure households in receipt of social assistance payments endured significant financial stress, with a large proportion co-currently experiencing "fuel" or "energy" poverty. Our results support calls by a range of Australian non-government organisations, politicians, and academics for a comprehensive review of the Australian social security system.

Keywords: food insecurity; access to food; social assistance payments; social security; Newstart allowance

1. Introduction

In Australia, conservative estimates show food insecurity attributable to financial constraints is experienced by 4–5% of the population, with the rate significantly higher among Aboriginal and Torres Strait Islander people [1–3]. Addressing food insecurity in high-income countries such as Australia is important because of the deleterious consequences of exposure for individual health and wellbeing. A substantial and growing evidence base shows food insecurity is associated with symptoms of depression and anxiety, multimorbidity, lower levels of self-reported health status, poor nutrition, a greater likelihood of reporting social isolation, long-standing health problems and activity limitations, and a greater likelihood of reporting heart disease, diabetes, high blood pressure, or peripheral arterial disease [4–13]. Food insecurity experienced within households also has implications for the intergenerational transmission of health issues for children living in food-insecure households [14–16] and may also contribute to ongoing economic inequality [17]. Given these significant outcomes of food insecurity, many high-income countries have extensive social welfare safety nets to alleviate poverty which, in turn, reduces food insecurity at a population level.

However, studies have shown that welfare reforms over recent years have had a severe impact on vulnerable populations and increased the likelihood of food insecurity. For example, in the UK, increased sanctioning of unemployment claimants led to an increase in the rate of adults attending food banks [18]. In the U.S., welfare reforms limiting access to immigrant populations had the impact of significantly increasing levels of food insecurity [19]. In Australia, too, evidence from a recent qualitative study showed changes to welfare eligibility by low-income single parents increased the risk of food insecurity [20].

Australian studies have also shown significantly higher levels of food insecurity among the unemployed relative to other Australians [2,21]. Indeed, numerous Australian studies have underscored the strength of economic factors (e.g., income and labour force status) in explaining exposure to food insecurity. Temple's (2008) nationally representative study of food insecurity in Australia concludes that because of this strong association, policies must target improvements to economic wellbeing through revisiting the appropriateness of extant unemployment benefits and labour market programs [2].

Omitted from existing research on food insecurity and social assistance in Australia is an understanding of how the likelihood of food insecurity differs across the range of social assistance payments provided by the Federal Government. In this paper, newly released data from the 2016 ABS Household Expenditure Survey were used to investigate levels of food insecurity and financial wellbeing reported by recipients of a range of social assistance payments, broadly categorised as the Age Pension, Disability and Carer payments, Family Support payments, and Unemployment and Student allowances.

Background to Social Assistance Payments in Australia

The Australian social security system is intended to increase the wellbeing of the population by redistributing Government revenue collected in the tax system to individuals and families [22]. It is a broader part of a social protection system that includes direct expenditure on services and infrastructure (such as health, education, and community services), the superannuation system—which complements the age pension in Australia's retirement income system—and payments, services, and investment to promote the efficient and effective functioning of the economy, which underpins individual and national wellbeing [22].

Relative to other Organisation for Economic Co-Operation and Development (OECD) member countries, Australia's social security system is unique as (1) most social assistance cash payments are flat-rate entitlements funded by direct Government revenue, and (2) most benefits are heavily income- or asset-tested, with payment reducing as individual private resources increase [23]. This design enables Australia to have a relatively broad social safety net encompassing unemployment benefits and universal health care and assistance for vulnerable populations across the life course [24]. Concerns have been raised, however, about the erosion of the safety net and the particularly low levels of income support provided through social assistance payments, such as the Newstart Allowance—the key payment available for unemployed people of working age [25–27].

Previous Australian studies on food insecurity have focused on particularly vulnerable populations, many with an increased higher likelihood of receipt of some form of social benefit payments—for example, homeless or at-risk youth [28,29], students [30,31], refugees [32,33], Aboriginal and Torres Strait Islander peoples [3,34], older Australians [35,36] and those living in disadvantaged suburbs [37]. Despite this significant evidence base, there is a paucity of studies examining variations in food insecurity across a range of social assistance payments. This is important as variations in the prevalence of food insecurity by payment type may uncover populations at particular risk, which could be addressed through the existing social welfare system.

In this study, we examine food insecurity by receipt of social assistance payments, broadly classified at the household level as the Age Pension, Disability and Carer payments, Family Support payments, Unemployment and Student allowances, and other Government pensions and allowances.

At the individual level, we further analyse food insecurity by a number of specific social assistance payments. Among those discussed in this paper include [38]:

- Austudy: Available to persons aged 25 and over undertaking study or a full-time Australian apprenticeship. Basic rates start from $445 per fortnight for a single person with no dependent children.
- Abstudy: Available to persons of Aboriginal or Torres Strait Islander descent, undertaking an approved course on full-time Australian apprenticeship. Basic rates start from $445.80 per fortnight for a single person with no dependent children.
- Age pension: Available to persons aged 65 or over (if born before July 1952) to 67 and over (if born January 1957 and later). Basic rates start from $834.40 per fortnight for a single person. Subject to income and assets test.
- Carer payment: Available to persons providing constant care to 1 or more persons with a disability as determined by specific assessment tools and as a result of the carer role do not work. Basic rates start from $834.40 per fortnight for a single person. Subject to income and assets test.
- Disability support pension (DSP): Available to persons aged 16 or over, but less than Age Pension age, with a disability as defined by an impairment table, and who are unable to work or undertake training within the next two years. Basic rates start from $572.90 per fortnight for a single person (Independent).
- Newstart allowance: Available to Australian residents who are aged 22 or over (but less than age pension age) and unemployed. Basic rates range from $550 per fortnight for a single person depending on circumstances.
- Parenting payment: Available for parents who have a child under 6 (if partnered), or 8 (if single). Once the child is beyond these ages, the parent must enter into a job plan. Subject to stringent income and assets test. Basic rates of up to a maximum of $768 per fortnight, inclusive of a pension supplement.
- Youth allowance: Available to full-time students and Australian apprentices aged 16–24. Basic rates range from $244 to $768 per fortnight depending on household circumstances.

2. Materials and Methods

2.1. Survey Data

Data for this study were from the Household Expenditure Survey (HES) conducted by the Australian Bureau of Statistics (ABS) over the period July 2015 to June 2016. The purpose of the HES was to "facilitate the analysis and monitoring of the social and economic welfare or Australian residents in private dwellings. The main users are government and other social and economic analysts involved in the development, implementation and evaluation of social and economic policies" [39].

The HES is a repeated cross-section design, with nine surveys conducted since 1974–1975. Since 2003–2004, the HES sample was drawn alongside respondents of the ABS Survey of Income and Housing (SIH). Of the 17,768 households recorded in the SIH, 10,046 were included in the HES. Dwellings were sampled using a stratified, multistage cluster design across a 12-month enumeration period to account for seasonality effects on income and expenditure.

As the HES samples private dwellings, a number of populations are excluded from our analyses. These include persons residing in hotels, boarding schools, and institutions. Also excluded are households containing members of non-Australian Defence forces, diplomatic personnel as well as households in very remote areas of Australia. Apart from houses and flats, the ABS consider persons residing in caravans, garages, tents, and other structures used as residences to be private dwellings.

These data were collected by Australia's official statistical agency, and accordingly, the protection of participants and the provision of data to us is enshrined in legislation. Specifically, data for the Household Expenditure Survey were collected by the ABS under the provisions of the *Census and Statistics Act (CSA) 1905*. Prior to field operations, the survey was submitted to the Australian Privacy

Commissioner and tabled in the Australian Parliament. The confidentiality of these data is guaranteed under the Act and information was provided freely from respondents. Confidentialised data were made available to the authors for this study through the ABS and Universities Australia agreement.

2.2. Measurement

The measures of food insecurity used by the ABS have heretofore been confined to measures of financial attributions of running out of food. For example, two item questions in the National Nutrition Survey and National Health Survey ask: "In the past 12 months were there any time(s) when you ran out of food and couldn't afford to buy any more". Those who reported yes to this question are considered food-insecure. The measure used in the HES is comparable but is likely to identify a more at-risk group of food-insecure persons [3]. Respondents in the 2009/10 HES were asked: "Over the past year, have any of the following happened to (you/your household) because of a shortage of money?" Those reporting 'yes' to 'went without meals' are coded as food-insecure.

The HES also included a number of measures of financial wellbeing, consisting of measures of financial stress, income management, standard of living, and access to emergency funds. These measures provide a complimentary view of the financial position of food-insecure households in receipt of social assistance payments. Respondents were sought to identify whether in the previous 12 months, they had undertaken a number of financial stress behaviours, including seeking help from welfare or community organisations, pawning or selling something, seeking financial help from family or friends, or inability to heat their home or pay utility or other bills on time. As a summary measure of self-assessed financial wellbeing, respondents were further asked: "Thinking of your household's situation over the last 12 months, which of the following statements best describes your financial situation?" A prompt card was then displayed listing: Spend more money than we get, just break even most weeks or able to save money most weeks. Furthermore, respondents were prompted: "Which of these statements best describes your household's standard of living compared to 2 years ago?" A prompt card was then shown listing: Better than 2 years ago, the same as 2 years ago or worse than 2 years ago.

Finally, as a measure of financial resilience to unanticipated events, respondents were asked: "If all of a sudden your household had to get two thousand dollars for something important, could the money be obtained within a week"? Following a response, using a prompt card, respondents were asked to nominate the sources of the emergency funds from a list including: Savings, loan from bank/building society, loan from finance company, loan on credit card, loan from family or friends, loan from welfare or community organisation, sell something or from any other source.

In this descriptive study, we calculated the weighted prevalence of food insecurity by payment type with tests of proportions between groups.

3. Results

Table 1 cross-tabulates source of household income and main source of social assistance payments by food insecurity status. The first panel of Table 1 displays the proportion of each group (food-secure by receipt of benefits and food-insecure by receipt of benefits) by the main source of household income. In the second panel, the broad social assistance payment types are tabulated by food security status.

Approximately 80% of Australian households who report food insecurity received some form of social assistance payment in 2015–2016 (82.4%), with 75% of food-insecure households in receipt of social assistance benefits listing this as the main source of household income (74.8%). Food-insecure households receiving social assistance payments are predominately in receipt of Disability and Carer payments (38%) and Unemployment and Student allowances (28.7%)—Table 1. By contrast, food-secure households in receipt of social assistance payments are more likely to receive the Age Pension (36.6%), with less than 10% being in receipt of Unemployment and Student allowances. Approximately 20% of food-insecure and 24% of food-secure households are in receipt of Family benefits. Of households not in receipt of social assistance payments, almost 90% of both food-insecure and -secure households receive wages from employment. Approximately 2.8% of households reported food insecurity (as measured by going without a meal due to financial constraints).

Table 1. Food insecurity and receipt of social assistance, by main source of income and source of social assistance—households, weighted (%), 2016.

Food-Secure:	Yes		No [1]	
Receipt of Social Assistance Benefits:	**No**	**Yes**	**No**	**Yes**
Main Source of Income [2]				
Employee Income	85.7	43.2	89.4	23.8 ***
Own Business Income	4.8	3.5	6.8	0.4 ***
Government Pensions & Allowances	0.0	41.3	0.0	74.8 ***
Other Income	9.5	12.1	3.8	1.0 ***
Main Source of Social Assistance Payments [3]				
No Social Assistance	100	n.a.	100	n.a.
Age Pension	n.a.	36.6	n.a.	9.4 ***
Disability and Carer Payments	n.a.	12.2	n.a.	38.3 ***
Family Support Payments	n.a.	24.1	n.a.	19.7
Unemployment and Student Allowances	n.a.	9.7	n.a.	28.7 ***
Other Government Pensions/Allowances	n.a.	17.4	n.a.	4.0 ***
Unweighted _n_ [4]	3855	5884	38	263
Weighted % [5]	43.5	53.7	0.5	2.3

[1] Going without meals due to financial constraints in the previous 12 months; [2] Household main source of income in the previous 12 months; [3] Source of social assistance benefits at the household level; n.a. not applicable for households not in receipt of social assistance payments; [4] number of raw observations; [5] percentages weighted using survey weights to account for non-response. *** $p < 0.001$ for test of proportions. Test of proportions conducted between each social assistance benefit groups. That is, assistance benefit recipients (food-secure) compared with assistance benefit recipients (food-insecure) and for non-assistance benefits also (insignificant differences).

As indicators of financial wellbeing, the HES includes a number of measures of financial stress (Appendix Table A1), income management, standard of living (Appendix Table A2), and access to emergency funds (Appendix Table A3). About 60% of food-insecure households in receipt of social assistance payments reported seeking financial help from friends or family and about 43% had sought assistance from a welfare or community organisation (Appendix Table A1). Sixty per cent could not pay utility bills on time, about 35% had pawned or sold something, and 30% reported being unable to heat their home. Less than one per cent of households who are food-secure and not in receipt of social assistance payments were unable to heat their home or had pawned something, and <6% had difficulty paying for utilities. Almost half of food-insecure households receiving social assistance payments reported spending more money than they receive and just over half reported their standard of living as worse than 2 years ago (Appendix Table A2). By contrast, 82% of food-secure households not receiving benefits reported their standard of living as the same or better than two years ago and 60% of this group were able to save money most weeks.

Seventy three percent of food-insecure households in receipt of social assistance payments could not raise $2000 within a week, with very few options from capital markets with respect to raising funds (Appendix Table A3). The key source of emergency funds for this group was reported as loans from family or friends (20%). By contrast, only 6% of food-secure households with no social assistance payments and 16% of those with social assistance payments could not raise emergency funds, with a much broader range of emergency fund sources across capital markets and personal resources.

When these measures of financial stress (Appendix Table A1), income management, and standard of living (Appendix Table A2) and access to emergency funds (Appendix Table A3) are cross-tabulated by social assistance type, households in receipt of Disability and Carer payments as well as Unemployment and Student allowances are shown to be in a financially precarious position. In comparison, among social assistance recipients, households in receipt of the Age Pension appear to have lower levels of financial stress, higher self-assessed standard of living, and an improved access to emergency funds.

The specific social assistance benefit received by individuals who are members of food-insecure households in the HES is shown in Table 2. The higher prevalence of food insecurity reported by those receiving Unemployment, Student, and Disability payments is highlighted in these data. Prevalence was highest among people receiving Austudy/Abstudy (14%), Disability Support Pension (12%), Newstart Allowance (11%) and the Carer payment (11%). Age pension recipients were significantly less likely to report food insecurity (<1%), as were those receiving the DVA Disability pension.

Table 2. Food insecurity prevalence and percentage receiving social assistance payments—persons, weighted (%), 2016.

Social Assistance Benefit Type	Food Insecurity (%) [3]	Food-Insecure in Receipt of Benefit (%) [2]	n [1] =
Austudy/Abstudy	13.8 **	3.9 *	83
Age Pension	<1 ***	4.6 ***	3733
Carer Allowance	5.0 **	4.8 **	470
Carer Payment	10.9 ***	5.8 ***	255
Carer Supplement	5.9 **	6.9 **	565
Disability Pension (DVA)	<1	<1	101
Disability Support Pension	12.4 ***	18.9 ***	803
Family Tax Benefits	5.5 ***	17.3 ***	1284
Newstart Allowance	11.0 ***	14.6 ***	645
Parenting Payment	9.0 ***	5.7 ***	322
Youth Allowance	6.0 *	4.0 *	233
Any Social Assistance Payment?			
Yes	3.9	64.2	8545
No	1.3	35.8	10,660

[1] Unweighted sample size per benefit; [2] percentage of food-insecure persons in receipt of each social assistance payment. Tests of proportions for proportion of food-insecure in receipt of each benefit compared to food-secure in receipt of each benefit; [3] food insecurity prevalence. Tests of proportions for in receipt of each payment compared to those not in receipt; percentages weighted using survey weights to account for non-response; *** $p < 0.001$ ** $p < 0.01$ * $p < 0.05$ denoting significance tests for tests of proportions.

4. Discussion

International evidence shows that individuals in receipt of social assistance payments are at increased risk of food insecurity [40]. To date, there has been scant evidence on the prevalence of food insecurity by social assistance payment type in Australia. Of the information available, a 2013 study of people accessing Anglicare Australia's emergency relief centres in two states reported that 31% of food-insecure households were reliant upon the Newstart allowance and 44% on the disability support pension [41]. Using nationally representative data, this study confirms the significantly higher prevalence of food insecurity among recipients of Australian government social assistance payments—with about 80% of households reporting food insecurity receiving some form of social assistance payment.

Particularly high levels of food insecurity were found among households in receipt of Unemployment, Student, Carer, and Disability payments, suggesting the inadequacy of these transfers. Specifically, when examined at the level of specific payment types, individuals in receipt of Newstart Allowance (11%), Austudy/Abstudy (14%), Disability Support Pension (12%), the Carer Payment (11%), and Parenting Payment (9%) were at significantly higher risk of food insecurity compared to those in receipt of the Age Pension (<1%) or no payment (1.3%).

In 2018, the Australian Prime Minister indicated that his Government prioritises an increase to the Age Pension above any changes to the Newstart Allowance [42]. This is despite research underscoring the deleterious financial position of those in receipt of unemployment and student payments. For example, the Newstart Allowance has long been criticised for not providing a healthy living allowance, and the problem has compounded over time due to the method of indexation [26,27].

The current study findings are consistent with research showing that the standard of living experienced by older Australians has increased considerably over the past decade, with higher levels of income and wealth relative to previous generations of older persons [43–45]. The basic rate for the Age Pension is currently AUD \$834 per fortnight compared with AUD \$550 per fortnight for Newstart Allowance recipients. Further, the Australian Council of Social Services (2018) reported that the poverty gaps (the average depth of poverty for those living below the poverty line) among people aged 65 years and over in income support households were much lower than those across the whole population [45]. The mismatch between indicated government policy for older and younger and working age people and research evidence is concerning.

Apart from Newstart Allowance recipients, the higher levels of food insecurity reported by those in receipt of Disability Support Pension are consistent with recent research on disabilities, health conditions, and food insecurity in Australia and internationally [46,47]. Temple (2018) found that the onset of serious disability (OR 2.3 $p < 0.01$) or mental illness (OR 2.9 $p < 0.001$) more than doubled the odds of experiencing food insecurity in Australia [21]. Although the Disability Support Pension has a higher basic rate of payment than the Newstart Allowance, almost one in five food-insecure respondents in this current study are in receipt of the disability support pension. The findings are consistent with UK research, which shows that households with a disability are almost three times more likely to be foodbank users [48].

This study also identified those on Parenting and Carer payments were at an increased risk of food insecurity. These findings resonate with previous Australian research that found single parents were more likely to experience food insecurity due to factors such as income and housing instability [49,50]. Australia shifted its welfare policy context to 'Welfare to Work' in 2006, founded on the principle of mutual obligation where recipients must complete compulsory activities in order to access income support. Those receiving parenting benefits were transitioned to the lower-rate Newstart Allowance [50,51]. Single mothers relying on the Newstart Allowance experienced a struggle to buy basics such as food, reliance on foodbanks, and keeping children home from school as they were unable to provide food which met the school lunchbox policy [50]. The higher prevalence of food insecurity among persons in receipt of the Carer payment is consistent with recent evidence showing financial support is the greatest unmet need reported by Australian carers [52].

Our findings pointing to the higher prevalence of food insecurity on these payments is concerning given recent research on intergenerational transfer of disadvantage. Cobb-Clark (2017) has shown that households in receipt of Disability, Carer, and Parenting payments are at a strong risk of intergenerational persistence of disadvantage [53]. Of major concern is that children living in households dependent on these specific payments are more likely themselves to receive more intensive social assistance payments in their early adulthood and more likely to experience unemployment.

Finally, our findings underscore the deleterious financial position experienced by food-insecure households and those on specific social assistance payments in Australia. The high levels of 'fuel or energy poverty' faced by food-insecure Australians is of particular concern. About 30% of food-insecure households in receipt of social assistance payments reported being unable to heat their home, and 60% were unable to pay their utility bills on time.

UK and U.S. research has also drawn attention to the relationship between food insecurity and fuel or energy poverty. Anderson et al. (2012) described the experience of 'cold' homes in the UK where households faced with financial difficulty cut the range and quality of food while simultaneously cutting energy consumption [54]. Large reductions in food expenditure have been reported in low-income households during colder than expected winter conditions [55]. Poor families living in the US reduced their food expenditure commensurate to increases in fuel expenditures when cold-weather shocks occurred, suggesting that existing social programs were ineffectual in buffering against these shocks [56]. Canadian evidence shows energy price shocks at the turn of the century led to an increase in the population at risk of food insecurity [57].

Australia has experienced significant energy price inflation following the deregulation of energy markets [58]. The high levels of concurrent energy poverty facing the food-insecure can lead to further financial burden, for example, the cost of reconnection or default payments [59]. Australian households that were disconnected or at risk of disconnection experienced very difficult financial circumstances, in which they often struggled to afford necessities such as food and housing [59]. In a recent article, Nelson et al. (2019) suggested, among other solutions, increasing income support for particular groups (including those on Newstart) as well as the reform of state-based energy concessions to combat energy poverty [60].

These solutions, by reducing energy costs and increasing income support, would undoubtedly reduce the likelihood of vulnerable populations experiencing food insecurity. International evidence suggests that increases to social assistance payments reduce the prevalence and severity of food insecurity at a population level. For example, in Newfoundland and Labrador in Canada, the prevalence of food insecurity reduced dramatically from 2007–2011 due to welfare reforms [61]. Another Canadian study found that a one-off increase in social assistance benefits led to a significant decline in moderate and severe food insecurity among households on social assistance [62].

Study Limitations

In interpreting results from this study, it is important to recognise the limitations. Firstly, the measure of food insecurity in Australia comprising of measures of 'going without meals due to financial constraints' captures neither temporality nor severity [2]. However, currently, these are the only population-based measures available. Our study, however, does raise the question of the use of household expenditure data to improve measurement and understanding of food insecurity. Future research on this issue is currently underway by the authors.

The measurement issue is also important given the differences in food insecurity prevalence experienced by those of working age or younger populations compared to older persons in receipt of the age pension. Previous studies have note that food insecurity attributable to financial constraints tends to decrease in older age in Australia [2,35]. Part of this may reflect a measurement issue. Herein, we focus only on financially attributable food insecurity, but international studies show that storage, transportation, and functional barriers are all important in explaining food insecurity in older populations [63]. Thus, we are likely to be biasing downward the prevalence of food insecurity among older Australians. Moreover, the prevalence of food insecurity may be higher for age pension recipients who rent rather than own their home. Secondly, there is the role of selective mortality in these cross-sectional data. As individuals with higher economic and social resources are more likely to exhibit higher survival prospects relative to their financially disadvantaged peers, in cross-sectional data we may be observing these individuals in later life.

More generally, the HES data are cross-sectional, and it is not possible to draw any type of causal relationship between receipt of certain payments and food insecurity. Specifically, we do not know if prior to receipt of certain payments, they were food-insecure, or only insecure once on payments. However, recent evidence shows that experience of involuntary job loss (OR 2.6 $p < 0.001$) or difficulty finding employment (OR 2.5 $p < 0.001$) within the past 12 months increases the odds of food insecurity by about 2.5 times [21]. The purpose of this paper has been to present prevalence rates of food insecurity across a range of social benefit payment types. Further multivariable analyses, ideally with longitudinal data, should be conducted to provide further detail on the experiences of food insecurity faced by social assistance payment recipients in Australia.

5. Conclusions

This is the first Australian study to examine the differences in the prevalence of food insecurity across a wide range of social assistance payments. We found a high prevalence of food insecurity among those receiving Australian Government social assistance payments, including the Newstart Allowance, Austudy/Abstudy, Disability Support Pension, the Carer payment, and Parenting payment. The relatively higher levels of income support through the Age Pension payment may have had a protective effect on food insecurity and financial wellbeing, demonstrating the benefits of addressing income inadequacy that has been found in the international literature. Due to differences in indexing the respective payments, the level of the Newstart Allowance as a percentage of the age pension has fallen from 90% in the 1990s to 60% today [64].

Australian advocates for action to reduce poverty and inequality have called for the Government to 'raise the rate' of Newstart and related payments, noting that Newstart has not increased in real terms for 24 years [65]. Recent Australian modelling indicates that an increase in the Newstart Allowance to $800 per fortnight in Australia would significantly decrease the poverty gap in Australia by about 11% [66]. Our results support calls by a range of Australian non-government organisations, politicians, and academics calling for a comprehensive review of the Australian social security system [67]. Our findings, when combined with others in the Australian literature, suggest well designed increases in the Newstart, Disability, Student, Carer, and disability payments may improve the material resources of food-insecure households and thus ameliorate their food insecurity experience and potentially offset health and economic risks [4–17].

Author Contributions: Conceptualization, J.B.T., C.M.P., and S.B.; Formal Analysis, J.B.T.; Writing—Original Draft Preparation, J.B.T., S.B., and C.M.P.

Acknowledgments: Data for this study were provided to the authors by the Australian Bureau of Statistics (ABS) through the ABS Universities Australia agreement.

Appendix A

Table A1. Indicators of Financial Stress (%) by Food Insecurity Status and Receipt of Social Assistance, Households 2015/2016.

Receives Social Assistance Benefits:	Food Insecure				Main Source of Household Social Assistance Benefits in Cash					
	No		Yes		None	Age Pension	Disability and Carer Payments	Family Support Payments	Unemployment and Student Allowances	Other Pensions and Allowances
	No	Yes	No	Yes						
Sought assistance from welfare/community organisation	<1	2.7	1.1	42.7	<1	1.6	10.4	5.4	9.6	<1
Pawned or sold something	<1	2.3	12.9	34.7	1.1	<1	7.8	5.2	8.8	1
Sought financial help from friends or family	3.9	6.9	57.6	59.7	4.5	2.5	14.2	14	21.5	4.2
Unable to heat home	<1	2.1	22.8	30.4	1	1.9	6.9	2.6	8.3	1.1
Could not pay gas/electricity/telephone	5.6	10.5	55.9	59.3	6.1	4	19.6	22	20.9	6.1
Could not pay registration / insurance on time	2.3	3.8	35.2	31.6	2.7	1	6.7	8.6	12.1	2.3
Unweighted (n)	3855	5884	38	263	3894	2680	836	1177	528	926
Weighted (%)	43.5	53.7	0.5	2.3	44.0	19.9	7.4	13.4	5.9	9.5

Table A2. Management of Household Income and Standard of Living (%) by Food Insecurity Status and Receipt of Social Assistance, Households 2015/2016.

Receives Social Assistance Benefits:	Food Insecure				Main Source of Household Social Assistance Benefits in Cash					
	No		Yes		None	Age Pension	Disability and Carer Payments	Family Support Payments	Unemployment and Student Allowances	Other Pensions and Allowances
	No	Yes	No	Yes						
Management of Household Income										
Spend more money than we get	10	13.6	22	46.1	10.1	8.9	21	19.8	20.9	12.3
Just break even most weeks	33.2	49.6	60.2	48.8	33.5	49.5	50.1	52.3	55.1	41.1
Able to save money most weeks	56.8	36.8	17.8	5.1	56.4	14.6	28.9	27.4	24	46.6
Present Standard of Living										
Better than 2 years ago	41	22.3	15.2	22.9	40.7	13.1	22.9	31.6	27.9	25.1
The same as 2 years ago	40.9	50.6	32.5	24.9	40.8	62.6	43.6	39.3	30.6	50.6
Worse than 2 years ago	18.1	27.1	52.4	52.1	18.5	23.4	33.5	29.1	41.5	24.4
Unweighted (n)	3855	5884	38	263	3894	2680	836	1177	528	926
Weighted (%)	43.5	53.7	0.5	2.3	44.0	19.9	7.4	13.4	5.9	9.5

Table A3. Access to Emergency Funds (%) by Food Insecurity and Receipt of Social Assistance, Households 2015/2016.

Receives Social Assistance Benefits:	Food Insecure				Main Source of Household Social Assistance Benefits in Cash					
	No		Yes		None	Age Pension	Disability and Carer Payments	Family Support Payments	Unemployment and Student Allowances	Other Pensions and Allowances
	No	Yes	No	Yes						
Access to Emergency Funds										
Could not raise $2000 within a week	6.3	16.1	32.5	73.2	6.6	11.3	34.7	21.5	33.9	6.7
Source(s) of Emergency Funds										
Own Savings	77.9	65.1	19	10.4	77.3	74.5	45.4	51.9	41.9	78.6
Loan from a Bank, Building Society	14.3	9.9	8.9	<1	14.3	5.8	9.3	13.3	9	12.4
Loan from a Finance Company	4.3	1.8	0	1.1	4.2	<1	2.6	2.3	1.2	3.3
Loan on Credit Card	19.5	11.8	25.1	2.2	19.6	8.1	9.5	15.9	11.2	13.4
Loan from Family or Friends	19.4	15.9	26.7	19.7	19.5	8.5	15.3	25.3	20.5	16.6
Loan from Welfare or Community Organisation	<1	<1	<1	<1	<1	<1	2.4	1	<1	<1
Sell Something	9.1	4.9	6.7	4.3	9.1	1.7	3.8	7.8	7.1	6.7
Other Sources	2.4	2.8	3.1	<1	2.5	2.7	1.9	2.3	3.9	3.1
Unweighted (n)	3855	5884	38	263	3894	2680	836	1177	528	926
Weighted (%)	43.5	53.7	0.5	2.3	44.0	19.9	7.4	13.4	5.9	9.5

References

1. Australian Bureau of Statistics. *Australian Health Survey: Nutrition—State and Territory Results, 2011–2012 (Catalogue Number 4364.0.55.009)*; Australian Bureau of Statistics: Canberra, Australia, 2015.
2. Temple, J.B. Severe and moderate forms of food insecurity in Australia: Are they distinguishable? *Aust. J. Soc. Issues* **2008**, *43*, 649–668. [CrossRef]
3. Temple, J.B.; Russell, J. Food insecurity among older Aboriginal and Torres Strait Islanders. *Int. J. Environ. Res. Public Health* **2018**, *15*, 1766. [CrossRef]
4. Kendall, A.; Olson, C.; Frongillo, E. Relationship of hunger and food insecurity to food availability and consumption. *J. Am. Diet. Assoc.* **1996**, *96*, 1019–1024. [CrossRef]
5. Rose, D.; Oliveria, D. Nutrient intakes of individuals from food insufficient households in the United States. *Am. J. Public Health* **1997**, *87*, 1956–1961. [CrossRef] [PubMed]
6. Heflin, C.; Siefert, K.; Williams, D. Food insufficiency and women's mental health: Findings from a 3 year panel of welfare recipients. *Soc. Sci. Med.* **2005**, *61*, 1971–1982. [CrossRef] [PubMed]
7. Sharkey, J. Risk and presence of food insufficiency are associated with low nutrient intakes and multimorbidity among housebound older women who receive home-delivered meals. *J. Nutr.* **2003**, *133*, 3485–3491. [CrossRef]
8. Stuff, J.; Casey, P.; Szeto, K.; Gossett, G.; Robbins, J.; Simpson, P.; Connell, C.; Bogle, M. Household food insecurity is associated with adult health status. *J. Nutr.* **2004**, *134*, 2330–2335. [CrossRef]
9. Tarasuk, V. Household food insecurity with hunger is associated with women's food intakes, health and household circumstances. *J. Nutr.* **2001**, *131*, 2670–2676. [CrossRef]
10. Vozoris, N.; Tarasuk, V. Household food insufficiency is associated with poorer health. *J. Nutr.* **2003**, *133*, 120–126. [CrossRef]
11. Laraia, B.; Siega-Riz, A.; Gundersen, C.; Dole, N. Psychosocial factors and socioeconomic indicators are associated with household food insecurity among pregnant women. *J. Nutr.* **2006**, *136*, 177–182. [CrossRef]
12. German, L.; Kahana, C.; Rosenfeld, V.; Zabrowsky, I.; Wiezer, Z.; Fraser, D.; Shahar, D. Depressive symptoms are associated with food insufficiency and nutritional deficiencies in poor community-dwelling elderly people. *J. Nutr. Health Aging* **2011**, *15*, 3–8. [CrossRef] [PubMed]
13. Redmond, M.; Dong, F.; Goetz, J.; Jacobson, L.; Collins, T. Food insecurity and peripheral arterial disease in older adult populations. *J. Nutr. Health Aging* **2016**, *20*, 989–995. [CrossRef] [PubMed]
14. Cook, J.; Frank, D.; Berkowitz, C.; Black, M.; Casey, P.; Cutts, D.; Meyers, A.; Zaldivar, N.; Skalicky, A.; Levenson, S.; et al. Food insecurity is associated with adverse health outcomes among human infants and toddlers. *J. Nutr.* **2004**, *134*, 1432–1438. [CrossRef] [PubMed]
15. Jyoti, D.; Frongillo, E.; Jones, S. Food insecurity affects children's academic performance, weight gain, and social skills. *J. Nutr.* **2005**, *135*, 2831–2839. [CrossRef] [PubMed]
16. Alaimo, K.; Olson, C.; Frongillo, E. Family food insufficiency, but not low family income, is positively associated with dysthymia and suicide symptoms in Adolescents. *J. Nutr.* **2002**, *132*, 719–725. [CrossRef] [PubMed]
17. Hamelin, A.; Habicht, J.; Beaudry, M. Food insecurity: Consequences for the household and broader social implications. *J. Nutr.* **1999**, *129*, 525s–528s. [CrossRef] [PubMed]
18. Loopstra, R.; Fledderjohann, J.; Reeves, A.; Stuckler, D. Impact of welfare benefit sanctioning on food insecurity: A dynamic cross-area study of food bank usage in the UK. *J. Social Policy* **2018**, *47*, 437–457. [CrossRef]
19. Borjas, G.J. Food insecurity and public assistance. *J. Public Econ.* **2004**, *88*, 1421–1443. [CrossRef]
20. McKenzie, H.J.; McKay, F.H. Food as a discretionary item: The impact of welfare payment changes on low-income single mother's food choices and strategies. *J. Poverty Soc. Just.* **2017**, *25*, 35–48. [CrossRef]
21. Temple, J.B. The association between stressful events and food insecurity: Cross-sectional evidence from Australia. *Int. J. Environ. Res. Public Health* **2018**, *15*, 2333. [CrossRef]
22. Harmer, J. *Pension Review Report*; Department of Families, Housing, Community Services and Indigenous Affairs: Canberra, Austria, 2009.
23. Davidson, P.; Whiteford, P. *An Overview of Australia's System of Income and Employment Assistance for the Unemployed*; OECD Social, Employment and Migration Working Papers, No. 129; OECD: Paris, France, 2012.

24. Pollard, C.; Begley, A.; Landrigan, T. The Rise of Food Inequality in Australia. In *Food Poverty and Insecurity: International Food Inequalities*; Caraher, M., Coveney, J., Eds.; Springer: Cham, Switzerland, 2016.

25. Friel, S. A fair go for health? Not at the moment. *Aust. N. Z. J. Public Health* **2014**, *38*, 302–303. [CrossRef] [PubMed]

26. Saunders, P.; Bedford, M. New minimum healthy living budget standards for low-paid and unemployed Australians. *Econ. Labour Rel. Rev.* **2018**. [CrossRef]

27. Saunders, P. Using a budget standards approach to assess the adequacy of Newstart allowance. *Aust. J. Soc. Issues* **2018**, *53*, 4–17. [CrossRef]

28. Crawford, B.; Yamazaki, R.; Franke, E.; Amanatidis, S.; Ravulo, J.; Steinbeck, K.; Ritchie, J.; Torvaldsen, S. Sustaining dignity? Food insecurity in homeless young people in urban Australia. *Health Prom. J. Aust.* **2014**, *25*, 71–78. [CrossRef] [PubMed]

29. Booth, S. Eating rough: Food sources and acquisition practices of homeless young people in Adelaide, South Australia. *Public Health Nutr.* **2006**, *9*, 212–218. [CrossRef] [PubMed]

30. Hughes, R.; Serebryanikova, I.; Donaldson, K.; Leveritt, M. Student food insecurity: The skeleton in the university closet. *Nutr. Diet* **2011**, *68*, 27–32. [CrossRef]

31. Micevski, D.A.; Thornton, L.E.; Brockington, S. Food insecurity among university students in Victoria: A pilot study. *Nutr. Diet* **2014**, *71*, 258–264. [CrossRef]

32. Gallegos, D.; Ellies, P.; Wright, J. Still there's no food! Food insecurity in a refugee population in Perth, Western Australia. *Nutr. Diet.* **2008**, *65*, 78–83. [CrossRef]

33. McKay, F.H.; Dunn, M. Food security among asylum seekers in Melbourne. Australian and New Zealand. *J. Public Health* **2015**, *39*, 344–349. [CrossRef]

34. McCarthy, L.; Chang, A.; Brimblecombe, J. Food insecurity experiences of Aboriginal and Torres Strait Islander Families with young children in an urban setting: Influencing factors and coping strategies. *Int. J. Environ. Res. Public Health* **2018**, *15*, 2649. [CrossRef]

35. Temple, J.B. Food insecurity among older Australians: Prevalence, correlates and well-being. *Aust. J. Ageing* **2006**, *25*, 158–163. [CrossRef]

36. Russell, J.; Flood, V.; Yeatman, H.; Mitchell, P. Prevalence and risk factors of food insecurity among a cohort of older Australians. *J. Nutr. Health Aging* **2014**, *18*, 3–8. [CrossRef] [PubMed]

37. Nolan, M.; Rikard-Bell, G.; Mohsin, M.; Williams, M. Food insecurity in three socially disadvantaged localities in Sydney, Australia. *Health Prom. J. Aust.* **2006**, *17*, 247–253. [CrossRef]

38. DHS. *A Guide to Australian Government Payments*; Department of Human Services: Canberra, Australia, 2018. Available online: https://www.humanservices.gov.au/organisations/about-us/publications-and-resources/guide-australian-government-payments (accessed on 1 November 2018).

39. ABS. *Household Expenditure Survey and Survey of Income and Housing, User Guide, Australia, 2015–2016*; Catalogue Number 6503.0; Australian Bureau of Statistics: Canberra, Australia, 2017.

40. Tarasuk, V.; Mitchell, A.; Dachner, N. *Household Food Insecurity in Canada*; PROOF: Toronto, ON, Canada, 2014; Available online: https://proof.utoronto.ca/ (accessed on 1 November 2018).

41. King, S.; Bellamy, J.; Kemp, B.; Mollenhauer, J. Hard Choices—Going without in a Time of Plenty. A Study of Food Insecurity in NSW and the ACT. 2013. Available online: https://www.anglicare.org.au/media/2850/anglicaresydney_hardchoicesfoodinsecurity_2013.pdf (accessed on 1 December 2018).

42. Banger, M.; McCulloch, D. Increase Pension before Newstart: Morrison. Australian Associated Press. 2 November 2018. Available online: https://www.news.com.au/national/breaking-news/morrison-ridicules-raising-newstart-rate/news-story/04df1d4237f9e609435362de5153c15b (accessed on 1 November 2018).

43. Temple, J.B.; Rice, J.M.; McDonald, P.F. Mature age labour force participation and the life cycle deficit in Australia: 1981–82 to 2009–10. *J. Econ. Ageing* **2017**, *10*, 21–33. [CrossRef]

44. Temple, J.B.; McDonald, P.F.; Rice, J.M. Net assets available at age of death in Australia: An extension of the National Transfer Accounts methodology. *Popul. Rev.* **2017**, *56*. [CrossRef]

45. Davidson, P.; Saunders, P.; Bradbury, B.; Wong, M. *Poverty in Australia*; ACOSS/UNSW Poverty and Inequality Partnership Report No. 2; ACOSS: Sydney, Australia, 2018.

46. Gorton, D.; Bullen, C.R.; Mhurchu, C.N. Environmental influences on food security in high-income countries. *Nutr Rev.* **2010**, *68*, 1–29. [CrossRef] [PubMed]

47. Huang, J.; Guo, B.; Kim, Y. Food insecurity and disability: Do economic resources matter? *Soc. Sci. Res.* **2010**, *39*, 111–124. [CrossRef]

48. Loopstra, R.; Lalor, D. *Financial Insecurity, Food Insecurity, and Disability: The Profile of People Receiving Emergency Food Assistance from The Trussell Trust Foodbank Network in Britain*; The Trussell Trust, University of Oxford, King's College London: London, UK, 2017.

49. Stevens, C.A. Exploring food insecurity among young mothers (15–24 years). *J. Spec. Pediatric Nurs.* **2010**, *15*, 163–171. [CrossRef]

50. Good Shepherd Australia New Zealand. Outside Systems Control My Life: Single Mothers' Stories of Welfare and Work. 2018. Available online: https://goodshep.org.au/media/2188/outside-systems-control-my-life_single-mothers-stories-of-welfare-to-work.pdf (accessed on 1 December 2018).

51. Brady, M. Targeting single mothers? Dynamics of contracting Australian employment services and activation policies at the street level. *J. Soc. Policy* **2018**, *47*, 827–845. [CrossRef]

52. Temple, J.B.; Dow, B. The unmet support needs of carers of older Australians: Prevalence and mental health. *Int. Psychoger.* **2018**. [CrossRef]

53. Cobb-Clark, D.; Dahman, S.; Salamanca, N.; Zhu, A. *Intergenerational Disadvantage: Learning about Equal Opportunity from Social Assistance Receipt*; IZA Discussion Paper No. 11070; IZA Institute of Labour Econmics: Bonn, Germany, 2017.

54. Anderson, W.; White, V.; Finney, A. Coping with low incomes and cold homes. *Energy Policy* **2012**, *49*, 40–52. [CrossRef]

55. Beatty, T.; Blow, L.; Crossley, T. Is there a 'heat-or-eat' trade-off in the UK? *J. R. Stat. Soc. A* **2014**, *177*, 281–294. [CrossRef]

56. Bhattacharya, J.; DeLeire, T.; Haider, S.; Currie, J. Heat or eat? Cold-weather shocks and nutrition in Poor American Families. *Am. J. Public Health* **2003**, *93*, 1149. [CrossRef] [PubMed]

57. Emery, J.; Bartoo, A.; Matheson, J.; Ferrer, A.; Kirkpatrick, S.; Tarasuk, V.; McIntyre, L. Evidence of the association between household food insecurity and heating cost inflation in Canada 1998–2001. *Can. Public Policy* **2012**, *38*, 181–215. [CrossRef]

58. Valadkhani, A.; Nguyen, J.; Smyth, R. Consumer electricity and gas prices across Australian capital cities: Structural breaks, effects of policy reforms and interstate differences. *Energy Econ.* **2018**, *72*, 365–375. [CrossRef]

59. Urbis. South Australian Disconnection Project: Final Report. 2014. Available online: https://www.sacoss.org.au/sites/default/files/public/140828_South%20Australian%20Disconnection%20Project.pdf (accessed on 1 December 2018).

60. Nelson, T.; McCracken-Hewson, E.; Sundstrom, G.; Hawthorne, M. The drivers of energy-related financial hardship in Australia–understanding the role of income, consumption and housing. *Energy Policy* **2019**, *124*, 262–271. [CrossRef]

61. Loopstra, R.; Dachner, N.; Tarasuk, V. An exploration of the unprecedented decline in the prevalence of household food insecurity in Newfoundland and Labrador, 2007–2012. *Can. Public Policy* **2015**, *41*, 191–206. [CrossRef]

62. Li, N.; Dachner, N.; Tarasuk, V. The impact of changes in social policies on household food insecurity in British Columbia, 2005–2012. *Prev. Med.* **2016**, *93*, 151–158. [CrossRef]

63. Wolfe, W.; Frongillo, E.; Valois, P. Understanding the experience of food insecurity by elders suggests ways to improve its measurement. *J. Nutr.* **2003**, *133*, 2762. [CrossRef]

64. Phillips, B.; Gray, M.; Webster, R. Cut the Pension, Boost Newstart. What Our Algorithm Says I the Best Way to Get Value for Our Welfare Dollars. *The Conversation.* 2018. Available online: https://theconversation.com/cut-the-pension-boost-newstart-what-our-algorithm-says-is-the-best-way-to-get-value-for-our-welfare-dollars-108417 (accessed on 10 December 2018).

65. ACOSS. Raise the Rate. 2018. Available online: https://www.acoss.org.au/raisetherate/ (accessed on 10 December 2018).

66. Phillips, B.; Webster, R.; Gray, M. Optimal Policy Modelling: A Microsimulation Methodology for Setting the Australian Tax and Transfer System. CSRM Working Paper N. 10/2018, Centre for Social Research and Methods; The Australian National University. 2018. Available online: http://csrm.cass.anu.edu.au/sites/default/files/docs/2018/12/Optimal-policy-modelling-setting-Australian-tax-and-transfer-system-10-2018-CSRM-working-paper_0.pdf (accessed on 10 December 2018).

67. Whiteford, P.; Phillips, B.; Bradbury, B. It's Not Just Newstart. Single Parents Are \$271 per Fortnight Worse off. *Labor Needs an Overarching Welfare Review.* *The Conversation.* 2018. Available online: https://theconversation.com/its-not-just-newstart-single-parents-are-271-per-fortnight-worse-off-labor-needs-an-overarching-welfare-review-107521 (accessed on 10 December 2018).

11

Food Reference Budgets as a Potential Policy Tool to Address Food Insecurity

Elena Carrillo-Álvarez [1],*[ID], Tess Penne [2], Hilde Boeckx [3], Bérénice Storms [4] and Tim Goedemé [5]

[1] Blanquerna School of Health Sciences—Universitat Ramon Llull-Global Research on Wellbeing—GRoW Research group, Padilla, 08025 Barcelona, Spain
[2] Research Foundation—Flanders, Herman Deleeck Centre for Social Policy—University of Antwerp, 2000 Antwerp, Belgium; tess.penne@uantwerpen.be
[3] Thomas More Kempen, 2440 Malle, Belgium; hilde.boeckx@thomasmore.be
[4] Herman Deleeck Centre for Social Policy—University of Antwerp, 2000 Antwerp, Belgium; bereniceML.storms@uantwerpen.be
[5] Institute for New Economic Thinking at the Oxford Martin School and Department of Social Policy and Intervention, University of Oxford, Oxford OX2 6ED, UK; tim.goedeme@uantwerp.be
* Correspondence: elenaca@blanquerna.url.edu

Abstract: The aim of this article is to present the development of cross-country comparable food reference budgets in 26 European countries, and to discuss their usefulness as an addition to food-based dietary guidelines (FBDG) for tackling food insecurity in low-income groups. Reference budgets are illustrative priced baskets containing the minimum goods and services necessary for well-described types of families to have an adequate social participation. This study was conducted starting from national FBDG, which were translated into monthly food baskets. Next, these baskets were validated in terms of their acceptability and feasibility through focus group discussions, and finally they were priced. Along the paper, we show how that food reference budgets hold interesting contributions to the promotion of healthy eating and prevention of food insecurity in low-income contexts in at least four ways: (1) they show how a healthy diet can be achieved with limited economic resources, (2) they bring closer to the citizen a detailed example of how to put FBDG recommendations into practice, (3) they ensure that food security is achieved in an integral way, by comprising the biological but also psychological and social functions of food, and (4) providing routes for further (comparative) research into food insecurity.

Keywords: reference budgets; food insecurity; cost of a healthy diet; Food-based dietary guidelines

1. Introduction

In a moment in which 18.8% of the global burden of disease has been attributed to unhealthy eating [1], and in the context of growing inequalities in many countries [2–6], policy-makers face the challenge of developing strategies that are sufficiently powerful to revert long-standing patterns of unhealthy eating.

While ecologic approaches and upstream actions have been argued to be indispensable to effectively tackle the situation, actions addressed to the individual are still timely [7–9]. Food-Based Dietary Guidelines (FBDG) constitute the closest set of nutritional standards for the population and are primarily intended for consumer information and education. Starting from the available evidence on the most relevant diet-disease relationships for the targeted population, FBDG are science-based policy recommendations in the form of guidelines that describe dietary patterns that can facilitate the adherence to eating habits that maintain and promote health [10,11].

Since there exists a strong link between diet and the most prevalent diseases in developed societies, the development and implementation of FBDG has the potential to substantially influence the burden of disease within its citizenship, to the extent that the quality of such tools may accentuate or blur diet-related health inequalities between and within countries [10,12–14]. As the EFSA explains in its 'Scientific Opinion on establishing Food-Based Dietary Guidelines' [10], the development of pan-European detailed and effective FBDG is not possible due to wide cross-country variations in nutritional priorities, which are the result of differences in terms of nutrient intake [15], eating habits and traditions [16] and diet-related health situation [14].

In 1996, the FAO and WHO published a set of recommendations on the development of FBDG that remains a point of reference for policy makers on the field [11]. In Europe, additionally, this work was taken further by the EURODIET project, which proposed an updated framework for the development of FBDG in the European Union [17]. Their main recommendations can be summarized in five points: (1) FBDG must start from recognized public health problems; (2) FBDG are prepared for a particular socio-economic context and must reflect the particularities of the territory with regard to food availability and consumption patterns; (3) FBDG should be updated systematically, ideally every 5 years, to adapt to the evolution of consumption patterns and food availability; (4) FBDG must reflect patterns of consumption, rather than numerical goals in terms of nutrients; and (5) they must be relatively consistent with prevailing patterns of consumption (otherwise they will hardly be accepted). A sixth point was added by Roth and Knai in a report issued in 2003 by the WHO Regional Office for Europe, concerning the need for government endorsement of FBDG to further articulate health policies coherent with dietary recommendations [13]. At that moment, only 25 of the 48 countries participating in the study reported having national, government-endorsed food-based dietary guidelines.

Fifteen years later, we conducted a similar research to the EURODIET project, in which the FBDG available in 26 EU Member States were analysed in the light of the previously mentioned guidelines (Carrillo et al., submitted for publication). Our findings were consistent with the conclusions of previous studies [18–20], indicating little advancement on the topic in the last two decades. Among the different findings, we highlight the fact that none of the FBDG includes any specific recommendation for low-income groups, for which regular FBDG have been described as insufficient, as they do not address one of the main factors conditioning food decisions in this population: the cost of a diet [21,22].

In this paper, we present food reference budgets (RBs) for 26 EU Member States, as a tool that can complement regular FBDG to better orientate the dietary intake of low-income groups. RBs are defined as illustrative priced baskets of goods and services that represent the minimum necessary resources for well-described types of families that allow for an adequate diet. In this context, not only the biological function of food is taken into account, but also the social, hedonistic and gastronomic role that food has in current societies [23]. While food reference budgets have been published for individual countries [24,25], to the best of our knowledge, this is the first attempt to document and illustrate in a comparative perspective the cost of a healthy diet in the European Union.

The aim of this article is to discuss the development of cross-country comparable food reference budgets in 26 European countries, as well as their added-value for FBDG for tackling food insecurity in low-income groups.

2. Materials and Methods

The research that we describe here is part of the pilot project for the development of a common methodology on Reference Budgets in Europe. The pilot project was funded by the European Commission's DG Employment, Social Affairs and Inclusion to develop a common methodology to construct high-quality comparable reference budgets in all EU Member States [26] (participating countries: AT, Austria; BE, Belgium; BG, Bulgaria; CY, Cyprus; CZ, Czech Republic; DE, Germany; DK, Denmark; EE, Estonia; EL, Greece; ES, Spain; FI, Finland; FR, France; HR, Croatia; HU, Hungary; IT, Italy; LT, Lithuania; LU, Luxembourg, LV, Latvia; MT, Malta; NL, Netherlands; PL, Poland; PT, Portugal; RO, Romania; SE, Sweden; SK, Slovakia; SI, Slovenia). For the purpose of this project, a common method was developed, along with food baskets for 26 EU Member States that illustrate what families need to access a diet that allows for adequate social participation. Being able to participate adequately means that people would have the essentials to play their various social roles in a particular society [26]. This is why, in the concrete context of food, we started from a broader perspective on the functions of food, beyond the necessities of a healthy diet, strictly speaking. The research was carried out by 26 country teams and coordinated by the Herman Deleeck Centre for Social Policy at the University of Antwerp together with three domain coordinators. The geographical coverage is the European Union, except for Ireland and the United Kingdom. Each country team collaborated with a nutritionist and started from the existing national FBDG. The choice to start from FBDG rather than, for instance, common nutritional guidelines from the WHO, was motivated by the fact that FBDG represent the country-specific recommendations on what people need to eat to achieve and/or maintain a good health, while at the same time respecting the cross-national differences in food habits and health priorities. The underlying assumption is that the overall objective of FBDG is the same across countries: facilitating a healthy diet, based on relevant insights from the scientific literature, while respecting local conditions. Finally, each country team organised three focus group discussions in order to test the completeness and acceptability of the food baskets. The items in the food basket were priced in accessible and affordable shops in the capital city.

For the construction of the food baskets we focused primarily on the required budget that should enable people to consume a healthy diet. Although we also considered the other functions of food (e.g., psychological and social) and the necessities for a minimum level physical activity, as recommended in many FBDG, in this paper we report only on the part related to having access to a healthy diet. The main reason is that the nature of collecting robust budgets for the other functions of food and physical activity required more time and resources than were available in our project. As a result, the budgets for the other functions of food and physical activity are not sufficiently robust and comparable. Obviously, in order to be able to afford a healthy diet, one should also have access to kitchen equipment, clean water, and energy to cook. However, due to the specific requirements to estimate their cost, also these are not considered here (see [26] for a discussion of kitchen equipment and energy costs).

Given the large variation in needs between individuals and households, and our objective to construct cross-country comparable baskets that represent what is needed at the minimum, in all countries the food baskets were developed for household types with the same specific characteristics:

(1)   a single man [35–45-years-old]
(2)   a single woman [35–45-years-old]
(3)   a couple [man, woman; 35–45-years-old]
(4)   a single woman [35–45-years-old] + 2 children [primary school boy, 10-years-old + secondary school girl, 14-years-old].
(5)   a couple [35–45-years-old] + 2 children [primary school boy, 10-years-old + secondary school girl, 14-years-old].

Furthermore, for assessing and pricing the concrete lists of items, the following assumptions were made:

-    The household types are assumed to live in the capital city of each participant country. This point is particularly relevant in terms of the pricing of the items and the frequency in which people rely on the production of food for own consumption.
-    All meals are prepared and eaten at home. All food is acquired, prepared and consumed in the most economical way possible. This means families are well-informed about prices and are able to shop in the most economic retailers that are accessible with public transport. However, we do not assume that people can always buy all their ingredients in the cheapest available supermarket. Hence, we allowed for a certain freedom of choice to shop within a range of cheap retailers.

- All household members are in good health and do not have specific dietary requirements. The reason for this assumption is not so much that this is the most common health condition, but rather that the cost of a diet varies depending on the kind and severity of health problems, each having different implications for the needs of the person affected.
- The ingredients should give families access to healthy, tasty and well varied meals. The food basket should be acceptable for citizens with different background characteristics provided that the healthy aspect is not compromised.
- Finally, we assume that the budget for food is allocated to each household member in accordance with her/his needs.

By making these assumptions, we focus on the minimum below which a healthy diet in accordance with the FBDG is not possible. In real-life situations, though, more resources will usually be needed because resources are not always spent in the most economical way, people could be confronted with diseases or special needs, people might lack the necessary capacities or information to buy and prepare healthy food at economical prices, and some household members may consume a share of the food budget that is not in proportion to their needs. The procedure that the various country teams followed was structured in five standardized steps or milestones.

(1) For the first milestone, the national experts provided a clear description of the scientific basis (DRVs) of the national FBDG, the results of the last food consumption survey and the model of health education in their country.

(2) In the following step, in cooperation with a nutritionist, country teams translated the FBDG into a concrete list of food items, including the necessary amounts for each hypothetical household.

(3) For the third milestone, three different focus groups were organized in the capital city. Several focus group trainings were organized and instructions were developed by the coordinating team to make sure that the focus groups were conducted and analysed in a standardized way (cf. Annex 1 in [26]). The national partners recruited for each focus group 5–11 participants of active age (30–50), through a questionnaire for recruitment ensuring a mix of different family situations, and a variety of socio-economic backgrounds. Involving people with different backgrounds increases the variation of opinions, the quality of discussions (in terms of argumentation) and validity of the outcome [27–29]. The recruitment of different socio-economic backgrounds was measured based on three variables: activity status, level of education and burden of housing costs as a proxy for income. Because of the limited number of focus groups, it was difficult to make sure ethnic minorities were equally involved. Therefore, this pilot project aimed in the first place at capturing the dominant cultural patterns through FG discussions, acknowledging that more research is necessary to reveal the cultural variety within cities. Each focus group followed a predefined topic list, with an estimated time of three hours. The first half of the discussion was devoted to evaluating the broader theoretical framework (the assessment of needs and essential social roles) and the underlying assumptions we made (characteristics of the reference family), and the second half was used to discuss the acceptability, feasibility and completeness of the food basket, the kitchen equipment and the other non-physical functions of food—as well as the related purchasing patterns. For the purpose of this article, we only make use of the second part of the focus group discussions, which had an average duration of approximately 90 min. To facilitate the discussion, an illustrative weekly menu was developed by the nutritionist, in accordance with the proposed food basket. The results were analysed by the country teams in accordance with a common template of analysis. Each focus group was recorded, and, during the discussion, an assistant wrote down the various arguments in a structured template. For each topic a final column was completed with the overall conclusions and general remarks on interaction processes, proxemics and paralinguistic information. In literature they call this a micro-interlocutor analysis [30], which allows to focus on the group as well as on the individual data while taking into account group dynamics. The purpose of the focus

groups was not to decide on specific quantities but rather to assess the nature, the origin and the construction of the arguments regarding why items are needed or not and what is acceptable and feasible within a given socio-cultural context.

(4) Next, the food baskets had to be adapted in function of feasibility and acceptability, based on the arguments put forward during focus group discussions. This was done in accordance with a common decision procedure that country teams had to follow to ensure that the healthy character of the diet was respected and to facilitate the consistency and robustness of the results across countries (cf. Annex 2 in [26]).

(5) The last milestone consisted of estimating the minimum feasible cost of the food basket. Again, several common assumptions were made. First of all, the food budget should represent the minimum resources that people need to get access to all essential food items. Further, people should have a minimum acceptable degree of freedom in the choice of shops and products. Thirdly, market prices are used, unless other purchasing patterns are common practice, but no sales prices are used. Another important guideline was that economies of scale in buying and preparing food should be taken into account. For the choice of shops to buy food, the national teams had to choose a few retailors or markets which were suggested by the participants in the focus groups. The retailers had to meet the following criteria: (1) they offer a wide variety of food items of acceptable quality at low prices, (2) the shops are well spread over the city, (3) the shops are well accessible by public transport. Being well spread over the country was another criterion that could be considered, as this could facilitate the future pricing of reference budgets developed for other regions. All countries priced the food baskets between March and April 2015 (exceptions are the food baskets for Luxembourg, Denmark and Slovakia which were priced in December 2014, July 2015 and October 2015, respectively). Prices were collected on the basis of a small-scale survey, carried out by researchers from each country team, making use of a standardised excel sheet (with the exception of Luxembourg, where the country team had access to the official price survey). To price pre-packaged food, the lowest price of suitable products had to be chosen. With regard to fresh food and food categories which contain a large variety of products, country teams had to follow a specific predefined pricing procedure, such that a weighted price could be estimated which takes into account the available range of relevant products. The food categories for which a weighted price procedure had to be used are the following: fresh fruit, canned fruit, fruit puree, frozen fruit, dried fruit, fresh vegetables, frozen prepared & unprepared vegetables, canned vegetables, fresh fish, frozen fish, canned fish, lean meat, fat meat, charcuterie and cheese. For instance, the cost of fresh fruit is based on a weighted average of all fresh fruit available in the shop, taking from each type of fruit the cheapest alternative of sufficient quality (e.g., the cheapest apple, the cheapest pear, etc.). The cheapest products are weighted 5/7, whereas the average weight of the more expensive items is given a weight of 2/7, while discarding the 10% most expensive fruits. This procedure aims to meet the dual objective of identifying the minimum cost to prepare healthy menus that still offer sufficient variation (see Annex 3 in [26] for the detailed instructions for assessing the cost of the food basket).

The applied pricing procedure was explicitly designed to balance standardisation, sensitivity to the local context, cross-national variations in purchasing patterns and considerations of acceptability. At the same time, it is clear that the procedure is open for improvement. More in particular, the number of shops frequented was generally low and the price survey typically shows a snapshot of the prices at one particular moment in time, collected by a single observer. A much more extensive price survey would be very useful and facilitate representativeness and reliability. In this context, building on the official price survey, especially for assessing the cost of food, could result in a significant improvement of the quality of the pricing procedure.

3. Results

3.1. The Contents of the Food Basket

What Constitutes a Healthy Diet?

Although there is little difference in the main food groups included in the country-specific FBDG, the type of foods and the recommended amounts within these main food groups differ substantially across countries [10]. These differences follow a clear geographical pattern which may be understood to be mainly a reflection of cultural background and food availability. For instance, in Eastern and Southern European countries the recommended quantities for protein-based foods such as meat or fish are higher compared to Western Europe. Nonetheless, the cross-national variation in FBDG can not only be explained by the differences in cultural habits. Also other factors play a role, including variations in health priorities and the availability of food products between EU member states, as well as the fact that the FBDGs have been updated at different points in time, by different institutions and aimed at different kind of age groups. Furthermore, the interpretation of international recommendations differs across EU Member States, which is reflected in differences in concrete guidelines. Figure 1 shows the content of the national healthy food baskets for a single woman expressed in daily food amounts (mg, and mL for liquids).

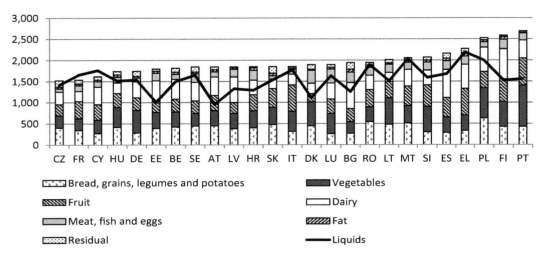

Figure 1. Daily food (mg/mL) amounts for a single woman, healthy food basket, 2015. Country abbreviations: AT, Austria; BE, Belgium; BG, Bulgaria; CY, Cyprus; CZ, Czech Republic; DE, Germany; DK, Denmark; EE, Estonia; EL, Greece; ES, Spain; FI, Finland; FR, France; HR, Croatia; HU, Hungary; IT, Italy; LT, Lithuania; LU, Luxembourg, LV, Latvia; MT, Malta; NL, Netherlands; PL, Poland; PT, Portugal; RO, Romania; SE, Sweden; SK, Slovakia; SI, Slovenia.

The amounts included in the graph refer to the quantity of food in the healthy food baskets that were developed by the country teams, taking account of the edible portions and typical wastes. Net amounts of fresh fruits, vegetables, potatoes, fish, fatter meat and eggs as recommended in the FBDG were increased with a waste percentage of respectively 22%, 28%, 10%, 30%, 20% and 12%. All countries have used the same edible portions, following guidelines that have originally been developed for Belgium [31]. An exception is Portugal, where –slightly different- national criteria were applied.

With regard to the amount of *vegetables* and *fruits*, country teams included on average between 300–400 g per day for each group. As explained above, the source of variation in the amounts relates to various factors, such as cultural differences (e.g., inclusion of vegetarian meals) or to differences in FBDG, e.g., some countries differentiate between fruit and vegetables while others formulate a joint recommendation. The amount of *dairy products* varies more across countries, ranging from 215 g in Latvia to 710 g in Finland. Also, for the group of *meat, fish and eggs*, variations fluctuate between less than 100 g per day (CZ, DE) to 339 g per day (LU). These variations reflect not only differences in guidelines but also, for instance, cultural differences in the composition of the meals. Countries with higher amounts usually include a portion of these foods in two of their meals per day, while others only include them for one daily meal. For the *liquids* group, the large variation is partly due to whether or not countries included wine and beer, and by the varying amounts of coffee and tea across countries. Water was the basic beverage in all countries and products like fruit juices or sodas were not included in this group, as they are not recommended on a regular basis. Milk was placed in the dairy group.

For some food groups, the variation can also be explained by the differences in the type of foods. For example, the food group *grains* includes foods such as bread, rice, pasta, pulses and potatoes. Nutritionally these items are considered as exchangeable, but the size of the portion in a daily meal varies considerably (e.g., for an adult: 70–100 g rice compared to 150–250 g potatoes). The *fat* group mainly includes cooking oil/fat. The Mediterranean countries nuts were also included in this group following some national guidelines. The type of fat included varies across countries. In Mediterranean countries the main source of recommended fat is olive oil and nuts, while in most of the other countries, butter and other spreadable fats are the most common type of fat. Hence, it is important to bear in mind that comparing food group amounts among the different countries does not necessarily provide information about the nutritional value of the baskets, since food items belonging to the same food group may have a different nutritional composition and/or different portion size.

The *residual* group is the food group with the highest variations, with amounts ranging from 25 g to 155 g. These differences are likely to be a consequence of the lack of guidelines with regard to these kind of products. All the countries include some salt, sugar and spices, but also sauces (such as mayonnaise and ketchup), dressings and sweets, especially for children, albeit with large variations.

3.2. The Cost of the Food Baskets

In this section, we present the results of the food baskets, priced in the capital cities in March-April 2015. Figure 2 shows the total food baskets for a single woman in EUR/month. The baskets represent the budget a single person needs to have a healthy diet.

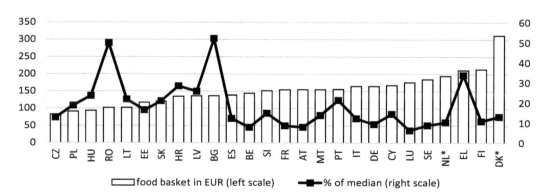

Figure 2. Total food baskets for a single woman in EUR / month (left axis) and as a percentage of the national median equivalent disposable household income (right axis). Results refer to the capital city of each country. Prices 2015. * Pricing procedure for DK and NL is not fully comparable. Source: [26] and Eurostat online database (median income).

When we compare the total food baskets, we observe large variations between EU Member States. The highest price can be found in Denmark, while the lowest cost can be observed for the Czech Republic. In Denmark a single woman needs about three times as much (312 EUR) for eating healthily as compared to a single woman in the Czech Republic (82 EUR). Even if we leave out Denmark (in which the pricing procedure was somewhat different), the difference between the most expensive food basket (Finland) and the cheapest one remains quite large. This substantial variation between countries is mainly a combination of differences in dietary guidelines on the one hand and price differences on the other hand.

At the same time, it is well known that the level of average household incomes varies a lot between EU Member States. In the context of food security, it is therefore relevant to consider the cost of a healthy diet also in relation to the level of incomes. Therefore, Figure 2 also depicts the food basket for a single person as a percentage of the median equivalent disposable household income in each country, as measured in the EU survey on Income and Living Conditions (EU-SILC) of 2016 (the source of the data on disposable household incomes is the Eurostat online database, last accessed 7 December 2018). This representative household survey collects on a yearly basis information on household incomes (including taxes, social contributions and benefits) in the previous calendar year [32]. We express the budgets as a percentage of the median disposable income (after taxes and transfers), adjusted for household size. This reveals a very different pattern of the relative cost of the food basket: it is lowest in Luxembourg (about 6% of the median income) and the highest in Romania (50%) and Bulgaria (52%), implying that in the latter countries, at the median income, households in the capital city would have to spend half of their income on food in order to have a diet in accordance with their national FBDG. Also, in Greece the relative cost of the food basket is remarkably high. Obviously, the implications for variations in food security require a much more in-depth analysis, with a focus on households with the lowest incomes, but this falls outside the scope of the present paper. In any case, this preliminary analysis shows that the cost of a healthy diet is a non-negligent factor to better understand patterns of food insecurity across the European Union.

4. Discussion

In the text above, we have described the process of development and the content of the Food Reference Budgets for 26 European countries, as constructed in the framework of the European Commission's DG Employment, Social Affairs and Inclusion funded *Pilot Project for the development of a common methodology on Reference Budgets in Europe.* We follow a normative perspective [33], and use guidelines and expert opinions to establish what is needed for an adequate diet. However, such an exercise is only helpful for health promotion if the resulting food baskets are sufficiently acceptable and feasible. Therefore, focus group discussions played a central role for assessing the acceptability and feasibility baskets.

The process of building food reference budgets is confronted with several limitations. First, there are a number of unavoidable arbitrary choices that condition the final budgets, such as the decision of not including promotions or discounts, the assumption that people are sufficiently informed and skilled to follow a healthy diet, or have enough time to do so. While we are aware that skills and capability to shop and cook healthily as well as time availability are important constraints towards a healthy eating [34,35], and that some studies describe that these aspects are even more critical in vulnerable groups [36–38], the decision to develop RBs for these types of family was consistent with the need of having a common and clear family type to facilitate the robustness of the results and the focus on the minimum required resources for an adequate diet. It would be worthwhile to expend the results of this pilot project to household types based on other assumptions regarding time constraints and competences, to reveal the importance of these personal factors in having access to a healthy diet. At the same time, we are convinced that the current food budgets, with their specific assumptions, can already be used in tailored nutrition education programs, as has been done in some countries [39,40]. Second, although the Supplementary materials (Table S1) contain the budgets for additional household types, the budgets have been developed for a limited number of types only and cannot be extrapolated to the entire population. Moreover, since food RBs start from FBDG, in their current form they only represent the *official* healthy way of eating, while they leave out a myriad of other possible ways of following a healthy diet. In this sense, future research should be able to take into account a greater variation of reference situations in terms of age, cultural background, personal choices and health conditions. Fourth, the pricing procedure that was applied could be further improved to increase representativeness and reliability by working with a larger, random sample of food products. Fifth, due to their detailed character, the budgets risk to be used in a prescriptive way. Given previously mentioned limitations, food reference budgets do not pretend to *define* what people should eat, but to illustrate a way in which an adequate diet can be achieved, and how much that would cost at the minimum. Finally, when using the food budgets for comparative research, researchers should be aware of the limits to their comparability that we have highlighted above. In particular, it should be clear that is the healthy food basket is comparable only in the sense that it reflects everywhere the state of affairs of FBDG in 2015. We are well aware that the extent to which the FBDG are an adequate cultural and scientific reflection of what a healthy diet should be in different national contexts can be criticised [41].

Notwithstanding these limitations, we are convinced that food reference budgets hold interesting contributions to the promotion of healthy eating and prevention of food insecurity in low-income contexts in at least four ways: First, because they show how a healthy diet can be achieved with limited economic resources, they constitute not only a guideline in terms of budgeting, but also offer policy-makers more insight into the cost of a healthy diet and how this may be a hurdle to achieve a healthy eating pattern.

Second, food reference budgets also bring closer to the citizen a detailed example of how to put general recommendations (as the ones contained in FBDG) into practice. Several studies show that the main motivators in the choice of food differ depending on the socioeconomic and educational level. We know that even though the price is a great determinant of the intake, culinary skills and food knowledge is also a determining factor among low-income people [36,37]. FBDG are designed to be easy to interpret and to translate into physical dishes and food preparations. However, in a moment in which most population is losing culinary referents and less and less familiar with cooking [42], much people do not have the necessary knowledge to translate dietary recommendations into daily eating practices (this is what the nutritionist on each country team did). Hence, a guide that shows how to cook a healthy diet with very few resources is most useful.

Third, if, when ensuring food security, we really aim at promoting a bio-psycho-social understanding of the person, healthy eating promotion must compulsorily include foods to share, foods to enjoy and foods to celebrate. This is something the focus groups laid bare. In all countries, FG participants stressed how food is not only about being in a good health, but it is an essential part of cultural and social life. Eating and drinking is playing a crucial role for social activities and gatherings with family, friends and colleagues in all different cultural contexts. The people in FGs emphasize the importance of cooking and dining together but also of eating out in order to maintain social relations and to socialize. Food can be a means to show care and respect, to create hospitality and to create a feeling of belonging. Further, the FG participants often mentioned the role of food in the preservation of traditions and in the expression of a certain cultural, religious or personal identity. These foods and activities are not essential for a healthy diet, nevertheless, they are seen as important to participate adequately in society. As mentioned above, in this project, the inclusion of these items was not done in a very standardized and cross-nationally comparable way, which is why we did not report their estimated levels. Nevertheless, we should acknowledge the importance of these functions in order to create more acceptable and complete food baskets that allow for adequate social participation in the different EU countries. Ultimately this is the only pathway to work toward narrowing diet-related health inequalities in a comprehensive and empowering manner. Therefore, it would be worthwhile to spend more time and resources on collecting high quality information on this aspect of an adequate diet.

Finally, it is worthwhile pointing out that although there is quite some variation between countries in the cost of a healthy diet, this variation is much smaller than the variation in median disposable household incomes we find in the EU. For instance, while the cost of a healthy diet is about 214 EUR/month in Finland as compared to just 102 EUR per month in Romania, its median equivalent disposable household income in EUR is about ten times higher [43]. As a result, it is clear that people living in countries with a relatively low median disposable will have a much harder time spending sufficient income to ensure a healthy diet. Furthermore, the ranking in the cost of a healthy diet differs from the ranking of countries in terms of their median disposable household income. For instance, even though Romania clearly is the EU country with the lowest median household incomes, the cost of a healthy diet in Bucarest is clearly higher than the cost of a healthy diet in, for instance, the Czech Republic, which in terms of household incomes is considerably less poor. This has clear implications for policies, especially at the EU level, but it also shows the potential of the food reference budgets for further research into better understanding patterns of food insecurity across the EU.

5. Conclusions

In this paper, food reference budgets are presented and their potential utility as a complement for FBDG in low-income contexts is discussed. These reference budgets are built upon cross-nationally comparable food baskets which reflect the minimum cost for a healthy diet, taking national food patterns and recommendations into account by starting from national FBDG. Food baskets were constructed for the capital city in 26 countries, including all EU Member States except Ireland and the United Kingdom. In Denmark and the Netherlands, the procedure that was applied was not fully comparable. The figures show that even though cross-national differences in the minimum cost of a healthy diet are large, they vary much less than net disposable median incomes. We are convinced that the part of the food baskets which relates to having a healthy diet is comparable across countries in the sense that it reflects dominant institutionalized expectations regarding what constitutes a healthy diet, as embedded in national FBDG, and so will be useful for further comparative research.

The procedure we set up for developing and pricing the cost of a healthy diet has been conceived to optimise the balance between the following objectives: (1) It should allow for a healthy diet in line with recommendations in the applicable food-based dietary guidelines; (2) It should be the most economical option possible, while allowing some room for choice; and (3) It should be acceptable, tasty and feasible for the wider public, that is, it should be in line with local food habits. This setup seemed to work well and led to reasonable outcomes. However, further efforts should be undertaken to develop strategies to also collect comparable information on the cost of other functions of food, kitchen equipment and national recommendations regarding physical activity.

We are strongly convinced that the food reference budgets offer a useful tool for the promotion of healthy eating and prevention of food insecurity in low-income contexts in at least four ways: (1) help with budgeting for a healthy diet and making the financial hurdles for realising a healthy diet visible to policy makers; (2) educational illustration of how to cook in accordance with national food recommendations as embedded in the FBDGs; (3) showing that also other functions of food matter, apart from having access to a healthy diet; (4) providing routes for further (comparative) research into food insecurity.

While the results of this pilot project have proven to be very useful, we have also pointed to several limitations that indicate the potential for further improvement. Overcoming these limitations is strongly dependent on having access to better data, including price data and comparable food consumption surveys in all EU Member States. Also, to make the food baskets more comparable in the sense of the minimum necessary for an adequate diet, it would be welcome to have up-to-date high quality FBDGs everywhere.

Author Contributions: All authors contributed equally to this paper.

Acknowledgments: We are very grateful to two anonymous reviewers for very constructive comments and suggestions and to all national experts who contributed to the development of the national food baskets. A complete list of the research teams involved in the Pilot Project can be found in ref. 26.

References

1.   GBD 2016 Risk Factors Collaborators. Global, regional, and national comparative risk assessment of 84 behavioural, environmental and occupational, and metabolic risks or clusters of risks, 1990–2016: A systematic analysis for the global burden of disease study 2016. *Lanct* **2017**. [CrossRef]

2.   Thomson, K.; Hillier-Brown, F.; Todd, A.; McNamara, C.; Huijts, T.; Bambra, C. The effects of public health policies on health inequalities in high-income countries: An umbrella review. *BMC Public Health* **2018**, *18*, 869. [CrossRef] [PubMed]

3.   World Health Organization. *World Health Statistics 2017. Monitoring Health for the SDGs*; World Health Organization: Geneva, Switzerland, 2017.

4.   OECD. *It Together: Why Less Inequality Benefits All*; OECD Publishing: Paris, France, 2015.

5.   Brian, N. *Inequality and Inclusive Growth in Rich Countries: Shared Challenges and Contrasting Fortunes*; Oxford University Press: Oxford, UK, 2018.

6.   Milanovic, B. *Global Inequality. A New Approach for the Age of Globalization*; Harvard University Press: Cambridge, MA, USA, 2016.

7.   Roberto, C.A.; Swinburn, B.; Hawkes, C.; Huang, T.T.-K.; Costa, S.A.; Ashe, M.; Zwicker, L.; Cawley, J.H.; Brownell, K.D. Patchy progress on obesity prevention: Emerging examples, entrenched barriers, and new thinking. *Lancet* **2015**, *385*, 2400–2409. [CrossRef]

8.   Carrillo-Álvarez, E.; Riera-Romaní, J. Childhood obesity prevention: Does policy meet research? Evidence-based reflections upon the Spanish case. *MOJ Public Heal.* **2017**, *6*, 1–14. [CrossRef]

9.   Kumanyika, S.; Libman, K.; Garcia, A. Strategic Action to Combat the Obesity Epidemic. Available online: http://www.wish.org.qa/wp-content/uploads/2018/02/27425_WISH_Obesity_Report_web14.pdf (accessed on 14 December 2018).

10. EFSA Panel on Dietetic Products, Nutrition, and Allergies (NDA). Scientific opinion on establishing food-based dietary guidelines. *EFSA J.* **2010**, *8*, 1–42. [CrossRef]

11. FAO/WHO. *Preparation and Use of Food-Based Dietary Guidelines*; WHO: Nicosia, Cyprus, 1996.

12. Stockley, L. Toward public health nutrition strategies in the European Union to implement food based dietary guidelines and to enhance healthier lifestyles. *Public Health Nutr.* **2001**, *4*, 307–324. [CrossRef] [PubMed]

13. Roth, N.; Knai, C. *Food Based Dietary Guidelines in the Who European Region*; WHO: Geneva, Switzerland, 2003.

14. WHO. *Global Status Report on Noncommunicable Diseases 2014*; WHO: Geneva, Switzerland, 2014.

15. Pomerleau, J.; McKee, M.; Lobstein, T.; Knai, C. The burden of disease attributable to nutrition in Europe. *Public Health Nutr.* **2003**, *6*, 453–461. [CrossRef]

16. Naska, A.; Fouskakis, D.; Oikonomou, E.; Almeida, M.; Berg, M.; Gedrich, K.; Moreiras, O.; Nelson, M.; Trygg, K.; Turrini, A.; et al. Dietary patterns and their socio-demographic determinants in 10 European countries: Data from the DAFNE databank. *Eur. J. Clin. Nutr.* **2006**, *60*, 181–190. [CrossRef]

17. Gibney, M.; Sandstrom, B. A framework for food-based dietary guidelines in the European Union. *Public Health Nutr.* **2000**, *4*, 293–305. [CrossRef]

18. European Food Information Council Food Based Dietary Guidelines in Europe. Available online: www.eufic.org/en/healthy-living/article/food-based-dietary-guidelines-in-europe (accessed on 14 December 2018).

19. Montagnese, C.; Santarpia, L.; Buonifacio, M.; Nardelli, A.; Caldara, A.R.; Silvestri, E.; Contaldo, F.; Pasanisi, F. European food-based dietary guidelines: A comparison and update. *Nutrition* **2015**, *31*, 908–915. [CrossRef]

20. Brown, K.A.; Timotijevic, L.; Barnett, J.; Shepherd, R.; Lähteenmäki, L.; Raats, M.M. A review of consumer awareness, understanding and use of food-based dietary guidelines. *Br. J. Nutr.* **2011**, *106*, 15–26. [CrossRef] [PubMed]

21. Drewnowski, A.; Eichelsdoerfer, P. Can low-income Americans afford a healthy diet? *Nutr. Today* **2010**, *44*, 246–249. [CrossRef] [PubMed]

22. Schönfeldt, H.C.; Hall, N.; Bester, M. Relevance of food-based dietary guidelines to food and nutrition security: A South African perspective. *Nutr. Bull.* **2013**, *38*, 226–235. [CrossRef]

23. Poulain, J.-P. *The Sociology of Food: Eating and the Place of Food in Society*; Bloomsbury: New York, NY, USA; ISBN 9781472586209.

24. Chrysostomou, S.; Andreou, S.N.; Polycarpou, A. Developing a food basket for fulfilling physical and non-physical needs in Cyprus. Is it affordable? *Eur. J. Public Health* **2017**, *27*, 553–558. [CrossRef] [PubMed]

25. Carrillo Álvarez, E.; Cussó-Parcerisas, I.; Riera-Romaní, J. Development of the Spanish Healthy Food Reference Budget for an adequate social participation at the minimum. *Public Health Nutr.* **2016**, *19*. [CrossRef] [PubMed]

26. Goedemé, T.; Storms, B.; Penne, T.; Van den Bosch, K. *Pilot Project for the Development of a Common Methodology on Reference Budgets in Europe. Final Report*; European Commission: Antwerp, Belgium, 2015; ISBN 9789279540912.

27. Deeming, C. The historical development of family budget standards in britafrom the 17th century to the present. *Soc. Policy Adm.* **2010**. [CrossRef]

28. Vranken, J. Using Reference Budgets for Drawing up the Requirements of a Minimum Income Scheme and Assessing Adequacy. Available online: https://ec.europa.eu/social/main.jsp?catId=1024&langId=en&newsId=1392&moreDocuments=yes&tableName=news (accessed on 14 December 2018).

29. Devuyst, K.; Storms, B.; Penne, T. *Methodologische Keuzes Bij De Ontwikkeling Van Referentiebudgetten: Welke Rol Voor Focusgroepen?* Aromede: Antwerp, Belgium, 2014.

30. Onwuegbuzie, A.J.; Dickinson, W.B.; Leech, N.L.; Zoran, A.G. A Qualitative Framework for Collecting and Analyzing Data in Focus Group Research. *Int. J. Qual. Methods* **2009**. [CrossRef]

31. Gezondheidsraad, H. *Maten en Gewichten: Handleiding Voor Een Gestandaardiseerde Kwantificering Van Voedingsmiddelen [Measures and Weights: Manual for Standardized Quantification of Foods]*; Belgische Hoge Gezondheidsraad: Brussels, Belgium, 2005.

32. Atkinson, T.; Guio, A.C.; Marlier, E. Monitoring Social Inclusion in Europe. Available online: https://ec.europa.eu/eurostat/web/income-and-living-conditions/publications/-/asset_publisher/zdEOYZhr9af3/content/KS-05-14-075/3217494?inheritRedirect=false (accessed on 14 December 2018).

33. Storms, B.; Goedemé, T.; Van den Bosch, K.; Penne, T.; Schuerman, N.; Stockman, S. Pilot Project for a Development of a Common Methodology on Reference Budgets in Europe. Review of Current State of Play on Reference Budget Practices at National, Regional and Local Level. Available online: http://www.referencebudgets.eu/ (accessed on 25 July 2014).

34. Sobal, J.; Bisogni, C.A. Constructing food choice decisions. *Ann. Behav. Med.* **2009**, *38*, 37–46. [CrossRef]

35. Leng, G.; Adan, R.A.H.; Belot, M.; Brunstrom, J.M.; de Graaf, K.; Dickson, S.L.; Hare, T.; Maier, S.; Menzies, J.; Preissl, H.; et al. The determinants of food choice. *Proc. Nutr. Soc.* **2017**, *76*, 316–327. [CrossRef]

36. Antentas, J.M.; Vivas, E. Impacto de la crisis en el derecho a una alimentación sana y saludable. Informe SESPAS 2014. *Gac. Sanit.* **2014**, *28*, 58–61. [CrossRef]

37. Darmon, N.; Drewnowski, A. Does social class predict diet quality? *Am. J. Clin. Nutr.* **2008**, *87*, 1107–1117. [CrossRef] [PubMed]

38. Tiwari, A.; Aggarwal, A.; Tang, W.; Drewnowski, A. Cooking at home: A strategy to comply with U.S. Dietary guidelines at no extra cost. *Am. J. Prev. Med.* **2017**, *52*, 616–624. [CrossRef] [PubMed]

39. Cornellis, I.; Vandervoort, B. *Een Hele Dag Lekker en Gezond Eten Voor 5 Euros*; Borgerhoff & Lamberigst: Ghent, Belgium, 2013.

40. Muro, P.; Carrillo-Álvarez, E.; Marzo, T. Empoderar en hábitos saludables a familias vulnerables. In *REPS 2018: Políticas sociales ante horizones de incertidumbre y desigualdad*; Red Española de Política Social: Zaragoza, Spain, 2018.

41. Carrillo-Álvarez, E.; Boeckx, H.; Penne, T.; Palma, I.; Goedemé, T.; Storms, B. Promoting healthy eating in Europe: A comparison of European countries FBDG. 2019. In press.

42. Sainz García, P.; Carmen Ferrer Svoboda, M.; Sánchez Ruiz, E.; Pedro Sainz García, C. Competencias culinarias y consumo de alimentos procesados o preparados en estudiantes universitarios de barcelona. *Rev. Esp. Salud. Pública* **2016**, *90*, 1–13.

43. Eurostat Eurostat Online Database. Available online: https://ec.europa.eu/eurostat/data/database (accessed on 14 December 2018).

12

Cost and Affordability of Diets Modelled on Current Eating Patterns and on Dietary Guidelines, for New Zealand Total Population, Māori and Pacific Households

Sally Mackay [1],* (iD), Tina Buch [2], Stefanie Vandevijvere [1], Rawinia Goodwin [1], Erina Korohina [3], Mafi Funaki-Tahifote [2], Amanda Lee [4] and Boyd Swinburn [1]

[1] School of Population Health, University of Auckland, Auckland 1142, New Zealand;
     s.vandevijvere@auckland.ac.nz (S.V.); rawiniagoodwin@icloud.com (R.G.);
     boyd.swinburn@auckland.ac.nz (B.S.)
[2] The Heart Foundation of New Zealand, Auckland 1051, New Zealand; TinaB@heartfoundation.org.nz (T.B.);
     mafift@heartfoundation.org.nz (M.F.-T.)
[3] Toi Tangata, Auckland 1010, New Zealand; erina@toitangata.co.nz
[4] The Australian Prevention Partnership Centre, The Sax Institute, Sydney 1240, Australia;
     amanda.lee@saxinstitute.org.au
*   Correspondence: sally.mackay@auckland.ac.nz

Abstract: The affordability of diets modelled on the current (less healthy) diet compared to a healthy diet based on Dietary Guidelines was calculated for population groups in New Zealand. Diets using common foods were developed for a household of four for the total population, Māori and Pacific groups. Māori and Pacific nutrition expert panels ensured the diets were appropriate. Each current (less healthy) diet was based on eating patterns identified from national nutrition surveys. Food prices were collected from retail outlets. Only the current diets contained alcohol, takeaways and discretionary foods. The modelled healthy diet was cheaper than the current diet for the total population (3.5% difference) and Pacific households (4.5% difference) and similar in cost for Māori households (0.57% difference). When the diets were equivalent in energy, the healthy diet was more expensive than the current diet for all population groups (by 8.5% to 15.6%). For households on the minimum wage, the diets required 27% to 34% of household income, and if receiving income support, required 41–52% of household income. Expert panels were invaluable in guiding the process for specific populations. Both the modelled healthy and current diets are unaffordable for some households as a considerable portion of income was required to purchase either diet. Policies are required to improve food security by lowering the cost of healthy food or improving household income.

Keywords: INFORMAS; diet prices; food affordability; Pacific diets; Māori diets; food security

1. Introduction

Dietary risks and a high body mass index are major risk factors contributing to health loss globally and in New Zealand (NZ) with dietary risk factors contributing to the highest proportion of total disability-adjusted life years in 2015 compared to other risk factors [1]. New Zealanders consume too much saturated fat, sodium and sugar and not enough dietary fibre, fruit and vegetables [2]. NZ has high rates of obesity with 32.2% of all adults, 50.2% of Māori adults and 68.7% of Pacific adults, obese [3]. For children (aged 2 to 14), 11% of the total population, 18.1% of Māori and 29.1% of Pacific children are obese [3]. Māori and Pacific people are more likely than non-Māori and non-Pacific to experience food insecurity [2].

An 'obesogenic' environment is 'the sum of influences that the surroundings, opportunities, or conditions of life have on promoting obesity in individuals or populations' [4]. A focus on creating healthy food environments is required to move populations towards diets that meet food-based dietary guidelines [5]. It is fundamental to consider cultural factors when discussing environmental influences on obesity [6].

Non-Māori are more advantaged than Māori across socioeconomic indictors related to education, employment, income and household crowding [7]. Inequities in health outcomes for Māori are influenced by the negative experiences of colonisation, institutional racism, alienation of land and thus identity and historical trauma [8]. In NZ, the Pacific Island community is a large and diverse ethnic group. Pacific communities, while being an integral part of New Zealand's society, continue to face challenges with lower levels of education and qualifications, lower incomes and a higher unemployment rate than the total population [9].

The International Network for Food and Obesity/NCDs Research, Monitoring and Action Support (INFORMAS) aims to monitor key aspects of food environments related to obesity and non-communicable diseases (NCDs) [10]. The INFORMAS food price module provides a framework to examine the price differential of healthy and unhealthy foods, meals and diets with this research focusing on the diet component.

Food prices are a major influence on household food purchases [11]. When the household budget is limited, fixed costs are prioritized so the money allocated for food reduces, which often results in food insecurity with potential health consequences [12].

Researchers have successfully used expert or focus panels to develop diets and select pricing outlets to ensure the costing of diets reflects intakes [13,14]. This is important in this research as eating patterns of Māori and Pacific households in NZ are influenced by traditional foods and eating patterns.

The relative difference in the affordability of a diet modelled to meet dietary guidelines compared with a modelled current (less healthy) diet has not been measured before in NZ, and there are few international studies. A systematic review by Rao et. al. (2013) concluded that healthier diets cost more than less healthy diets, though this depended on whether the cost of the total diet or cost per 2000 kcal was compared [15].

The affordability of a healthy diet compared to the current diet can be used to estimate the affordability component of food security for households on different income levels, for social planning and to advocate for fiscal policies and examine the influence on diet cost of taxes and subsidies on foods [16,17].

This study aims to assess the affordability of diets modelled on current eating patterns (current diet) and on dietary guidelines (healthy diet), for the total population, Māori and Pacific households, and to explore the feasibility of using expert panels to guide the process.

2. Materials and Methods

The methodology follows the guidelines set out in the INFORMAS food prices foundation paper [10] and the INFORMAS food prices module (www.INFORMAS.org). Māori and Pacific expert panels provided guidance for the selection of common foods, menus and price collection methods appropriate to the population group. Figure 1 illustrates the phases in assessing the cost of a modelled healthy versus the current diet. The diets for the total population were developed by a Registered Nutritionist (SM) rather than an expert panel.

The research was approved by the University of Auckland Human Participant Ethics Committee on 22 June 2016 for the Pacific diets (reference 017579) and on 26 September 2016 for the Māori diets (reference 018028). All expert panel participants provided written informed consent prior to participation.

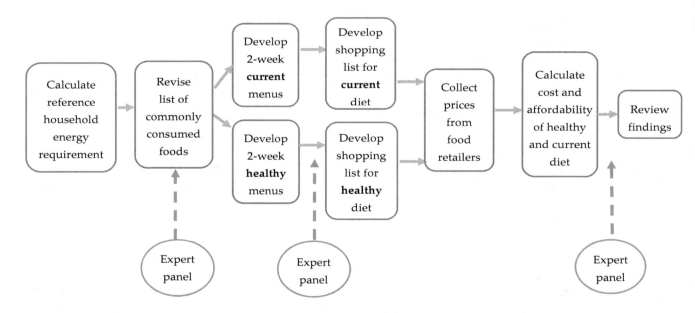

Figure 1. Phases in assessing the cost of a healthy and the current diet.

2.1. Expert Panels

The members of the Māori (four members) and Pacific (six members) expert panels were health professionals knowledgeable about foods and dietary patterns of their communities. The members were selected on the advice of Māori and Pacific non-governmental health organisations.

Phase 1: The expert panel reviewed a list of commonly consumed foods for Māori or Pacific people, provided feedback on menus for the diets and suggested the type and location of retailers for price collection. The initial discussion was face-to-face. The revised commonly consumed foods list and menu plans were emailed to the experts for review.

Phase 2: The results were presented to each expert panel who provided input into the interpretations and implications of the findings.

2.2. Common Foods

Commonly consumed foods were identified from the micro-data of the 2008/09 Adult Nutrition Survey [18] for the total population and for Māori and Pacific separately. Within each of the major food groups (33), the minor groups (395) with the most people consuming the item, or the most grams consumed were identified. Foods consumed by at least 5% of people were considered frequent. The amount consumed of a minor group depended on the food, for example, bread was consumed in higher amounts than butter.

A list of 109/107 common foods was presented to the Maori and the Pacific expert panels respectively. Items were then added or excluded based on the consensus of the expert panel on whether the foods were frequently consumed by the respective population group [Table S1]. The revised Māori common food list included traditional foods such as watercress and mussels. The revised Pacific common food list included taro, green bananas, cabin bread, canned corned beef, mutton flaps, panipopo (sweet coconut buns) and coconut cream.

The number of foods included on the list needed to be manageable for price collection, while ensuring sufficient variety for a two-week menu. The initial revised lists were too extensive so were refined by expert consensus, with some foods acting as proxies for similar foods e.g., jam represented all sweet spreads. The final selection contained 106 foods for the total population, 120 foods for Māori and 127 foods for Pacific populations.

2.3. Household Energy Requirements

The reference household used was that recommended in the INFORMAS food prices module: 45-year old man, 45-year old woman, 14-year old boy, 7-year old girl. The energy requirement for the adults for the healthy diet was calculated using the Body Weight Planner [19] based on a weight derived from a Body Mass Index (BMI) of 23 kg/m^2 calculated from mean population height [20] for moderate physical activity [Table S2]. The energy requirement for children for the healthy diet was based on the recommended energy requirements per KJ/kg per day by FAO/WHO/UNU [21] for moderate physical activity. The target weight was calculated from the 50th percentile BMI from the Centres for Disease Control and Prevention growth charts [22] using mean height [20].

The energy requirement for the current diet for adults was based on the current BMI [Table S2]. The average physical activity level (PAL) was unknown for the population, but approximately half of NZ adults met the physical activity guidelines [20] so a moderate physical activity level was selected. The energy requirement for the current diet for children was based on actual weight [20] and moderate physical activity as most children met the NZ physical activity guidelines [23]. The additional energy required for the actual weight was calculated using a validated equation for the excess energy intake per unit excess weight in childhood [24].

2.4. Diet Constraints

The current diets were modelled to reflect the median intake of the macronutrients (percentage of energy), fibre and total sugar, serves of fruits, vegetables, grains, meat and alternatives and dairy products reported in the 2008/09 Adult Nutrition Survey [2] and the Children's Nutrition Survey 2002 [25] [Tables S3 and S4]. The estimated intakes of sodium were from a later survey using a 24-h urine collection [26]. The current diets met Recommended Dietary Intakes (RDIs) and Adequate Intakes (AIs) for micronutrients except for iodine for all household members, and calcium, iron or Vitamin A for some household members.

The healthy diets were modelled to meet the NZ Eating and Activity Guidelines food group recommendations for number of servings [27] [Table S3] and the acceptable macronutrient distribution range, adequate intake for fibre and the upper limit for sodium (2.3 g per day) from the Nutrient Reference Values and the RDIs and AIs for micronutrients [28] [Table S4]. The intake of iodine could not be assessed due to incomplete food composition data on this micronutrient. The RDI for iron was not met by the adult female of each population group. Foods recommended by the Eating and Activity Guidelines (for example, whole-grain bread, lean meat, reduced-fat milk) were selected. There were no discretionary foods (high in added salt, sugar, saturated fat) in the standard healthy diets. An additional scenario was modelled which replaced 6% of energy from a wide range of foods with discretionary foods and alcohol (adult's diets) to compare a realistic healthy diet rather than an aspirational diet with the current diet.

Additional healthy foods were added to the list of common foods to enable the NZ Eating and Activity Guidelines recommendations for whole-grains, low-fat dairy and legumes to be met; for example, unsalted peanuts, reduced fat corned beef, brown rice, hummus, canned beans. The additional foods were selected based on frequency of consumption in the nutrition surveys and advice from the expert panels.

2.5. Gifting and Gathering of Food

The Māori expert panel identified the gifting and gathering of kai (food) as an important part of accessing food. Foods commonly gifted and/or gathered were seasonal fruit and vegetables and seafood. An additional scenario was analysed where the foods commonly gifted or gathered were priced in the original diet at $0 (mandarins, fresh fish, mussels, puha and watercress).

2.6. Menu Development

A fortnightly menu was developed for the current and healthy diets for each household member separately using the commonly consumed foods for breakfast, lunch, dinner, snacks and beverages. The expert panels advised on the menu structure. For example, the Pacific expert panel highlighted that on Sunday there is a large shared church feast so people only have a cup of tea and cabin bread for breakfast. The Māori expert panel considered it important to include sauces and spreads in the healthy diet to ensure the diet was realistic. The nutrient content of the menus was analysed using FoodWorks [29] with the NZ Food Composition Database. The nutrient composition of some Pacific foods were entered as additional foods, sourced from the Pacific Island Food Composition Tables [30]. Modifications were made to ensure diets met the constraints.

2.7. Price Collection

The amount to purchase for the household, allowing for inedible portion, yield and retention factors, [31] was calculated [Tables S5 and S6]. The expert groups advised that households would select the cheapest brand. Therefore, the brand with the cheapest price was collected from each store, including discount prices and generic brands. For items sold per unit, for example head of broccoli or a donut, three units were weighed and averaged to calculate the price per 100 g.

For the total population, prices were collected from a convenience sample of twelve supermarkets representing the three major supermarket chains and twelve neighbouring fresh produce stores in greater Auckland in November 2016 over two weeks. The prices for takeaway items were sourced from the INFORMAS meals cost study [32]. All items were available.

The Māori expert panel advised to collect prices from urban and rural grocery stores because price and access may be a barrier in rural areas. Prices were collected from three supermarkets (two large, one small) in an urban area and from three supermarkets (one large, two small) in rural areas and takeaway outlets in the Waikato region. Price collection was for one week in July 2017. Six items were not available in some of the smaller grocery stores, mainly fresh fish and meat.

The Pacific expert panel advised that prices should be collected in South Auckland to ensure specific Pacific foods were available. Prices were collected from three supermarkets (each major chain), three neighbouring fruit and vegetable shops, three bakeries and takeaway outlets. Price collection was for two weeks in September 2016. Not all items were available in stores such as mutton flaps, wholemeal pasta, light coconut cream and taro leaves.

2.8. Analysis

The cost of the household diet was calculated for the healthy and current diet (Table 1) for the three populations. A scenario was calculated with the 15% Goods and Services Tax (GST) removed from core foods (fruits, vegetables, less processed meat, seafood, poultry, legumes, nuts, dairy, healthy oils, grains).

To assess affordability of the diets, the percentage of household income required to purchase each diet was calculated for three scenarios:

Scenario 1: Median disposable income [33]

Scenario 2: Household receiving income support

- Jobseeker Support [34]
- Accommodation Supplement (area 2) [34]
- Family tax credit [35]

Scenario 3: Minimum wage [36]

- 60 h per week = one adult 40 h + one adult 20 h Jobseeker Support [34]
- Family tax credit calculated online using gross wages [35]

3. Results

3.1. Energy Requirements

The household energy requirement for the modelled healthy diet is 39.9 MJ and for the current diet is 43.6 MJ for the total population, 46 MJ for Māori and 47.3 MJ for Pacific. The current diet has 8.5% more energy than the healthy diet for the total population household, 13.3% for Māori and 15.6% for Pacific households.

3.2. Cost of Diets

The cost of the diets, and composite food groups, for each population group is outlined in Table 1. For the total population and Pacific Island households, the cost of a modelled healthy diet per fortnight is slightly less than the current diet by 3.5% and 4.5%, with a cost differential over one year of $588 and $575 respectively. For the Māori household, the cost of a healthy and current diet is similar (0.57% difference). When the diets are equivalent in energy, the healthy diet is more expensive than the current diet for all population groups (by 8.5% for the total population, 13.3% for Māori, and 15.6% for Pacific). When 6% of energy in the healthy diet is replaced by discretionary foods and alcohol, the healthy diet reduces in cost by 0.5% ($3.23 per fortnight).

Discretionary foods, beverages and takeaways comprise 36%, 46% and 41% respectively of the current diet costs for the total population, Māori and Pacific Islander populations. The healthy diets have more protein foods, vegetables, grains, fruit and dairy foods than the current diets, and no takeaways, discretionary foods, alcohol, or sugary beverages.

Table 1. Percentage of diet cost of each food group.

Food Group	Healthy Diet	Current Diet	Healthy Diet	Current Diet	Healthy Diet	Current Diet
	All	All	Māori	Māori	Pacific	Pacific
Fruits	18.1%	9.4%	13.6%	8.0%	14.1%	7.0%
Vegetables	17.6%	11.8%	20.8%	10.4%	25.2%	12.9%
Grains	13.8%	6.9%	14.0%	5.5%	15.4%	6.8%
Dairy	11.0%	5.5%	11.2%	6.8%	12.4%	5.2%
Protein	37.9%	31.4%	37.9%	22.0%	30.1%	26.6%
Fats and Oils	1.5%	1.3%	0.7%	1.4%	1.50%	0.9%
Sauces and Spreads	0	2.0%	1.6%	2.3%	0	3.0%
Snacks, sweets	0	6.9%	0	11.5%	0	8.0%
Processed meats	0	4.4%	0	5.3%	0	5.2%
Beverages	0	3.3%	0	5.2%	0	3.8%
Takeaway	0	10.8%	0	15.9%	0	14.9%
Alcohol	0	6.4%	0	5.7%	0	5.8%
Proportion less healthy food	0	35.5%	1.6%	45.9%	0	40.7%
Total cost	$649.06	$671.69	$558.50	$561.68	$526.92	$550.52

3.3. Affordability of Diets

The percentage of income required to purchase either diet is outlined in Table 2. When the 15% Goods and Services Tax (GST) is removed from core foods, affordability for a household improves more for the healthy diet than the current diet.

Table 2. Percentage of household income required to purchase diets.

	Standard Diet		GST off Core Foods	
	Healthy Diet % Income	Current Diet % Income	Healthy Diet % Income	Current Diet % Income
Median Household income ($1733 per week)				
Total population	18.7%	19.4%	16.3%	17.7%
Māori	16.1%	16.2%	14.0%	15.1%
Pacific	15.2%	15.9%	13.2%	15.2%
Minimum Wage ($1115 per week)				
Total population	32.8%	33.9%	28.5%	31.0%
Māori	28.2%	28.3%	24.5%	26.3%
Pacific	26.6%	27.8%	23.1%	26.6%
Income support ($636 per week)				
Total population	51.0%	52.8%	44.4%	48.2%
Māori	43.9%	44.2%	38.2%	41.0%
Pacific	41.4%	43.3%	36.0%	41.4%

3.4. Cost Scenarios

For Māori, six items were identified as foods typically gathered or gifted rather than purchased. The modelled healthy diet reduces in cost more than the current diet when these foods are gifted, as all these foods were healthy. In rural areas, the healthy diet cost reduces by $28.34 per week and the current diet cost reduces by $15.00 while in urban areas these figures were $27.23 and $14.20 respectively. Both the healthy and current diets are cheaper in the urban area compared to the rural area, with the healthy diet costing 9.4% more and the current diet 7.6% more in rural areas.

4. Discussion

This study showed that in NZ, a diet modelled on dietary guidelines is not more expensive than the current, less healthy diet, however when the diets are equivalent in energy the healthy diet is more expensive than the current diet for all population groups. For the total population and Pacific, the cost of a healthy diet is slightly cheaper than the current, less healthy diet. The current diets are higher in energy than the healthy diets because household energy requirement is determined by the average current BMI for the current diet, which is higher than the BMI used for the healthy diet to maintain weight at a healthy BMI.

The input from the Māori and Pacific expert panels was invaluable to identify some popular foods and practices, the type of food to price, meal patterns, common type of retailers and the importance of gathered and gifted food.

An Australian pilot study using similar methodology found the modelled healthy diet cost approximately 12% less than the modelled current diet for a household of four [37]. The healthy diet had 9.6% less energy than the current diet. The energy requirement of the healthy diet was that required to maintain the current BMI and physical activity level of the population. In the New Zealand study, the energy requirement of the healthy diet was determined by a healthy BMI. In Australia, there is no GST on basic, healthy foods but 10% GST on discretionary foods, which contributed to the healthy diet being cheaper than the current diet.

The Otago Food Cost Survey [38] collects the price of a diet that meets the NZ Eating and Activity Guidelines and contains some less healthy snack foods but no alcohol or takeaways. The cost of three diets is calculated: basic (cheapest), moderate and liberal (most expensive, most variety). For a similar household of four, the costs of the healthy diets for Māori ($559) and Pacific ($527) in this study were between the cost of the basic ($482) and moderate ($628) diets in the Otago study, while the cost for the total population ($649) was slightly higher than the moderate diet.

There is no accepted benchmark for affordability of a healthy diet internationally, though other researchers consider a household is suffering from food stress if more than 25% of disposable income is spent on food [39]. Therefore, NZ households receiving the minimum wage or income support would be suffering from food stress with some households requiring half of their income to purchase a healthy diet. The percentage of household income required for other major costs such as housing and utilities also determines the income available for food. Affordability was similar for the healthy and current diets for Māori. The healthy diet was slightly more affordable for Pacific and the total population. However, for a household of four receiving income support or minimum wage, a considerable portion of household income is required to purchase either diet. Food insecurity is a concern with 7.3% of NZ households classified as having low food security in the 2008/09 national nutrition survey [2]. In NZ, all foods have 15% GST added [40]. If GST was removed from basic healthy foods, this would improve affordability more for the healthy diet than the current diet.

4.1. Strengths

Few reported studies have compared the cost of a hypothetical healthy diet and a current diet, particularly for different population groups. The current diet is based on the common foods reported by the population in a national nutrition survey. The healthy diet is developed to meet food-based dietary guidelines and Nutrient Reference Values. The energy requirement for the current diet reflected the actual BMI of the population rather than using the mean reported energy intake in the survey, which is always under-reported [41]. Takeaway foods and alcohol were included in the current diet as these are common. Overall, the healthy diet met more of the micronutrient recommendations than the current diet though the diet for the adult female (total population only) met the RDI for iron on the current diet but not the healthy diet. This study demonstrated that an expert panel is a useful method for gaining cultural input into the commonly consumed foods, dietary patterns and selection of retail outlets used by Māori and Pacific households. As the national nutrition surveys were not recent, the expert panels offered an up-to-date view on commonly consumed foods.

4.2. Limitations

Arbitrary decision points occur at all stages of the process from selecting common foods, selecting items to represent other foods, the amount of each food in the diets, the energy requirement, the definition of a healthy diet, sampling retail outlets and the price selected. The nutrient intake of the current diet was based on older nutrition surveys (2008/09, 2002/03) so may not reflect the nutrient intake of the current diet, however no other data were available.

There is a range of healthy menus that could fit the food-based dietary guidelines and recommended dietary intakes. Only one healthy and one current diet was developed for each population group, so this may not be representative of the average cost if a range of diets were priced. The healthy diet was modelled to be aspirational but when limited discretionary foods were added the cost was similar.

There are other inputs to the cost of producing a household meal, aside from food prices, which could underestimate diet cost, particularly for healthy diets, which may require more preparation. Inputs include time, cooking fuel, transport for groceries, storage, preparation, cooking utensils, cooking space and skills [10].

The cost of the diets was calculated using food prices collected at supermarkets, rather than actual household expenditure that may take into account brand loyalty or purchases from multiple stores. The prices for the different population groups were collected at different times and seasons: Pacific in September 2016, total population in November 2016, Māori in July 2017. The Food Price Index indicated that the price of foods increased by 3.0% from July 2016 to July 2017, particularly fruit and vegetables (8.2%) [42]. Therefore, the relative difference between the healthy and current diets of the different population groups was compared, not the absolute amount. The higher price of fruit and vegetables could be a factor in explaining why the Māori healthy and current diets were a similar price, rather than the healthy diet being slightly cheaper for the Pacific and total population diets. Seasons affect fruit and vegetable prices with fresh fruit and vegetables more expensive in July and September, and close to the average monthly price in November [42], therefore it is expected that the cost differences between the healthy and current diets would persist in seasons where prices are lower.

4.3. Implications

A diet modelled on dietary guidelines is not more expensive than the current diet when the reference household also shifts from the estimated current energy intake to the recommended energy intake. This is particularly important for those on low incomes because food costs are typically between a quarter and a half of household budgets indicating they are suffering from food stress. There is a perception that healthy diets are more expensive than those currently consumed [43,44]. However, this research and similar research in Australia [37] indicates it is possible to shift to a healthy diet (that does not exceed energy requirements) from the current, healthy diet without additional cost. Price is only one barrier to healthy eating. Other key influences are taste, traditions, convenience, knowledge and cooking skills [43]. Gathering and gifting food is important in reducing diet costs.

This paper describes the collection of the baseline data. After further price collections, it can be seen whether the healthy diet is increasing in cost at a different rate than the current diet. An analysis of foods in the NZ Food Price Index [45] over ten years indicates the price of healthy foods rose at a similar rate compared to unhealthy foods.

It is recommended that work be conducted with the expert panels on how to translate these findings into a practical health promotion tool for Pacific, Māori and low-income households. Monitoring the price and affordability of diets provides robust data and benchmarks to inform economic and fiscal policies [10]. As demonstrated in this study, having information on the prices of the current and healthy diets is invaluable to demonstrating the impact taxes and subsidies will have on diets.

5. Conclusions

Expert panels were invaluable in guiding development of the diets to be costed for specific population groups. In NZ, a lower-energy healthy diet is not necessarily more expensive than the current diet, but discretionary foods make up 36–41% of food costs in the current diet. Strategies to switch current spending on discretionary food and takeaways to healthy food need not cost more. However, overall food security is of concern as a considerable portion of income is required to purchase either a healthy or the current diet in NZ, especially for households receiving minimum wage or income support. In order to consume a healthy diet, policies are required to lower the cost of healthy food or ensure that households have sufficient income after fixed expenses to purchase nutritious, acceptable and safe food.

Supplementary Materials:
. Table S1: Common foods added and removed from diets by Māori and Pacific expert panels, Table S2: Individual and household energy requirements for each population group, Table S3: Number of serves of each food group per week for each household member for healthy and current diets, Table S4: Nutrient intake of household members for healthy and current diets for each population group, Table S5: Edible amount of each common food in the current diet per fortnight for each population group, Table S6: Edible amount of each common food in the healthy diet per fortnight for each population group.

Author Contributions: S.M., A.L., S.V. and B.S. conceived and designed the study; S.M., T.B. and R.G. performed the study and analyzed the data; S.M. wrote the paper. E.K. and M.F.-T. provided expert advice and contributed to performing the study; All authors critically revised the manuscript.

Acknowledgments: This research was funded by a grant from the Health Research Council (3704724).

References

1. GBD 2016 Risk Factor Collaborators. Global, regional, and national comparative risk assessment of 79 behavioural, environmental and occupational, and metabolic risks or clusters or risks, 1990–2015: A systematic analysis for the Global Burden of Diseases Study 2015. *Lancet* **2016**, *388*, 1659–1724.

2. University of Otago and Ministry of Health. *A Focus on Nutrition: Key Findings of the 2008/09 New Zealand Adult Nutrition Survey*; Ministry of Health: Wellington, New Zealand, 2011.

3. Ministry of Health. New Zealand Health Survey 2016/17. Available online: https://www.health.govt. nz/nz-health-statistics/national-collections-and-surveys/surveys/current-recent-surveys/new-zealand-health-survey#published (accessed on 20 November 2017).

4. Swinburn, B.; Egger, G.; Raza, F. Dissecting obesogenic environments: The development and application of a framework for identifying and prioritizing environmental interventions for obesity. *Prev. Med.* **1999**, *29*, 563–570. [CrossRef] [PubMed]

5. Swinburn, B.; Sacks, G.; Vandevijvere, S.; Kumanyika, S.; Lobstein, T.; Neal, B.; Barquera, S.; Friel, S.; Hawkes, C.; Kelly, B.; et al. INFORMAS (International Network for Food and Obesity/non-communicable diseases Research, Monitoring and Action Support): Overview and key principles. *Obes. Rev.* **2013**, *14* (Suppl. 1), 1–12. [CrossRef] [PubMed]

6. Kumanyika, S.K. Environmental influences on childhood obesity: Ethnic and cultural influences in context. *Physiol. Behav.* **2008**, *94*, 61–70. [CrossRef] [PubMed]

7. Ministry of Health; Kahukura, T. *Māori Health Chart Book 2015*, 3rd ed.; Ministry of Health: Wellington, New Zealand, 2015.

8. Berghan, G.; Came, H.; Coupe, N.; Doole, C.; Fay, J.; McCreanor, T.; Simpson, T. Tiriti-Based Health Promotion Practice. STIR: Stop Institutional Racism. 2017. Available online: https://trc.org.nz/treaty-waitangi-based-practice-health-promotion (accessed on 7 February 2018).

9. Sorensen, D.; Jensen, S.; Rigamoto, M.; Pritchard, M. *Pacific People in New Zealand: How Are We doing?* Pasifika Futures Ltd.: Auckland, New Zealand, 2015.

10. Lee, A.; Ni Mhurchu, C.; Sacks, G.; Swinburn, B.; Snowdon, W.; Vandevijvere, S.; Hawkes, C.; L'Abbé, M.; Rayner, M.; Sanders, D.; et al. Monitoring the price and affordability of foods and diets globally. *Obes. Rev.* **2013**, *14* (Suppl. 1), 82–95. [CrossRef] [PubMed]

11. Ni Mhurchu, C.; Eyles, H.; Dixon, R.; Matoe, L.; Teevale, T.; Meagher-Lundberg, P. Economic incentives to promote healthier food purchases: Exploring acceptability and key factors for success. *Health Promot. Int.* **2012**, *27*, 331–341. [CrossRef] [PubMed]

12. Lloyd, S.; Lawton, J.; Caraher, M.; Singh, G.; Horsley, K.; Mussa, F. A tale of two localities: Healthy eating on a restricted income. *Health Educ. J.* **2011**, *70*, 48–56. [CrossRef]

13. Bowyer, S.; Caraher, M.; Eilbert, K.; Carr-Hill, R. Shopping for food: Lessons from a London borough. *Br. Food J.* **2009**, *111*, 452–474. [CrossRef]

14. Goedemé, T.; Storms, B.; Van den Bosch, K. *Pilot Project: Developing a Common Methodology on Reference Budgets in Europe*; European Commission: Brussels, Belgium, 2015.

15. Rao, M.; Afshin, A.; Singh, G.; Mozaffarian, D. Do healthier foods and diet patterns cost more than less healthy options? A systematic review and meta-analysis. *BMJ Open* **2013**, *3*, e004277. [CrossRef] [PubMed]

16. Kettings, C.; Sinclair, A.; Voevodin, M. A healthy diet consistent with Australian health recommendations is too expensive for welfare-dependent families. *Aust. N. Z. J. Public Health* **2009**, *33*, 566–572. [CrossRef] [PubMed]

17. Nathoo, T.; Shoveller, J. Do healthy food baskets assess food security? *Chronic Dis. Can.* **2003**, *24*, 65–69. [PubMed]

18. Statistics New Zealand. *Adult National Nutrition Survey 2008/09 Confidentialised unit Record Files*; Statistics New Zealand: Wellington, New Zealand, 2011.

19. National Institute of Diabetes and Digestive and Kidney Diseases. Body Weight Planner. Available online: https://www.niddk.nih.gov/health-information/weight-management/body-weight-planner (accessed on 6 April 2017).

20. Ministry of Health. Annual Update of Key Results 2013/14: New Zealand Health Survey. Available online: https://www.health.govt.nz/publication/annual-update-key-results-2013-14-new-zealand-health-survey (accessed on 20 November 2017).

21. FAO; WHO; UNU. *Report on Human Energy Requirements*; Food and Agricultural Organization; World Health Organization; United Nations University Expert Consultation: Rome, Italy, 2004.

22. CDC Growth Charts 2010. Available online: http://www.cdc.gov/growthcharts/index.htm (accessed on 11 January 2016).

23. Clinical Trials Research Unit and Synovate. *A National Survey of Children and Young People's Physical Activity and Dietary Behaviours in New Zealand: 2008/09: Key Findings*; Ministry of Health: Wellington, New Zealand, 2010.

24. Hall, K.; Butte, N.; Swinburn, B.; Chow, C. Dynamics of childhood growth and obesity: Development and validation of a quantitative mathematical model. *Lancet Diabetes Endocrinol.* **2013**, *10*, 97–105. [CrossRef]

25. Ministry of Health. *NZ Food NZ Children: Key Results of the 2002 National Children's Nutrition Survey*; Ministry of Health: Wellington, New Zealand, 2003.

26. Skeaff, S.; McLean, R.; Mann, J.; Williams, S. *The Impact of Mandatory Fortification of Bread with Iodine*; MPI Technical Paper No: 2013/025; Ministry of Primary Industries: Wellington, New Zealand, 2013.

27. Ministry of Health. Eating and Activity Guidelines for New Zealand Adults. 2015. Available online: https://www.health.govt.nz/publication/eating-and-activity-guidelines-new-zealand-adults (accessed on 20 November 2017).

28. NHMRC. *Nutrient Reference Values for Australia and New Zealand*; National Health and Medical Research Council: Canberra, Australia, 2006.

29. Xyris Software (Australia) Pty Ltd. *FoodWorks 7 Professional [computer program]*; Xyris Software (Australia) Pty Ltd.: Brisbane, Australia, 2012.

30. Dignan, C.; Burlingame, B.; Kumar, S.; Aalbersberg, W. *The Pacific Island Food Composition Tables*; Food and Agriculture Organization of the United Nations: Rome, Italy, 2004.

31. New Zealand Institute of Plant and Food Research. *FOODfiles 2013*; The New Zealand Institute of Plant and Food Research and the New Zealand Ministry of Health: Palmerston North, New Zealand, 2013.

32. Mackay, S.; Vandevijvere, S.; Xie, P.; Lee, A.; Swinburn, B. Paying for convenience: Comparing the cost of takeaway meals with their healthier home-cooked counterparts in New Zealand. *Public Health Nutr.* **2017**, *20*, 2269–2276. [CrossRef] [PubMed]

33. OECD Income Distribution and Poverty. 2016. Available online: http://stats.oecd.org/Index.aspx?DataSetCode=IDD (accessed on 30 May 2016).

34. Ministry of Social Development. Benefit Rates at 1 April 2016. Available online: http://www.workandincome.govt.nz/products/benefit-rates/benefit-rates-april-2016.html#null (accessed on 4 May 2016).

35. Inland Revenue. Estimate Your Working for Families Tax Credits 2016. Available online: http://www.ird.govt.nz/calculators/keyword/wff-tax-credits/calculator-wfftc-estimate-2016.html (accessed on 30 May 2016).

36. Employment New Zealand. The Minimum Wage. 1 April 2016. Available online: https://www.employment.govt.nz/hours-and-wages/pay/minimum-wage/ (accessed on 30 May 2016).

37. Lee, A.J.; Kane, S.; Ramsey, R.; Good, E.; Dick, M. Testing the price and affordability of healthy and current (unhealthy) diets and the potential impacts of policy change in Australia. *BMC Public Health* **2016**, *16*, 315. [CrossRef] [PubMed]

38. Department of Human Nutrition. *Information Package for Users of the New Zealand Estimated Food Costs 2016*; University of Otago: Dunedin, New Zealand, 2016.

39. Landrigan, T.; Kerr, D.; Dhaliwal, S.; Savage, V.; Pollard, C. Removing the Australian tax exemption on healthy food adds food stress to families vulnerable to poor nutrition. *Aust NZ J Public Health* **2017**. [CrossRef] [PubMed]

40. New Zealand Legislation. Goods and Services Tax Act 1985. Available online: http://www.legislation.govt.nz/act/public/1985/0141/latest/DLM81035.html (accessed on 30 August 2016).

41. Poslusna, K.; Ruprich, J.; de Vries, J.; Jakubikova, M.; van't Veer, P. Misreporting of energy and micronutrient intake estimated by food records and 24 h recalls, control and adjustment methods in practice. *Br. Nutr.* **2009**, *101* (Suppl. 2), S73–S85. [CrossRef] [PubMed]

42. Statistics New Zealand. Food Price Index: July 2017. Available online: http://www.stats.govt.nz/browse_for_stats/economic_indicators/prices_indexes/FoodPriceIndex_HOTPJul17.aspx (accessed on 10 October 2017).

43. Andajani-Sutjahjo, S.; Ball, K.; Warren, N.; Inglis, V.; Crawford, D. Perceived personal, social and environmental barriers to weight maintenance among young women: A community survey. *Int. J. Behav. Nutr. Phys. Act.* **2004**, *1*, 15. [CrossRef] [PubMed]

44. Funaki-Tahifote, M.; Fung, M.; Timaloa, Y.; Langi, T.; Lafuloa, S.; Manuopangai, V.; Johnston, O. *Better Quality and Reduced Quantity in Food/Drinks in Pacific Settings*; Health Promotion Agency: Wellington, New Zealand, 2016.

45. Statistics New Zealand. Food Price Index Selected Monthly Weighted Average Prices for New Zealand. 2017. Available online: http://www.stats.govt.nz/infoshare/SelectVariables.aspx?pxID=e3632d54-64c5-45c0-80f5-721bc77c2bca (accessed on 30 May 2017).

13

The Overlooked Burden of Food Insecurity among Asian Americans

Monideepa B. Becerra [1,*] (iD), **Salome Kapella Mshigeni** [1] and **Benjamin J. Becerra** [2]

[1]   Department of Health Science and Human Ecology, California State University, 5500 University Parkway, San Bernardino, CA 92407, USA; salome.mshigeni@csusb.edu

[2]   School of Allied Health Professions, Loma Linda University, 24951 North Circle Drive, Loma Linda, CA 92350, USA; bbecerra@llu.edu

*   Correspondence: mbecerra@csusb.edu

Abstract: *Objective*: Food insecurity remains a major public health issue in the United States, though lack of research among Asian Americans continue to underreport the issue. The purpose of this study was to evaluate the prevalence and burden of food insecurity among disaggregated Asian American populations. *Methods*: The California Health Interview Survey, the largest state health survey, was used to assess the prevalence of food insecurity among Asian American subgroups with primary exposure variable of interest being acculturation. Survey-weighted descriptive, bivariate, and multivariable robust Poisson regression analyses, were conducted and alpha less than 0.05 was used to denote significance. *Results*: The highest prevalence of food insecurity was found among Vietnamese (16.42%) and the lowest prevalence was among Japanese (2.28%). A significant relationship was noted between prevalence of food insecurity and low acculturation for Chinese, Korean, and Vietnamese subgroups. Language spoken at home was significant associated with food insecurity. For example, among Chinese, being food insecure was associated with being bilingual (prevalence ratio [PR] = 2.51) or speaking a non-English language at home (PR = 7.24), while among South Asians, it was associated with speaking a non-English language at home was also related to higher prevalence (PR = 3.62), as compared to English speakers only. Likewise, being foreign-born also related to being food insecure among Chinese (PR = 2.31), Filipino (PR = 1.75), South Asian (PR = 3.35), Japanese (PR = 2.11), and Vietnamese (PR = 3.70) subgroups, when compared to their US-born counterparts. *Conclusion*: There is an imperative need to address food insecurity burden among Asian Americans, especially those who have low acculturation.

Keywords: Asian Americans; California Health Interview Survey; food security; Supplemental Nutrition Assistance Program (SNAP); acculturation; English language use

1. Introduction

The Asian American population is one of the fastest growing minority groups in the United States [1], yet, little research on health disparities exists for the group. One potential reason has been attributed to the model minority myth, which assumes Asians have unparalleled achievements in education and success [2], thus leading to the assumption that the population suffers little health disparities. Yet, studies demonstrate that such a myth has led to internalized racialism, further resulting in negative attitudes towards seeking mental health care and increased psychological distress [3].

Furthermore, Asian American data has been historically aggregated to present a homogeneous representation, resulting in the masking of more vulnerable subpopulations. Recent policy implementations, such as the White House Initiative for Asian Americans and Pacific Islanders [4], and the body of literature, demonstrates the importance of addressing the heterogeneity in the population. For example, Sakamoto, in evaluating the American Community Survey, demonstrated that when compared to whites, Asian Indians, Japanese, and Filipinos were less likely to be living in poverty, while Chinese, Koreans, Vietnamese, and several other Asian American subgroups were more likely to be in poverty [5]; hence contradicting the model minority myth. In an evaluation of hemorrhagic stroke risk among Asian Americans and other ethnic groups, Klatsky et al. [6] noted that while Asian Americans reported a higher risk of such stroke compared to whites, the rate was only explained by Japanese and Filipinos; thus demonstrating the heterogeneity in chronic disease risk among the Asian American population. Similarly, heterogeneity among Asian Americans has been noted in regards to health behaviors and chronic illnesses [7–9]. For example, results from a study addressing physical activity among Asian American subgroups utilizing CHIS data showed Chinese and Vietnamese subgroups who were bilingual were more likely to meet American College of Sport Medicine recommendations of physical activity level, as compared to those who reported only speaking a non-English language at home [10]. Undoubtedly, disaggregated research in the Asian American population is key to ensuring healthier outcomes of the nation's population, as set forth by Healthy People 2020.

In recent years, food insecurity has gained national attention. Food insecurity, defined by the U.S. Department of Agriculture (USDA) as consistent access to and availability of enough food for all members of a household to lead an active and healthy lifestyle. The USDA further defines reduced quality, variety, or desirability of diet as low food security, which was historically called food insecurity without hunger, while the same characteristics with disrupted eating patterns reduction in food intake is considered very low food security, or historically known as food insecurity with hunger [11]. In 2016, 12.3% of U.S. households (42.2 million Americans), were reported to be food insecure. Furthermore, rates of food insecurity were found to be more prevalent among Hispanic and non-Hispanic Black households and those residing below the 185% poverty threshold [12]. Food insecurity has also been associated with negative health outcomes, including poor cognitive development [13,14], poor dietary choices [15,16], and mental illness [17,18]. For example, Weigel and group found higher rate of mental illness (including depression) among food insecure migrant and seasonal farmworkers [19]. Likewise, food insecurity with hunger was found to be substantially related to serious psychological distress among African-Americans [20], while low household food insecurity has been associated with adherence to physical activity guidelines among both children and adults [21]. Despite such empirical evidence, no current research exists on the burden of food insecurity among Asian Americans. As such, in this study we aimed to address this gap in the literature, by evaluating the period prevalence of food insecurity among disaggregation Asian American population using the largest state health survey.

Furthermore, we emphasized the role of acculturation in food insecurity among the population. The literature has identified acculturation, the process by which immigrants adapt to the host nation, as a major determinant of health disparities. For example, Tsunoda et al. [22] demonstrated that while Japanese adults in Japan perceived the time spent with children as appropriate for also drinking alcohol, Japanese Americans in Hawaii and California, on the other hand, perceived such a situation to be inappropriate. Ma and colleagues [23] further noted that cigarette smoking in homes was positively associated with being a new immigrant while less with increasing acculturation to the United States. Likewise, being more acculturated has been associated with higher fast food consumption among South Asian population in California [24]. While studies on the role of acculturation and food insecurity does not exist among Asian Americans, studies among other ethnic groups highlight putative relationship. For example, a study noted among West African refugees [25] noted that low acculturation was substantially related to higher rates of food insecurity, with similar trend noted among Puerto Ricans as well [26]. Despite such empirical evidence, studies on food insecurity and its potential relationship to acculturation is lacking. In fact, a recent study evaluating the burden of food insecurity, excluded Asian Americans from the study due to low sample [27]; thus further limiting the body of literature on the burden of food insecurity among the population. As such, our study addresses this critical gap in the literature. We hypothesize that the prevalence of food insecurity will be substantially different across the Asian American subgroups and less acculturated groups will likely have higher rates, putatively due to their limited knowledge or accessibility to food aid services.

2. Methods

2.1. Data Source

The public-use files of California Health Interview Survey (CHIS) adult section (2001, 2003, 2005, 2007, 2009, and 2011/2012) were used in this study. The study population was limited to Asian American subgroups: Chinese, Filipino, South Asian, Japanese, Korean, and Vietnamese.

2.2. Measures

The primary dependent variable was CHIS-provided variable on food insecurity, categorized in this study as food insecure versus food secure. CHIS provided a combined poverty and food insecurity variable as: at or above 200% federal poverty level (FPL), below 200% FPL and food secure, below 200% FPL and food insecure without hunger, below 200% FPL and food insecure with hunger. CHIS does not ask those at 200% or above their food security status. In this study, to ensure consistency with USDA guidelines, we refer to food insecure without hunger as low food security and food insecure with hunger as very low food secure. To assess food security level, CHIS researchers asked respondents the following questions: [1] "The food that (I/we) bought just didn't last, and (I/we) didn't have money to get more" [2] "(I/We) couldn't afford to eat balanced meals," [3] "In the last 12 months, did you or other adults in your household ever cut the size of your meals or skip meals because there wasn't enough money for food?" [4] "How often did this happen—almost every month, some months but not every month, or only in 1 or 2 months?" [5] "In the last 12 months, did you ever eat less than you felt you should because there wasn't enough money to buy food?" and [6] "In the last 12 months, were you ever hungry but didn't eat because you couldn't afford enough food?", with the last variable assessing hunger. In this study, to ensure adequate sample size, we collapsed low food security and very low food security variables and refer to them as food insecure.

Primary independent variables included acculturation proxies of language spoken at home (Non-English only, English and another, English only) and country of birth (foreign-born vs. U.S.-born). Such measures have shown validity in the literature as proxies of acculturation and thus makes our results comparable to the empirical body of evidence on acculturation among Asian Americans. For example, Van Wieren and others [28] used CHIS data to explore acculturation and cardiovascular behaviors among the Latino population in California, and acculturation was assessed by country of birth. Likewise, An et al. [29] also utilized CHIS to assess how acculturation was related to cigarette smoking behaviors among Asian Americans where acculturation was assessed using language spoken at home.

Control variables included in regression analyses were: age (18–44 years, 45 years or more), sex (male or female), marital status (currently married or not currently married), education (high school or less, some college, bachelor's degree or higher), employment status (currently employed or not currently employed), self-reported general health status (fair or poor vs. excellent, very good, or good), and zip code-based urban or rural residence, as such location may impact food insecurity due to availability of food items. Such variables were categorized based on CHIS-provided groups and/or natural breakpoints in the distribution. Additionally, body mass index (BMI) categories (overweight or obese, not overweight or obese) based on Asian BMI cutoffs [30] and survey year were included as controls. We chose to include BMI, though it is not a commonly utilized sociodemographic characteristics, as some studies have noted that BMI is related to food insecurity status among other populations [31,32]. Given that Supplemental Nutrition Assistant Program (SNAP) may alleviate food insecurity, we further assessed SNAP participation prevalence among the subgroups by citizenship status as a dichotomized variable.

2.3. Data Analysis

STATA v14 (StataCorp; College Station, TX, USA) was used for all analyses. Appropriate CHIS-provided jackknife survey weights were applied using the "svy" command to compute standard errors and obtain weighted prevalence estimates based on California population control totals. Chi-square analyses utilizing survey design-based *F* values were used to determine if there were significant differences in food insecurity prevalence among aforementioned control variables for each Asian American subgroup, in addition to SNAP participation by such subgroup stratified by citizenship status due to residential requirements for such federal aid programs. Survey-weighted Poisson regression, which utilizes a robust estimator by default in STATA [33], was run to estimate the adjusted prevalence ratios, according to Petersen and Deddens [34], of food insecurity by each Asian American subgroup as well as differences in SNAP participation by such subgroups. Finally, we also compared the food insecurity rates to the overall CHIS population for the study years. An alpha less than 0.05 was set for all analyses. The study was approved by the Institutional Review Board of California State University (approval number: 13086).

3. Results

A total of 24,803 Asian Americans, representing an average annual population estimate of 18,975,978, were included in this study. As displayed in Table 1, the highest period prevalence of food insecurity was noted among the Vietnamese subgroup (16.42%) and lowest among the Japanese subgroup (2.28%). Prevalence of speaking only a foreign language at home (acculturation proxy) was also highest among the Vietnamese subgroups (52.36%) and lowest among the Japanese (4.95%). Similarly, highest percent of foreign-born individuals (acculturation proxy) was noted among Vietnamese households (88.59%), with the lowest rate for foreign-born individuals among Japanese households (27.02%). Additional population characteristics are further displayed in Table 1.

Table 1. Study population characteristics by Asian American subgroup.

	Chinese	Filipino	South Asian	Japanese	Korean	Vietnamese
Food insecure						
No	6859 (92.4)	3506 (91.74)	2443 (96.86)	2325 (97.72)	3887 (93.43)	3732 (83.58)
Yes	488 (7.60)	259 (8.26)	90 (3.14)	52 (2.28)	308 (6.57)	854 (16.42)
Language spoken at home						
Non-English only	3204 (45.93)	563 (13.39)	351 (14.38)	135 (4.95)	2235 (44.3)	2791 (52.36)
English and another	2788 (38.31)	2008 (53.81)	1792 (70.88)	596 (26.51)	1600 (45.1)	1611 (42.22)
English only	1355 (15.76)	1194 (32.8)	390 (14.74)	1646 (68.54)	359 (10.6)	184 (5.424)
Country of birth						
Foreign-born	5790 (78.05)	2945 (72.69)	2289 (86.78)	652 (27.02)	3838 (82.62)	4370 (88.59)
U.S.-born	1557 (21.95)	820 (27.31)	244 (13.22)	1725 (72.98)	357 (17.38)	216 (11.41)
Age (years)						
18–44	3245 (54.39)	1782 (56.45)	1696 (74.79)	653 (33.61)	1760 (57.35)	1881 (56.77)
45 or more	4102 (45.61)	1983 (43.55)	837 (25.21)	1724 (66.39)	2435 (42.65)	2705 (43.23)
Sex						
Male	3103 (45.41)	1484 (45.87)	1352 (57.24)	926 (40.95)	1568 (39.00)	2263 (49.48)
Female	4244 (54.59)	2281 (54.13)	1181 (42.76)	1451 (59.05)	2627 (61.00)	2323 (50.52)
Marital status						
Not currently married	2647 (38.23)	1492 (42.62)	655 (29.42)	1096 (39.68)	1402 (39.67)	1595 (40.93)
Currently married	4700 (61.77)	2273 (57.38)	1878 (70.58)	1281 (60.32)	2793 (60.33)	2991 (59.07)

Table 1. *Cont.*

	Chinese	Filipino	South Asian	Japanese	Korean	Vietnamese
Education						
High school or less	1980 (31.9)	718 (23.58)	274 (12.14)	488 (26.54)	1334 (30.76)	2478 (51.93)
Some college	1162 (15.07)	927 (25.72)	263 (10.55)	632 (25.17)	570 (13.87)	833 (19.89)
Bachelors or higher	4205 (53.03)	2120 (50.7)	1996 (77.31)	1257 (48.3)	2291 (55.37)	1275 (28.18)
Employment status						
Currently employed	4598 (62.74)	2643 (70.07)	1857 (73.87)	1259 (54.34)	2097 (58.93)	2337 (59.20)
Currently unemployed	2749 (37.26)	1122 (29.93)	676 (26.13)	1118 (45.66)	2098 (41.07)	2249 (40.80)
Self-rated general health status						
Fair or poor	1574 (20.03)	605 (15.68)	189 (5.548)	296 (11.91)	1250 (22.89)	2249 (40.43)
Excellent, very good, or good	5773 (79.97)	3160 (84.32)	2344 (94.45)	2081 (88.09)	2945 (77.11)	2337 (59.57)
Asian-specific BMI category						
Not overweight or obese	3814 (53.37)	1272 (32.62)	978 (40.95)	993 (41.11)	2116 (53.97)	2430 (60.1)
Overweight or obese	3533 (46.63)	2493 (67.38)	1555 (59.05)	1384 (58.89)	2079 (46.03)	2156 (39.9)
Urban/rural status						
Urban	7162 (97.57)	3541 (95.12)	2427 (96.4)	2220 (95.04)	4092 (97.37)	4539 (99.27)
Rural	182 (2.43)	224 (4.88)	106 (3.60)	157 (4.96)	95 (2.63)	34 (0.73)

As shown in Table 2, a significant relationship was found between prevalence of food insecurity and acculturation proxies for Chinese, Korean, and Vietnamese subgroups. For example, prevalence of food insecurity was reported to be 13.72% among non-English speaking Chinese households, as compared to 1.04% among English-only speaking households. Likewise, prevalence of food insecurity was higher among foreign-born Chinese households than those born in the United States (8.90% vs. 3.00%). Among Koreans, prevalence of food insecurity was significantly higher among non-English speaking households than their English-speaking counter parts (9.55% vs. 2.41%), with a similar trend noted for Vietnamese subgroup as well (23.46% vs. 4.84%). Similarly, when compared to those born in the U.S., food insecurity was more prevalent among foreign-born Vietnamese households (18.03% vs. 3.93%). As further noted in Table 2, several other characteristics were associated with food insecurity; and thus all variables were included in the full survey weighted multivariable regression analyses.

Table 2. Association between prevalence of food insecurity and study population characteristics, by Asian American subgroups, results of chi-square analysis.

	Chinese	Filipino	South Asian
Language spoken at home	<0.0001	0.316	0.0722
English only	1.04 (0.56, 1.94)	6.55 (4.04, 10.45)	1.12 (0.46, 2.69)
English and another	2.97 (2.19, 4.01)	9.04 (7.20, 11.29)	3.24 (2.35, 4.45)
Non-English only	13.72 (11.26, 16.59)	9.30 (6.59, 12.96)	4.73 (2.37, 9.22)
Country of birth	0.001	0.422	0.2622
U.S.-born	3.00 (1.52, 5.83)	6.91 (3.97, 11.75)	2.20 (1.16, 4.13)
Foreign-born	8.90 (7.40, 10.65)	8.76 (7.26, 10.54)	3.29 (2.42, 4.45)
Age	0.0032	0.1556	0.0428
18–44 years	5.57 (3.87, 7.96)	7.29 (5.30, 9.95)	2.66 (1.90, 3.73)
45 years or more	10.02 (8.42, 11.89)	9.51 (7.80, 11.54)	4.57 (2.94, 7.04)
Sex	0.9977	0.1846	0.3004
Male	7.60 (5.50, 10.43)	9.40 (6.94, 12.61)	2.73 (1.79, 4.17)
Female	7.60 (6.24, 9.22)	7.29 (5.86, 9.04)	3.69 (2.53, 5.36)
Marital Status	0.4084	0.0272	0.0036
Currently married	8.03 (6.38, 10.04)	6.74 (5.18, 8.71)	2.35 (1.62, 3.37)
Not currently married	6.91 (5.24, 9.06)	10.31 (7.84, 13.44)	5.06 (3.37, 7.54)
Education	<0.0001	<0.0001	<0.0001

Table 2. *Cont.*

	Chinese	Filipino	South Asian
Bachelors or higher	2.69 (1.75, 4.11)	4.25 (3.15, 5.71)	1.42 (0.89, 2.25)
High school or less	16.69 (13.57, 20.34)	17.19 (12.80, 22.69)	10.25 (6.28, 16.29)
Some college	5.67 (4.15, 7.70)	7.97 (5.76, 10.91)	7.62 (4.59, 12.39)
Employment status	0.0005	0.0001	0.0899
Currently employed	5.59 (4.08, 7.62)	6.15 (4.83, 7.81)	2.68 (1.89, 3.78)
Currently unemployed	10.98 (8.85, 13.54)	13.19 (9.90, 17.36)	4.46 (2.75, 7.15)
General health status	<0.0001	<0.0001	<0.0001
Excellent, very good, good	5.49 (4.22, 7.12)	6.80 (5.30, 8.69)	2.57 (1.88, 3.50)
Fair or poor	16.01 (12.67, 20.02)	16.11 (12.05, 21.20)	12.93 (7.65, 21.00)
Asian-specific BMI category	0.7872	0.0666	0.1769
Not overweight/obese	7.77 (6.00, 10.00)	6.57 (5.04, 8.53)	2.49 (1.56, 3.93)
Overweight/obese	7.41 (5.86, 9.32)	9.07 (7.19, 11.39)	3.60 (2.58, 5.00)
Urban/rural status	0.0163	0.3464	0.0589
Urban	7.72 (6.46, 9.20)	8.14 (6.71, 9.84)	2.96 (2.21, 3.97)
Rural	3.15 (1.47, 6.60)	10.57 (6.16, 17.54)	7.96 (2.90, 20.04)

	Japanese	Korean	Vietnamese
Language spoken at home	0.358	0.0005	<0.0001
English only	2.06 (1.22, 3.47)	2.41 (1.08, 5.29)	4.84 (1.66, 13.28)
English and another	2.45 (1.31, 4.54)	4.63 (2.89, 7.35)	9.18 (6.85, 12.19)
Non-English only	4.46 (1.86, 10.29)	9.55 (7.73, 11.75)	23.46 (20.81, 26.33)
Country of birth	0.0863	0.0932	<0.0001
U.S.-born	1.87 (1.08, 3.24)	3.02 (1.04, 8.44)	3.93 (1.74, 8.60)
Foreign-born	3.38 (2.14, 5.32)	7.32 (5.96, 8.97)	18.03 (15.99, 20.26)
Age	0.2102	<0.0001	<0.0001
18–44 years	3.05 (1.68, 5.47)	4.02 (2.72, 5.89)	12.46 (9.96, 15.47)
45 years or more	1.89 (1.15, 3.10)	10.01 (7.92, 12.57)	21.63 (19.09, 24.39)
Sex	0.2766	0.0221	0.0019
Male	2.88 (1.59, 5.17)	4.86 (3.65, 6.45)	13.30 (10.91, 16.11)
Female	1.87 (1.12, 3.10)	7.66 (5.87, 9.94)	19.48 (16.72, 22.56)
Marital Status	0.26	0.0245	0.5668
Currently married	1.87 (1.03, 3.38)	5.32 (4.21, 6.71)	16.88 (14.61, 19.41)
Not currently married	2.91 (1.75, 4.78)	8.47 (6.07, 11.70)	15.76 (12.85, 19.17)
Education	0.0335	<0.0001	<0.0001
Bachelors or higher	1.20 (0.71, 2.02)	2.43 (1.73, 3.41)	6.74 (4.39, 10.20)
High school or less	3.73 (1.97, 6.96)	13.18 (10.17, 16.91)	23.06 (20.57, 25.75)
Some college	2.84 (1.39, 5.72)	8.43 (4.93, 14.03)	12.80 (8.48, 18.86)
Employment status	0.3548	<0.0001	<0.0001
Currently employed	1.91 (1.00, 3.60)	3.99 (2.92, 5.44)	11.65 (9.26, 14.55)
Currently unemployed	2.73 (1.73, 4.29)	10.27 (7.92, 13.21)	23.34 (20.51, 26.43)
General health status	0.2197	<0.0001	<0.0001
Excellent, very good, good	2.10 (1.35, 3.25)	3.93 (2.91, 5.29)	10.22 (8.06, 12.86)
Fair or poor	3.63 (1.65, 7.76)	15.47 (11.89, 19.87)	25.56 (22.50, 28.88)
Asian-specific BMI category	0.7825	0.5507	0.0316
Not overweight/obese	2.42 (1.54, 3.79)	6.21 (4.67, 8.22)	14.72 (12.22, 17.62)
Overweight/obese	2.19 (1.22, 3.89)	7.00 (5.26, 9.25)	18.98 (16.34, 21.92)
Urban/rural status	0.192	0.1162	0.2329
Urban	2.34 (1.57, 3.48)	6.67 (5.42, 8.18)	16.45 (14.54, 18.55)
Rural	1.08 (0.34, 3.38)	2.48 (0.66, 8.84)	6.68 (1.16, 30.43)

As shown in Table 3 (data on prevalence ratio [PR] for control variables is not shown), both acculturation proxies were associated with food insecurity among Asian Americans, though the relationships varied between subgroups. For example, speaking a language other than English at home was associated with 7.24 times higher prevalence of being food insecure, as compared to speaking English only, among the Chinese subgroup. Similarly, speaking English and another language was associated with nearly three times higher prevalence of food insecurity compared to only speaking English in the same population. South Asians speaking a non-English language at home also had over three and a half times higher prevalence of food insecurity, compared to those who reported speaking English only at home. Furthermore, prevalence food insecurity was significantly associated with being foreign-born among Chinese (prevalence ratio [PR] = 2.31), Filipino (PR = 1.75), Japanese (PR = 2.11), South Asian (PR = 3.35), and Vietnamese (PR = 3.70) subgroups.

Table 3. Prevalence ratio of food insecurity by acculturation status, among Asian American subgroup, results of multivariable robust Poisson regression analysis.

	Language Spoken at Home [a] PR (95% CI)			Country of Birth [b] PR (95% CI)	
	English Only (Reference)	English and Another	Non-English only	U.S.-Born (Reference)	Foreign-Born
Chinese	Ref.	2.51 (1.28, 4.94) **	7.24 (3.68, 14.24) ***	Ref.	2.31(1.17, 4.54) *
Filipino	Ref.	1.55 (0.98, 2.47)	1.56 (0.95, 2.55)	Ref.	1.75 (1.06, 2.87) *
South Asian	Ref.	2.53 (0.97, 6.64)	3.62 (1.04, 12.66) *	Ref.	3.35 (1.36, 8.20) **
Japanese	Ref.	1.24 (0.51, 3.00)	1.82 (0.71, 4.70)	Ref.	2.11 (1.09, 4.09) *
Korean	Ref.	1.57 (0.58, 4.23)	2.06 (0.73, 5.78)	Ref.	1.81 (0.67, 4.90)
Vietnamese	Ref.	1.56 (0.56, 4.40)	2.76 (0.99, 7.66)	Ref.	3.70 (1.58, 8.66) **

[a] Poisson regression model includes language spoken at home as the primary exposure variable and control variables of age, sex, martial status, education, employment, self-reported general health status, urban/rural, BMI, and survey year; [b] Poisson regression model includes country of birth as the primary exposure variable and control variables of age, sex, martial status, education, employment, self-reported general health status, urban/rural, BMI, and survey year; PR = prevalence ratio, CI = confidence interval, Ref. = reference category; * $p < 0.05$, ** $p < 0.01$, *** $p < 0.001$.

Table 4 further displays the SNAP participation rate by acculturation status among the six Asian American subgroups.

Table 4. Prevalence of SNAP participation among Asian American subgroups.

	Language Spoken at Home			Country of Birth		Citizenship Status	
	English only	English and Another	Non-English only	U.S.-Born	Foreign-Born	Citizen	Non-Citizen
Chinese	–	2.95	4.77	–	4.28	1.3397	3.4626
Filipino	–	2.88	1.75	–	2.64	0.5794	2.9532
South Asian	–	3.35	–	–	3.48	0.7457	1.0001
Japanese	–	–	–	–	–	–	–
Korean	–	1..85	3.16	–	2.94	1.2389	1.3562
Vietnamese	–	9.02	15.67	3.12	14.33	6.7969	17.4218

– The percent is not reported due to sample size being $n < 10$.

As noted, such participation is substantially low in the population over all. The highest rate based on language spoken at home was noted among Vietnamese who spoke a non-English only (15.67%) and were foreign-born (14.33%). Even when looking at by citizenship status, the prevalence was substantially low for all with the higher rates noted among non-citizens, especially among Vietnamese. For most subgroups, the participation rate was less than n = 10, thus resulting in lack of data reporting to ensure privacy of CHIS participants.

4. Discussion

While evaluation of the burden of food insecurity among minority populations is prevalent in the empirical body of literature, little assessment exists among the Asian American population. We thus studied the period prevalence of food insecurity among disaggregated Asian American subgroups in California, as well as whether acculturation was a determining factor of such disparities. The results of our study highlight several key findings: (1) food insecurity among Asian American subgroups is diverse, with lowest prevalence noted among Japanese (2.28%) and highest among Vietnamese (16.42%), (2) low acculturation is predominantly associated with higher prevalence of food insecurity among most Asian American subgroups, and (3) SNAP participation among the population remains substantially low.

Such results have several implications. In a previous study based in Los Angeles, Furness et al. noted that Whites, African-Americans, and Latinos had a higher prevalence of food insecurity compared to Asian/Pacific Islanders [35]. One plausible difference from such results to what is highlighted in our study is the disaggregation of data. Asian Americans are a diverse population with unique cultural and linguistic characteristics. Thus, the aggregation into one homogenous group can often mask true disparities among subgroups. Furthermore, in our study the highest prevalence of food insecurity was noted among the Vietnamese subgroup (16.42%), which is substantially higher than the other Asian American subgroup population as well as the entire CHIS population (11.80%). As such, consistent with the literature evaluating health disparities among Asian American, our study also demonstrate that Asian Americans remain a diverse population [36] with unique needs and thus disaggregation of data when assessing such social determinants of health are critical for public health efforts.

In addition, we noted that two proxies of acculturation were related to food insecurity among specific Asian American subgroups. This is similar to other studies that have shown Asian Americans who are less acculturated to suffer worse disparities. For instance, Tang et al. [37] noted that less acculturation was associated higher tobacco use while Jang and group [38] noted that alienation from heritage culture was associated with worse physical and mental health among Asian Americans.

One putative explanation for our results could be that less acculturated populations are more likely to adhere to Asian-based traditional food items, which are often more difficult to access due to cost [39], thus making such households more food insecure; however comprehensive assessment of Asian traditional food cost as compared to American food remains limited in the literature. In addition, in our study, we further see a substantially low SNAP participation in each Asian American subgroup, even among citizens. This could be potentially explained by culture-based stigma. For example, a report including Korean-speaking adults noted that most participants would not turn to a food assistance program for help and often considered them as a last option, often due to limitations of culturally appropriate food items [40] and culturally-associated stigma as such opportunities are often considered "handouts" [40]. The lack of any empirical evidence understanding the barriers to food aid participation among the Asian American population and the limitation of the aforementioned report to Korean population only, further highlights the imperative need for further research on understanding the barriers to ensuring food security among the Asian American population.

Finally, given the negative burden of food insecurity on health and behavioral outcomes, as noted in the literature, [18,21], the higher rates of food insecurity among less acculturated Asian American subgroups further shown in our study, the cumulative evidence warrants targeted public health efforts among the most at-risk groups. However, limited studies exist on what such public health efforts should include.

Herein also lies the opportunity for collaborative effort between the healthcare system and the community to ensure more positive outcomes. For example, in a proof of concept assessment of the efficacy of community health workers to improve childhood health outcomes, Martin et al. demonstrated the positive influence of home visitations on asthma control, emergency care utilizations, and inhaler usage [41]. While similar assessment on the efficacy of home visitation techniques on food insecurity remains limited, Tough et al. noted that home visitations improved nutrition counselling attendance among at-risk mothers, including those with language barriers [42]. As such, public health efforts to pilot test the efficacy of community health workers among Asian American subgroups and to create home visitation programs in order to assess food availability and increase participation in food assistance programs may help alleviate the burden of food insecurity among the most vulnerable Asian American populations.

Additionally, a critical point of contact for most populations remain the healthcare system. Means to identify Asian American subgroups at risk of food insecurity at healthcare facilities remains imperative. For example, the American Academy of Pediatrics notes the importance of a screening tool utilized during practice to identify children living in food insecure households; such as the Household Food Security Scale or the in-office 2-item screener [43]. A similar strategy can be utilized when screening adults, especially one tailored to Asian-specific languages.

Finally, as noted by Roncarolo and Potvin [44], simply providing access to food banks or food aid program is analogous to treating diseases with drugs. Instead, there is undoubtedly a need to identify the most at-risk populations early to prevent food insecurity from occurring. As such, to preventing the onset of food insecurity, if it were to be truly treated as a symptom of "social disease" [44], then governmental-level interventions, including that of local initiatives, are needed to improve continued access to healthy food options. For example, while farmers' markets continue to be considered a key component of improving access to food, often they lack culturally appropriate food items. In San Francisco, California, a collaborative effort among food stamp programs and public health and nonprofit organizations demonstrated feasibility of increased access to farmers' markets, especially through payment systems [45]. Similar strategies that incorporate partnerships between Asian American-based organizations and local public health agencies may provide a scope of improved access to food among such at-risk groups.

The results of our study should be interpreted in the context of some limitations inherent to the study design. The study sample is limited to California and thus cannot be generalized outside of the state. Furthermore, the proxies of acculturation utilized in this study may not encompass all feasible operationalization of acculturation. For example, studies note that acculturation can be bidimensional or unidimensional and these domains are not captured by the proxies. The self-report and recall biases inherent to surveys may further posit as limitations to interpretation of results. Nevertheless, such limitations do not negate the diversity in food insecurity prevalence noted in the Asian American subgroups, especially the disproportionately high levels noted among the Vietnamese subgroup.

5. Conclusions

Our study results demonstrate heterogeneity in the burden of food insecurity among the most vulnerable Asian American subgroups, especially those who are less acculturated. There is a significant gap in the literature addressing barriers to food aid among such populations and thus our results not only highlight the need for more comprehensive assessment, but also outreach to increase food aid participation for the most at-risk groups. There are also several strengths to this study. The sampling design of CHIS and survey-weighted analyses allow for generalization to Asian Americans in California, thus increasing the external validity of this study. Furthermore, the results provide one of the first assessments of food insecurity among Asian American subgroups, especially since there remains limited data to assess South Asian health, with CHIS being one of the few to provide public access to such data. As such, this study's results provide a valuable addition by providing the first comprehensive analyses of the burden of food insecurity among disaggregated Asian American populations.

Author Contributions: M.B.B. was the principal investigator of this study. S.K.M. conducted literature review. B.J.B. conducted data analysis. All authors contributed to data interpretation and manuscript development.

Acknowledgments: M.B.B. would also like to thank the Institute for Child Development and Family Relations and Faculty Center for Excellence for providing M.B.B. the time and resources for writing.

References

1. Colby, S.; Ortman, J. *Projections of the Size and Composition of the U.S. Population: 2014 to 2060, Current Population Reports, P25-1143*; U.S. Census Bureau: Washington, DC, USA, 2015.
2. Yi, V.; Museus, S.D. Model Minority Myth. In *The Wiley Blackwell Encyclopedia of Race, Ethnicity, and Nationalism*; John Wiley & Sons, Ltd.: Hoboken, NJ, USA, 2015.
3. Gupta, A.; Szymanski, D.M.; Leong, F.T.L. The 'model minority myth': Internalized racialism of positive stereotypes as correlates of psychological distress, and attitudes toward help-seeking. *Asian Am. J. Psychol.* **2011**, *2*, 101–114. [CrossRef]

4.   Initiative on Asian Americans and Pacific Islanders. 24 September 2014. Available online: https://www.whitehouse.gov/embeds/footer (accessed on 3 October 2016).

5.   Takei, I.; Sakamoto, A. Poverty among Asian Americans in the 21st Century. *Sociol. Perspect.* **2011**, *54*, 251–276. [CrossRef]

6.   Klatsky, A.L.; Friedman, G.D.; Sidney, S.; Kipp, H.; Kubo, A.; Armstrong, M.A. Risk of hemorrhagic stroke in Asian American ethnic groups. *Neuroepidemiology* **2005**, *25*, 26–31. [CrossRef] [PubMed]

7.   Sarwar, E.; Arias, D.; Becerra, B.J.; Becerra, M.B. Sociodemographic Correlates of Dietary Practices among Asian-Americans: Results from the California Health Interview Survey. *J. Racial Ethn. Health Disparities* **2015**, *2*, 494–500. [CrossRef] [PubMed]

8.   Becerra, M.B.; Becerra, B.J. Disparities in Age at Diabetes Diagnosis among Asian Americans: Implications for Early Preventive Measures. *Prev. Chronic. Dis.* **2015**, *12*, E146. [CrossRef] [PubMed]

9.   Palaniappan, L.; Wang, Y.; Fortmann, S.P. Coronary heart disease mortality for six ethnic groups in California, 1990–2000. *Ann. Epidemiol.* **2004**, *14*, 499–506. [CrossRef] [PubMed]

10.   Becerra, M.B.; Herring, P.; Marshak, H.H.; Banta, J.E. Social Determinants of Physical Activity among Adult Asian-Americans: Results from a Population-Based Survey in California. *J. Immigr. Minor. Health* **2014**, *17*, 1061–1069. [CrossRef] [PubMed]

11.   United States Department of Agriculture. *Definitions of Food Security*; United States Department of Agriculture: Washington, DC, USA, 2017.

12.   United States Department of Agriculture. *Economic Research Service, Key Statistics & Graphics*; United States Department of Agriculture: Washington, DC, USA, 2016.

13.   Wong, J.C.; Scott, T.; Wilde, P.; Li, Y.; Tucker, K.L.; Gao, X. Food Insecurity Is Associated with Subsequent Cognitive Decline in the Boston Puerto Rican Health Study. *J. Nutr.* **2016**, *146*, 1740–1745. [CrossRef] [PubMed]

14.   Alaimo, K.; Olson, C.M.; Frongillo, E.A. Food Insufficiency and American School-Aged Children's Cognitive, Academic, and Psychosocial Development. *Pediatrics* **2001**, *108*, 44–53. [PubMed]

15.   Becerra, M.B.; Hassija, C.M.; Becerra, B.J. Food insecurity is associated with unhealthy dietary practices among US veterans in California. *Public Health Nutr.* **2016**, *20*, 2569–2576. [CrossRef] [PubMed]

16.   Kaiser, L.L.; Lamp, C.L.; Johns, M.C.; Sutherlin, J.M.; Harwood, J.O.; Melgar-Quiñonez, H.R. Food Security and Nutritional Outcomes of Preschool-Age Mexican-American Children. *J. Am. Diet. Assoc.* **2002**, *102*, 924–929. [CrossRef]

17.   Pryor, L.; Lioret, S.; van der Waerden, J.; Fombonne, É.; Falissard, B.; Melchior, M. Food insecurity and mental health problems among a community sample of young adults. *Soc. Psychiatry Psychiatr. Epidemiol.* **2016**, *51*, 1073–1081. [CrossRef] [PubMed]

18.   Becerra, B.J.; Sis-Medina, R.C.; Reyes, A.; Becerra, M.B. Association between Food Insecurity and Serious Psychological Distress among Hispanic Adults Living in Poverty. *Prev. Chronic. Dis.* **2015**, *12*, E206. [CrossRef] [PubMed]

19.   Weigel, M.M.; Armijos, R.X.; Hall, Y.P.; Ramirez, Y.; Orozco, R. The Household Food Insecurity and Health Outcomes of U.S.–Mexico Border Migrant and Seasonal Farmworkers. *J. Immigr. Minor. Health* **2007**, *9*, 157–169. [CrossRef] [PubMed]

20.   Allen, N.L.; Becerra, B.J.; Becerra, M.B. Associations between food insecurity and the severity of psychological distress among African-Americans. *Ethn. Health* **2017**, *23*, 511–520. [CrossRef] [PubMed]

21.   To, Q.G.; Frongillo, E.A.; Gallegos, D.; Moore, J.B. Household food insecurity is associated with less physical activity among children and adults in the U.S. population. *J. Nutr.* **2014**, *144*, 1797–1802. [CrossRef] [PubMed]

22.   Tsunoda, T.; Parrish, K.M. The effect of acculturation on drinking attitudes among Japanese in Japan and Japanese Americans. *J. Stud. Alcohol* **1992**, *53*, 369. [CrossRef] [PubMed]

23.   Ma, G.X.; Shive, S.E.; Tan, Y.; Feeley, R.M. The Impact of Acculturation on Smoking in Asian American Homes. *J. Healthc. Poor Underserved* **2004**, *15*, 267–280. [CrossRef] [PubMed]

24.   Becerra, M.B.; Herring, P.; Marshak, H.H.; Banta, J.E. Generational differences in fast food intake among South-Asian Americans: Results from a population-based survey. *Prev. Chronic. Dis.* **2014**, *11*, E211. [CrossRef] [PubMed]

25.   Hadley, C.; Zodhiates, A.; Sellen, D.W. Acculturation, economics and food insecurity among refugees resettled in the USA: A case study of West African refugees. *Public Health Nutr.* **2007**, *10*, 405–412. [CrossRef] [PubMed]

26. Dhokarh, R.; Himmelgreen, D.A.; Peng, Y.-K.; Segura-Perez, S.; Hromi-Fiedler, A.; Perez-Escamilla, R. Food Insecurity is Associated with Acculturation and Social Networks in Puerto Rican Households. *J. Nutr. Educ. Behav.* **2011**, *43*, 288–294. [CrossRef] [PubMed]

27. Strings, S.; Ranchod, Y.K.; Laraia, B.; Nuru-Jeter, A. Race and Sex Differences in the Association between Food Insecurity and Type 2 Diabetes. *Ethn. Dis.* **2016**, *26*, 427–434. [CrossRef] [PubMed]

28. Van Wieren, A.J.; Roberts, M.B.; Arellano, N.; Feller, E.R.; Diaz, J.A. Acculturation and cardiovascular behaviors among Latinos in California by country/region of origin. *J. Immigr. Minor. Health Cent. Minor. Public Health* **2011**, *13*, 975–981. [CrossRef] [PubMed]

29. An, N.; Cochran, S.D.; Mays, V.M.; McCarthy, W.J. Influence of American acculturation on cigarette smoking behaviors among Asian American subpopulations in California. *Nicotine Tob. Res. Off. J. Soc. Res. Nicotine Tob.* **2008**, *10*, 579–587. [CrossRef] [PubMed]

30. WHO Expert Consultation. Appropriate body-mass index for Asian populations and its implications for policy and intervention strategies. *Lancet* **2004**, *363*, 157–163. [CrossRef]

31. Townsend, M.S.; Peerson, J.; Love, B.; Achterberg, C.; Murphy, S.P. Food Insecurity Is Positively Related to Overweight in Women. *J. Nutr.* **2001**, *131*, 1738–1745. [CrossRef] [PubMed]

32. Dinour, L.M.; Bergen, D.; Yeh, M. The Food Insecurity–Obesity Paradox: A Review of the Literature and the Role Food Stamps May Play. *J. Acad. Nutr. Diet.* **2007**, *107*, 1952–1961. [CrossRef] [PubMed]

33. StataCorp LLC. A Stata Press Publication, Stata Survey Data Reference Manual: Release 14, 2015. Available online: https://www.stata.com/manuals14/svy.pdf (accessed on 20 October 2017).

34. Petersen, M.R.; Deddens, J.A. A comparison of two methods for estimating prevalence ratios. *BMC Med. Res. Methodol.* **2008**, *8*, 9. [CrossRef] [PubMed]

35. Furness, B.W.; Simon, P.A.; Wold, C.M.; Asarian-Anderson, J. Prevalence and predictors of food insecurity among low-income households in Los Angeles County. *Public Health Nutr.* **2004**, *7*, 791–794. [CrossRef] [PubMed]

36. Holland, A.T.; Palaniappan, L.P. Problems with the Collection and Interpretation of Asian-American Health Data: Omission, Aggregation, and Extrapolation. *Ann. Epidemiol.* **2012**, *22*, 397–405. [CrossRef] [PubMed]

37. Tang, H.; Shimizu, R.; Chen, M.S. English Language Proficiency and Smoking Prevalence among California's Asian Americans. *Cancer* **2005**, *104*, 2982–2988. [CrossRef] [PubMed]

38. Jang, Y.; Park, N.S.; Chiriboga, D.A.; Kim, M.T. Latent Profiles of Acculturation and Their Implications for Health: A Study with Asian Americans in Central Texas. *Asian Am. J. Psychol.* **2017**, *8*, 200–208. [CrossRef] [PubMed]

39. Mekouar, D. Does Bias Impact Price of U.S. Ethnic Food?—All about America. VOA, 2016. Available online: https://blogs.voanews.com/all-about-america/2016/04/13/why-americans-will-pay-more-for-french-food-than-chinese-cuisine/ (accessed on 20 October 2017).

40. Gabor, V.; Williams, S.; Bellamy, H.; Hardison, B.; Health Systems Research, Inc. *Seniors' Views of the Food Stamp Program and Ways to Improve Participation—Focus Group Findings in Washington State*; Economic Research Service, U.S. Department of Agriculture: Washington, DC, USA, 2002.

41. Martin, M.A.; Rothschild, S.K.; Lynch, E.; Christoffel, K.K.; Pagán, M.M.; Rodriguez, J.L.; Barnes, A.; Karavolos, K.; Diaz, A.; Hoffman, L.M.; et al. Addressing asthma and obesity in children with community health workers: Proof-of-concept intervention development. *BMC Pediatr.* **2016**, *16*, 198. [CrossRef] [PubMed]

42. Tough, S.C.; Johnston, D.W.; Siever, J.E.; Jorgenson, G.; Slocombe, L.; Lane, C.; Clarke, M. Does Supplementary Prenatal Nursing and Home Visitation Support Improve Resource Use in a Universal Health Care System? A Randomized Controlled Trial in Canada. *Birth* **2006**, *33*, 183–194. [PubMed]

43. Council on Community Pediatrics. Commitee on Nutrition, Promoting Food Security for All Children. *Pediatrics* **2015**, *136*, e1431–e1438. [CrossRef] [PubMed]

44. Roncarolo, F.; Potvin, L. Food insecurity as a symptom of a social disease. *Can. Fam. Physician* **2016**, *62*, 291–292. [PubMed]

45. Jones, P.; Bhatia, R. Supporting Equitable Food Systems through Food Assistance at Farmers' Markets. *Am. J. Public Health* **2011**, *101*, 781–783. [CrossRef] [PubMed]

Permissions

The contributors of this book come from diverse backgrounds, making this book a truly international effort. This book will bring forth new frontiers with its revolutionizing research information and detailed analysis of the nascent developments around the world.

We would like to thank all the contributing authors for lending their expertise to make the book truly unique. They have played a crucial role in the development of this book. Without their invaluable contributions this book wouldn't have been possible. They have made vital efforts to compile up to date information on the varied aspects of this subject to make this book a valuable addition to the collection of many professionals and students.

This book was conceptualized with the vision of imparting up-to-date information and advanced data in this field. To ensure the same, a matchless editorial board was set up. Every individual on the board went through rigorous rounds of assessment to prove their worth. After which they invested a large part of their time researching and compiling the most relevant data for our readers.

The editorial board has been involved in producing this book since its inception. They have spent rigorous hours researching and exploring the diverse topics which have resulted in the successful publishing of this book. They have passed on their knowledge of decades through this book. To expedite this challenging task, the publisher supported the team at every step. A small team of assistant editors was also appointed to further simplify the editing procedure and attain best results for the readers.

Apart from the editorial board, the designing team has also invested a significant amount of their time in understanding the subject and creating the most relevant covers. They scrutinized every image to scout for the most suitable representation of the subject and create an appropriate cover for the book.

The publishing team has been an ardent support to the editorial, designing and production team. Their endless efforts to recruit the best for this project, has resulted in the accomplishment of this book. They are a veteran in the field of academics and their pool of knowledge is as vast as their experience in printing. Their expertise and guidance has proved useful at every step. Their uncompromising quality standards have made this book an exceptional effort. Their encouragement from time to time has been an inspiration for everyone.

The publisher and the editorial board hope that this book will prove to be a valuable piece of knowledge for researchers, students, practitioners and scholars across the globe.

List of Contributors

Teresa Borelli, Danny Hunter, Céline Termote and Johannes Engels
Alliance of Bioversity International and CIAT, via dei Tre Denari 472/a, 00054 Rome, Italy

Bronwen Powell
Center for International Forestry Research, Penn State University, State College, PA 16802, USA

Tiziana Ulian and Efisio Mattana
Royal Botanic Gardens Kew, Wakehurst, Ardingly, West Sussex RH17 6TN, UK

Lukas Pawera
Faculty of Tropical AgriSciences, Czech University of Life Sciences Prague, Kamýcká 129, 16500 Praha-Suchdol, Czech Republic
The Indigenous Partnership for Agrobiodiversity and Food Sovereignty, c/o Alliance of Bioversity International and CIAT, Via dei Tre Denari 472/a, 00054 Rome, Italy

Daniela Beltrame
Biodiversity for Food and Nutrition Project, Ministry of the Environment, Brasília-DF 70068-900, Brazil

Daniela Penafiel
Escuela Superior Politécnica del Litoral, Centro de Investigaciones Rurales–FCSH, Campus Gustavo Galindo-km. 30.5 vía Perimetral, Guayaquil 090112, Ecuador
Faculty of Medicine, Universidad de Especialidades Espíritu Santo, Samborondon 091650, Ecuador

Ayfer Tan
Aegean Agricultural Research Institute, Menemen, Izmir, Turkey

Mary Taylor
Environmental Studies, University of the Sunshine Coast, Maroochydore, QLD 4556, Australia

Anna K. Farmery, Jessica M. Scott, Tom D. Brewer, Dirk J. Steenbergen and Neil L. Andrew
Australian National Centre for Ocean Resource and Security, Faculty of Business and Law, University of Wollongong, Wollongong 2522, Australia

Hampus Eriksson
Australian National Centre for Ocean Resource and Security, Faculty of Business and Law, University of Wollongong, Wollongong 2522, Australia
WorldFish, Honiara, Faculty of Agriculture, Fisheries and Forestry, C/O Solomon Islands National University, Ranadi, Solomon Islands

Jillian Tutuo
WorldFish, Honiara, Faculty of Agriculture, Fisheries and Forestry, C/O Solomon Islands National University, Ranadi, Solomon Islands

Joelle Albert
Island Elements, Brisbane 4069, Australia

Jacob Raubani
Fisheries, Aquaculture and Marine Ecosystems Division, The Pacific Community, Noumea Cedex 98849, New Caledonia

Michael K. Sharp
Statistics for Development Division, The Pacific Community, Noumea Cedex 98849, New Caledonia

Sue Booth
College of Medicine and Public Health, Flinders University, Adelaide 5000, Australia

Christina Pollard
Faculty of Health Sciences, School of Public Health, Curtin University, Perth 6102, Australia

John Coveney
College of Nursing & Health Sciences, Flinders University, Adelaide 5000, Australia

Ian Goodwin-Smith
College of Business, Government and Law, Flinders University, Adelaide 5000, Australia

Leisa McCarthy
Menzies School of Health Research, 0870 Darwin, Australia

Anne B. Chang
Menzies School of Health Research, 0870 Darwin, Australia
Department of Respiratory Medicine, Queensland Children's Hospital, 4101 Brisbane, Australia
Children's Centre for Health Research, Queensland University of Technology; 4101 Brisbane, Australia

Julie Brimblecombe
Menzies School of Health Research, 0870 Darwin, Australia
Department of Nutrition, Dietetics and Food, School of Clinical Sciences, Monash University, 3168 Melbourne, Australia

Jeromey B. Temple
Demography and Ageing Unit, Melbourne School of Population and Global Health, University of Melbourne, Melbourne 3010, Australia

Joanna Russell
School of Health and Society, University of Wollongong, Wollongong 2522, Australia

Merryn Maynard
Meal Exchange Canada, Toronto, ON M5V 3A8, Canada

Lesley Andrade, Sara Packull-McCormick, Christopher M. Perlman, Cesar Leos-Toro and Sharon I. Kirkpatrick
School of Public Health and Health Systems, University of Waterloo, Waterloo, ON N2L 3G1, Canada

Sue Kleve, Zoe E. Davidson and Claire Palermo
Department of Nutrition, Dietetics and Food, School of Clinical Sciences, Faculty of Medicine, Nursing and Health Sciences, Monash University, Level 1, 264 Ferntree Gully Road, Notting Hill 3168, Australia

Danielle Gallegos
School of Exercise and Nutrition Sciences, Queensland University of Technology; Brisbane 4059, Australia
Center for Children's Health Research, Institute of Health and Biomedical Innovation, Queensland University of Technology, Brisbane 4101, Australia

Mariana M. Chilton
Department of Health Management and Policy, Dornsife School of Public Health, Drexel University, Philadelphia, PA 19104, USA

Amanda Lee
School of Public Health, Faculty of Medicine, The University of Queensland, Herston, Queensland 4006, Australia
The Australian Prevention Partnership Centre, The Sax Institute, Ultimo 2007, New South Wales, Australia
The Australian Prevention Partnership Centre, The Sax Institute, Sydney 1240, Australia

Meron Lewis
School of Public Health, Faculty of Medicine, The University of Queensland, Herston, Queensland 4006, Australia

Christina M. Pollard
Faculty of Health Sciences, School of Public Health, Curtin University, Perth 6102, Australia

Elena Carrillo-Álvarez
Blanquerna School of Health Sciences — Universitat Ramon Llull-Global Research on Wellbeing — GRoW Research group, Padilla, 08025 Barcelona, Spain

Tess Penne
Research Foundation — Flanders, Herman Deleeck Centre for Social Policy — University of Antwerp, 2000 Antwerp, Belgium

Hilde Boeckx
Thomas More Kempen, 2440 Malle, Belgium

Bérénice Storms
Herman Deleeck Centre for Social Policy — University of Antwerp, 2000 Antwerp, Belgium

Tim Goedemé
Institute for New Economic Thinking at the Oxford Martin School and Department of Social Policy and Intervention, University of Oxford, Oxford OX2 6ED, UK

Sally Mackay, Stefanie Vandevijvere, Rawinia Goodwin and Boyd Swinburn
School of Population Health, University of Auckland, Auckland 1142, New Zealand

Tina Buch and Mafi Funaki-Tahifote
The Heart Foundation of New Zealand, Auckland 1051, New Zealand

Erina Korohina
Toi Tangata, Auckland 1010, New Zealand

Monideepa B. Becerra and Salome Kapella Mshigeni
Department of Health Science and Human Ecology, California State University, 5500 University Parkway, San Bernardino, CA 92407, USA

Benjamin J. Becerra
School of Allied Health Professions, Loma Linda University, 24951 North Circle Drive, Loma Linda, CA 92350, USA

Index

Printed in the USA
CPSIA information can be obtained
at www.ICGtesting.com
JSHW051413091023
49903JS00006B/405